'This book explains the neuroscience behind canine-assisted psycho-therapy, detailing the mechanisms of change that produce regulation and resilience in children impacted by trauma. With over 35 years of co-producing significant clinical changes in conscientious partner-ships with dogs, Woolard consolidates substantial research, literature, and experience to produce a resource for clinicians.'

Ron Kotkin, *professor emeritus, University of California, Irvine*

'With impressive depth and breadth, Dr. Woolard brings together a vast amount of theory and research to explain how child maltreatment causes dysregulation of neural systems and can lead to severe psycho-pathology. She provides a cogent explanation of the neurobiological implications of canine-assisted psychotherapy for children suffering from developmental trauma. This book is an invaluable resource for theorists, researchers, and clinicians in their search for more effective ways to help these children.'

Nancy Parish-Plass, *author, clinician, researcher, and chairperson of the Israeli Association of Animal-Assisted Psychotherapy*

T0372868

Canine-Assisted Psychotherapy for Children with Trauma-Induced Dysregulation

This book provides mental health researchers and clinicians with valuable insight into the pathway that leads from developmental trauma to dysregulation and psychopathology.

Incorporating science that explains the impact of early trauma, this book details the theory, mechanisms, and applications of neurobiologically informed canine-assisted psychotherapy, using illuminating case studies that demonstrate the efficacy of the author's model.

Robbi Stevenson Woolard, PhD, has spent more than 35 years treating children, adolescents, and their families with traditional diagnoses and early childhood trauma. She has trained and incorporated dogs, horses, and other animals into treatment to restore regulation, function, and wellness in victims of interpersonal trauma. Woolard has been involved in the design and implementation of innovative programming and has developed and instituted crisis-response protocols for schools. She has also been involved in local, national, and international crisis and disaster response and collaborated in a multi-country, interagency initiative to develop a coordinated protocol for transportation disasters.

Canine-Assisted Psychotherapy for Children with Trauma-Induced Dysregulation

A Neurobiologically Infused Treatment

Robbi Stevenson Woolard

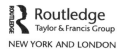

NEW YORK AND LONDON

Cover image credit: Cover image taken by Kate Maddux

First published 2024
by Routledge
605 Third Avenue, New York, NY 10158

and by Routledge
4 Park Square, Milton Park, Abingdon, Oxon, OX14 4RN

Routledge is an imprint of the Taylor & Francis Group, an informa business

Library of Congress Cataloging-in-Publication Data
Names: Woolard, Robbi Stevenson, author.
Title: Canine-assisted psychotherapy for children with trauma-induced dysregulation : a neurobiologically infused treatment / Robbi Stevenson Woolard.
Description: New York, NY : Routledge, 2023. | Includes bibliographical references and index.
Identifiers: LCCN 2023011614 (print) | LCCN 2023011615 (ebook) | ISBN 9781032108773 (hardback) | ISBN 9781032108759 (paperback) | ISBN 9781003217534 (ebook)
Subjects: MESH: Adverse Childhood Experiences | Animal Assisted Therapy | Dogs | Therapy Animals | Case Reports
Classification: LCC RM931.A65 (print) | LCC RM931.A65 (ebook) | NLM WS 105.5.A8 | DDC 615.8/5158--dc23/eng/20230705
LC record available at https://lccn.loc.gov/2023011614
LC ebook record available at https://lccn.loc.gov/2023011615

ISBN: 978-1-032-10877-3 (hbk)
ISBN: 978-1-032-10875-9 (pbk)
ISBN: 978-1-003-21753-4 (ebk)

DOI: 10.4324/9781003217534

Typeset in Times New Roman
by SPi Technologies India Pvt Ltd (Straive)

Contents

Acknowledgments and Dedications

Acknowledgments

The children, adolescents, and families who shared their lives with us have our utmost gratitude and respect. You enriched our world and remain in our hearts and memories. Your courage, commitment, and hard work were both inspiring and motivating, and a testament to your success. Thank you for allowing us to get to know you.

One of the first women to graduate from the University of Illinois in 1904, my Aunt Emma Ehly Williams was an incredible role model. She served as a missionary in China, wrote poetry and painted, and always encouraged me to be brave and try new things. Thanks to my parents, Pat and Wayne Stevenson who provided enormous energy, perseverance, and sacrifice to build our large family. They inspired my love for children and animals and encouraged me to write since I was very young. I am also grateful to Charles and Clariann Woolard who taught me so much about unconditional acceptance and the value of family and relationships.

Chuck, you have been a patient, supportive, and amazing husband for a very long time! When we first met, I recognized your incredible nature in the compassion you had for children and animals. I am truly grateful for your presence, advice, nourishing meals, and the adventures we continue to share. I am also thankful to you for our family, our sons, and daughters by love, CJ and Kate and Nick and Michelle, and the sweet grandchildren they share with us. Isabella and Cole: keep writing and creating; and Jackson and James, keep climbing to see what you can see. Aim high and never give up. I love and admire you all.

I have gained many new friends and colleagues who graciously supported me with advice and generous sharing of their wisdom and experience. I am especially grateful to Nancy Parish-Plass who was incredibly generous with her mentorship and time in reviewing, editing, and connecting me with resources. Rise VanFleet was also highly supportive, and willingly took the time to answer questions and expand my awareness and knowledge base.

Thanks to my brother Paul who believed, that 'dogs are people, too.' Thank you for your abundant encouragement and emotional support along with my sister and cousin, Beth and Sarah. I'm also grateful to other family and friends for their encouragement, advice, reading, editing, prayers, and ensuring my life remains full of joy and love. Thanks to Gwen, Marisa, Susan, Melanie, Beth, Adie, Joany, Dawn, and Meg.

Cover and chapter 3 photos: Kate Maddux. Chapter 5 photo credit: Amber Stevenson.

Dedications

If we are present and still, and open our hearts and minds, we can hear their messages. A great deal of wisdom is embedded in a source that through time has lost our admiration, appreciation, and even recognition of their value. Their instruction remains beneath the radar of consciousness, camouflaged by the roles we assign to them, and embedded beneath their cloaks of fur, scales, and even shells. Unlike most humans, animals have not forgotten the universal principles and codes of nature. They have maintained their indigenous connection with the Earth and we must pause to listen and take time to process the wisdom they share. This book is dedicated to the ones that share their lives, their love, and their lessons with those of us who need them.

This book is dedicated to Seamus, Bentley, Oliver, Kerbie, and Emma, who shared their deep compassion and infinite spirit with a multitude of children, comforting, restoring and healing their hidden wounds. Your ability to connect, communicate, and recognize needs was amazing to witness, and your ability to grow the relationship was a testament to your pure heart and authentic nature. You let them know it was safe to walk through the door and allow you into their hearts and lives. By reaching through the layers of fear and distress you uncovered the child they were meant to be.

I am also immensely grateful to those in my life that clearly sought to connect and synchronize before we even recognized the capabilities you possess. You continually surprised me as you demonstrated enormous capacity for relationships, social interaction, and healing. You all were teachers and opened our eyes to the potential for interspecies connection. You all served as ambassadors of the animal kingdom to hundreds of others whose lives you touched through the years, leaving an indelible print upon their hearts.

About the Author

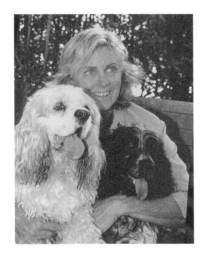

Our high school class was given a survey prior to graduation to identify a career option that fit our interests and abilities. The survey captured my essence yet resulted in a clear tie between two highly disparate choices. The two career recommendations were 'social worker/psychologist' *and* 'forest ranger.' One career was entirely about human–human interaction and the other was a human interface with animals and nature. While at that time I could not imagine how those two options could be combined, today it all makes sense.

My first position in the 1970s was as a therapist for adolescent girls who had been placed by the court into a residential facility. Each had devastating histories of multiple forms of abuse, and their emotion and behavior clearly reflected their pain. These innocent children had been interpersonally betrayed by the very people tasked with their care, their parents and families. These girls had not only suffered abuse and neglect; they suffered a 'deprivation of life.' They did not attend public schools or have birthday parties, friends, toys, or the typical experiences of other children. If their families did have a pet, it was often abused and neglected, as well. None of the girls trusted humans or even recognized dogs as possessing qualities of relatedness, support, and affection.

Though I never doubted my career choice, I found myself organizing a wilderness trip for the girls that involved camping in tents with no facilities and nighttime temperatures of 30 degrees. We loaded a station wagon with the girls, gear, and Kelly, our large dog and drove over ten hours to a forest that was devoid of any semblance of civilization. The girls had never been anywhere that lacked radios, television, other humans and the constant reminders that they were 'damaged goods.'

Captivated by this novel setting, the girls began to relax and within a few days they began to engage, explore, and cooperate with each other on an authentic level. Kelly followed them everywhere, and they began to talk to him, stroking his back, and showing affection. At night, the girls invited him into their tent to 'protect them.' Kelly slept soundly in the center of their tent with five bodies snuggled tightly around him.

Carrying buckets of water, building a fire, caring for Kelly, and washing in the snowmelt of the mountains gave the girls a newfound sense of pride and confidence. While what we did worked well, I was not yet aware that cold water immersion, nurturing safe touch, social support, and carrying heavy buckets of water improved vagal tone, increased oxytocin, and called on the parasympathetic nervous system which supports calm, wellbeing, and social connection. In the 1980s, most mental health professionals relied upon education, experience, and intuition to direct us in treatment. We lacked the science that explained how and why interventions work. While intuition has long been underrated, today there is science that explains what it is and how it works. Over the past two decades, momentum has been growing among clinicians and researchers to integrate the neurosciences with psychology, and the potential of that collaboration is profound.

Through the following years, I worked with inner-city children (and families) during the crack epidemic, and then children in other socioeconomic settings, witnessing a wide range of maltreatment, violence, and disrupted families. Involved with Head Start, abuse and neglect services, foster care, in- and out-patient programs, private practice, and all levels of schools, it became obvious that *all* children are vulnerable to the devastation of familial and societal adversity.

During that time period, increased community violence, drug use, and suicides raised concerns in school settings. This led to my involvement in district-wide programming and initiatives that created protocols for crisis response and training for traumatic events within schools. During that period, I also provided disaster response on a national level for the Red Cross and participated in an international collaboration of European governments and agencies for transportation disaster planning.

Involved with children, families, animals, nature, and outdoor sports since early childhood, I have had abundant opportunity to witness the beneficial effects of dogs, horses, the natural world, and movement-based activity on mental and physical health. These associations are not new discoveries and yet, interest, attention, and efforts have risen and fallen throughout history.

Profound advances in technology have improved human lifestyles, health, digital connectivity, and access to information across much of the world, yet the human cost of these advances has not been fully realized. Digital communication deprives the child and adolescent of the emotional information contained in facial expressions, vocal prosody and tone, and nonverbal gestures that are critical in social relationships. Even when humans are with other humans, eye contact and gaze has shifted away from faces to phones and laptops. The masking of faces due to the pandemic over the past three years is predicted to have delayed the normal social development of children across the world.

Concurrent with mass extinctions and loss of natural landscapes and resources, our species is also distancing from the animal and natural world which were primary sources that shaped our species. The social support, attachments, and comfort provided by our human–animal relationships are today desperately needed, as the world experiences increased violence, war, poverty, and decreased family and social support. These conditions cannot be rectified quickly, but improving the identification and treatment of children who have been victimized, deprived of healthy relationships, dysregulated, and disconnected is a step toward improving outcomes for all children.

The human and canine species have been shaped by their coevolution, and this distinct interspecies relationship can be a model for reconnection, healthy relationships, and healing. I have come to believe that there may be validity within interest surveys, as while it took some time to correctly interpret the results, they were right on. Humans and animals: that's a combination for the ages.

Abbreviations

AMA	American Medical Association
AAI	Animal-assisted interventions
AAP	Animal-assisted psychotherapy
AAT	Animal-assisted therapies
ABCD	Adolescent brain cognitive development
ACC	Anterior cingulate cortex
ACE	Adverse childhood experiences
ACTH	Adrenocorticotropic hormone
ADHD	Attention deficit hyperactivity disorder
ANS	Autonomic nervous system
ASD	Autism spectrum disorder
AVP	Vasopressin
BOLD	Blood Oxygen Level Dependent
CAP	Canine-assisted psychotherapy
CC	Corpus callosum
CD	Conduct disorder
CEN	Central executive network
CM	Child maltreatment
CNS	Central nervous system
CRH	Corticotropin-releasing hormone
CSF	Cerebrospinal fluid
CT	C-Tactile
DA	Disorganized attachment
DMN	Default mode network
DSM	Diagnostic and Statistical Manual of Mental Disorders
DT	Developmental trauma
DTD	Developmental Trauma Disorder
ED	Emotional dysregulation
EE	Enriched environment
EEG	Electroencephalogram
EF	Executive functions
ENS	Enteric nervous system
EQ	Encephalization quotient
ER	Emotion regulation

FC	Functional connectivity
HAB	Human–animal bond
HAI	Human–animal interaction
HCB	Human-canine bond
HCE	Human–canine coevolution
HCP	Human connectome project
HPA	Hypothalamus-pituitary-adrenal
HR	Heart rate
HRV	Heart rate variability
IAABC	The International Association of Animal Behaviour Consultants
IAHAIO	International Association of Human-Animal Interaction Organizations
IBS	Institute of Behavioral Science
ICN	Intrinsic connectivity networks
JAMA	Journal of the American Medical Association
lmPFC	Left medial prefrontal cortex
LS	Large-scale
MN	Mirror neurons
NCTSN	National Child Traumatic Stress Network
NIMH	National Institute of Mental Health
NIRS	Near-infrared spectroscopy
NMDA	myeloid cell nuclear differentiation antigen
ODD	Oppositional defiant disorder
OFC	Orbitofrontal Cortex
OT	Oxytocin
PACK	Positive Assertive Cooperative Kids
PCC	Posterior cingulate cortex
PET	Positron emission tomography
PFC	Prefrontal Cortex
PNS	Parasympathetic nervous systems
PP	Psychopathology
PT	Play therapy
PTSD	Post-traumatic stress disorder
PVT	Polyvagal theory
RB-RB	Right brain-to-right brain
RC	Regulatory competence
RDoC	Research domain criteria
RH	Right hemisphere
RNA	ribonucleic acid
SAM	Sympathetic-adrenal-medullary
SES	Social engagement system
SN	Salience network
SNS	Sympathetic nervous system

SPECT	Single photon emission computed tomography
SRS	Stress response system
TD	Trauma development
TLE	Temporal lobe epilepsy
ToM	Theory of mind
UCLA	University of California, Los Angeles
US	United States
WBS	William-Beurens Syndrome
WP	Working psychotherapy

Introduction

Samantha: 'The Theft of An Innocent Soul and the Broken Hearts Left Behind'

For several years, I was a volunteer member of the Red Cross disaster mental health team and provided services to victims of fires, weather disasters, and two major airline crashes. These events were challenging yet nothing like the assignment I received on a summer day in 2002.

A little girl was playing with her neighborhood friends in the shadow of their homes when a depraved predator drove into the complex and grabbed her. Five year old Samantha was kidnapped, assaulted, and murdered within the first few hours after she had disappeared. The loss of this courageous little girl devastated her family, her community, and all who came to know her story.

My supervisor from the Red Cross called and instructed me to immediately head up to the community. No protocol or guidelines existed for this type of response, and details were just emerging. I knew Samantha had suffered horrendous emotional and physical pain and that her family and community were shattered. We did not know what the neighborhood children knew of the circumstances, or what they may have witnessed or heard. I shuddered to even imagine their pain as I gathered myself and headed to my car. As I stepped into the garage however, I suddenly stopped. I didn't know why, but something in my gut made me turn around.

Opening the door, the apparent source of my hesitation was patiently sitting there, gazing up at me. Seamus and I had responded to a lot of difficult situations in the past and I had always had confidence in our work. This was different, though. How could I expect him to be comfortable when I was nervous? I studied his eyes, trying to read them. Seamus and I had an attuned, synchronous relationship, and when I quit over thinking and listened to my heart, I knew. We were a team, and he somehow knew I needed him. He jumped into the car, laid down, and fell asleep.

When we arrived, we exited the car and walked toward the apartment complex. I glanced down at the little guy and when he gazed back my uncertainty was replaced with a calm confidence. We were there to help and we were ready.

DOI: 10.4324/9781003217534-1

We entered the complex onto a grass lawn that was bordered by one-story residences. I quickly scanned the area and noticed multiple groups of residents, law enforcement personnel, and reporters, huddled in deep solemn conversation. Where were the children? As we walked further across the grass, they suddenly appeared. The children came from multiple directions and ran directly at us, as if they knew we were coming. They seemed driven by an overwhelming and unfamiliar state of arousal. Seamus knew the drill and dropped to the ground presenting his soft belly. He was quickly coated in a mass of little hands, as the children settled into the grass, encircling us. Taking in the scene of the confident little guy surrounded by these young friends and neighbors of Samantha, I realized this was right; this was what was needed.

Multiple voices tumbled over each other as they simultaneously spoke with an urgent cadence and pulsating prosody. Seamus just settled in and made no effort to move. He seemed relaxed and actually made eye contact with children as they spoke. The anxious messages just streamed out: 'I'm really afraid he'll come back.' 'I miss Samantha.' 'I can't sleep by myself.' 'I have a bunny.' 'My mom has been crying and hugging me too tight,' and 'what's his name?'

Seamus became a medium of connection and comfort for the children, providing a safe space to share their feelings and join with each other. The arrival of the children was unorchestrated and spontaneous, yet a joining had occurred. The kids were settled into the grass, still energized by a physiological agitation, yet they had come together as a group. They seemed to draw strength from each other by collectively connecting and sharing their grief, and Seamus was clearly a catalyst and hub of safety.

Most of the animal-assisted interventions (AAI) literature focuses on how animals benefit humans, and Seamus did provide these children with a much-needed sense of safety and connection. His confidence and compassion for the children reinforced my belief that he genuinely wanted to be present for them. Working psychotherapy dogs also function as a source of support for the clinician. Seamus seemed to know when he was needed and I was immensely grateful to him for his intuition, trust, and commitment.

The specific characteristics of many dogs that enable their efficacy in therapeutic situations also confer vulnerability. Sensitivity, attunement, and a willingness to be present can put them at risk for emotional contagion, fatigue, and stress. We need to be aware of the effects and impact of therapeutic experience on the animal. Are they merely tolerating human contact or do they truly enjoy their time together? What benefits might they experience and how do they give their consent? An animal with this degree of dedication deserves the respect, consideration, and attention of the clinician, as their participation can cause stress and harm to their health and well-being. Endowed with their incredible trust, we have an enormous responsibility to ensure their safety, health, and welfare.

Why the Dog?

Today, dogs share our homes, our beds, and our hearts, yet the majority of us are probably unaware of *why* they do so or *how* this relationship began. They have been beside us since early evolution. Humans and wolves (the ancestors of dogs) were brought together during the Pleistocene Epoch by a dramatic climate change known as the 'Ice Age.' The wolf was unknown to humans until this event thrust them together into a new habitat. Though morphologically disparate, humans and wolves converged, forming an alliance based on sociality, cooperation, and respect. Their alliance seeded a unique interspecies coevolution that profoundly influenced both species. Sociality in humans and canines continued to increase, and today both species are incredibly social and actually *require* healthy interpersonal interaction for early development, health, and well-being. Pertinent to current psychotherapy processes, neuroscientists, trauma scholars, and clinicians recognize that healing the consequences of maltreatment, dysregulation, and developmental trauma *also* require healthy relationships and the support of others.

Modern dogs are recognized for their unique and profound social interest in humans and capability for attunement, and these traits are not by chance. The emerging science behind this relationship is not only compelling, it validates the dog's potential to help heal and restore young humans. The potential of the working psychotherapy dog to help recalibrate and reregulate children and adolescents with dysregulation is supported by our coevolutionary history and the consolidation of recent paradigm-shifting research.

Dogs have developed an impressive proficiency for reciprocal communication with us. They are capable of recognizing our emotions, sensing our intentions, and can even predict our behavior. Current research reveals that humans and modern dogs share anatomical, neurobiological, and even genetic similarities, as a result of the coevolution. The convergence of our species has shaped who we are and our continuing relationship will perhaps shape who we will become, as evolution is not finished.

Several world leaders, including Mahatma Gandhi, believed that the measure of a country's morality and integrity could be determined by the way it treated their vulnerable populations. As children and animals reflect two of our most exploitable populations, perhaps this unique interspecies relationship *will* strengthen and improve the humanity of humans.

This book is about the distinctive capabilities of the canine species that support the therapeutic treatment of children with dysregulation, a state most commonly caused by early maltreatment and the consequential outcome of 'developmental trauma'. Through the integration of neurobiology and psychology, well-designed interventions can more precisely target the dysfunction, disconnection, and dysregulation that knock the child off a healthy developmental trajectory.

The Devastation of Childhood Maltreatment

Child maltreatment (CM) was identified as a public health crisis over 50 years ago and continues as a critical challenge today, in spite of increased focus on prevention programming. In 2020, 618,399 children were reported victims of maltreatment in the United States, with almost half under the age of five (U.S. Department of Health and Human Services, 2021). Maltreatment can be summarized as incidents of threat, harm, deprivation, and neglect (McLaughlin et al., 2014). Harm is abuse which can be physical, sexual, or emotional, and includes exposure to domestic violence. Neglect can be defined as the deprivation of care, nurturance, protection, and expected provisions of parenting.

A devastating paradox occurs for the young child when the caregiver who is tasked with their protection and care is the same individual who is perpetrating harm or deprivation. The deepest cut to the human psyche is the *interpersonal betrayal* by someone who is loved, trusted, and needed. Interpersonal betrayal robs the child of crucial requisites for development: safety, coregulation, and interpersonal relatedness. Maltreatment in the context of attachment impedes the child's mastery of critical developmental tasks such as acquiring autonomy, social and emotional skills, and emotion regulation (D'Andrea et al., 2012).

One of the most debilitating consequences of interpersonal betrayal is the generalization of distrust in the human perpetrator to other humans. This factor is an invisible elephant in the room that sabotages most forms of trauma treatment, as the success of most models is predicted by the therapeutic alliance between the clinician and client. A healthy relationship is fundamental in the success of early development, is predictive of future relationships and social function, and is the necessary context for healing children with dysregulation and disconnection. The evidence that supports the ideal fit of the canine into treatment of an interpersonally betrayed child is compelling and offers a solution to this clinical dilemma.

Child Maltreatment is Associated with Psychopathology

Severe and chronic childhood maltreatment (CM) confers a significant risk for disruption of the developmental trajectory of the child and is one of the most grievous causes of psychopathology (Jaffee, 2017; McCrory & Viding, 2015; van der Kolk, 2003). As the child is in the midst of development, the effects of early adversity can confer profound and widespread consequences, along with a lifelong vulnerability to further abuse and exploitation. A history of severe CM triples the risk of psychiatric disorders and is responsible for approximately 50% of diagnoses (Zeananah & Humphreys, 2018). Almost 75% of adults with enduring depressive disorders were found to have a history of moderate-to-severe maltreatment (Struck et al., 2020). A causal relationship between CM and psychopathology is well established, however, the mechanisms that link the two are not as well defined.

Dysregulation As a Link Between Maltreatment and Psychopathology

Robust research has shown that CM can induce alterations to neural structures, functions, and connectivity in the immature brain (Cross et al., 2017; deBellis & Zisk, 2014; McLaughlin et al., 2015). These alterations reflect *neural* dysregulation, and while changes function as adaptive responses to the immediate environment, they become maladaptive in a different environment.

The association between maltreatment and *emotional* dysregulation (ED) is well established and backed by substantial research conducted within the past 25 years (Beauchaine & Cicchetti, 2019). Emotional dysregulation is described as a compromised ability to tolerate negative emotion and difficulty processing and modulating affective states (Dvir et al., 2014). The distress of emotional dysregulation and the maladaptive processing, expression and communication of those states compromise goal-driven behaviors (Beauchaine, 2015).

Emotional dysregulation has been framed as a mediator of the relationship between maltreatment and consequential adverse behaviors and is linked to a lifelong risk for psychopathology (Cole et al., 2017). It is considered a transdiagnostic mechanism among multiple disciplines and across theoretical perspectives (Beauchaine & Cicchetti, 2019; Fernandez et al., 2016) including the research domain criteria (Beauchaine, 2015), a recently developed diagnostic system.

Another pathway by which CM can precipitate psychopathology that may precede ED is through its more direct effects upon the immature brain. Children are the most vulnerable of all populations as their protracted development renders them highly dependent upon the quality of adult protection and care. A large percentage of early brain development relies upon environmental conditions and experiences for healthy growth, integration, and organization. This development is accentuated by critical periods of heightened receptiveness called neuroplasticity. The knife cuts both ways, however, and increased neuroplasticity also increases susceptibility to relational and environmental adversity. Child maltreatment functions as a virulent toxin across the brain causing dysregulation that pervades neural structures, functions, and connectivity. Robust research has revealed consequences of CM that disrupt development, cause alterations to the brain, *and* seed dysregulation (Cross et al., 2017; DeBellis & Zisk, 2014; McLaughlin et al., 2015; Perry, 2000; Teicher et al., 2014).

More recently, other functional domains that become dysregulated have also come under consideration as possible mediators of the onset and maintenance of psychopathology, as all domains are vulnerable to dysregulation via the neural pathways that subserve functions. Consolidating literature and research, it can be predicted that neural dysregulation has the potential to impact all developmental domains, including emotion (Cole et al., 2017); behavior (McLaughlin et al., 2014); social cognition (Dvir et al., 2014); cognition (executive functions, memory, and attention) (Godsil et al., 2013); and intrapersonal (the self) and interpersonal (attachment and relationships) (van der Kolk, 2005). The increase in neuroimaging studies has produced strong evidence that neurobiology is, indeed, a primary domain that is impacted by dysregulation.

Numerous investigations seeking to identify a mechanistic link between maltreatment and psychopathology have focused upon the association between neural dysregulation of the stress response system and psychopathology (Heim et al., 2008). This theory, along with other emerging models, seems to imply that neurobiological dysregulation is at least partially responsible for other domain functional impairments. As every emotion, thought, and action is accompanied by a neural correlate, it makes sense that neurobiology is highly relevant to all functions (Grawe, 2007). Speculations and investigations of the neurobiology of early development, dysregulation, and developmental trauma are gaining momentum in multiple fields and a shift in perspectives is emerging.

Consolidating current literature and research, neural dysregulation is proposed as a linking mechanism between CM and psychopathology. Neural substrates serve all of the developmental domains, and dysregulation has been linked to almost all psychiatric disorders. Dysregulation of multiple domains also constitutes identifying criteria for the proposed developmental trauma disorder (Parish-Plass, 2021); Spinazzola et al., 2018).

The Integration of Neuroscience with Psychology

Louis Cozolino (2017) shared that psychotherapy emerged from neurology during the 19th century, and Sigmund Freud, initially a neuroscientist, may have been the first to envision an integration of these two fields. In spite of his foresight, however, the two disciplines diverged over the next century as psychologists pursued the interpretation of the mind and neuroscientists targeted the science of the brain. A century passed before the conceptualization was reintroduced and today, the incredible potential and value of an integration of neuroscience and psychology is being promoted by numerous scholars and scientists from multiple disciplines, including Cozolino, Eric Kandel, Allan Schore, Stephen Porges, Klaus Glawe, and Daniel Siegel.

There seems to be a shift from a dualism perspective that considers the mind, brain, and body as separate entities, to one of 'monosim', a term that conceptualizes these components as an integrated, complex, and interdependent system. This perspective will catalyze further collaboration between psychology and the neurosciences in research and clinical exploration providing the foundation of empirical evidence and knowledge that sanction and legitimize the field of animal-assisted therapy. Obtaining a clearer understanding of neurobiology also enables clinicians to draw from the precise principles and mechanisms of science that build the brain and subsidize development and function. Neurobiological theories also help explain dysfunction, dysregulation, and psychopathology. Many experts subscribe to the theory that emotion is seated in central nervous system processes and that psychopathology is likely caused by dysfunctional neuronal structures and systems (Hebb, 1949; van der Kolk, 2005). These principles and mechanisms will also inform the treatment of dysregulation, which functions well as a transdiagnostic target.

It is suggested that the future of psychotherapy will be directed by an increasing awareness of the neurobiological processes involved in early brain development, disruptions in the maturation process, dysregulation, and psychopathology. Even more exciting is that this knowledge and perspective can be applied to the design and application of treatments that restore regulation, heal trauma, and improve the functional success of the child. Changes in emotion, behavior, and regulation incurred through psychotherapy promote and shape neurobiological change (Cozolino, 2017; Kandel, 1998) which supports the longevity of functional improvements.

Treating Children with Dysregulation and Developmental Trauma

For much of the 20th century, behavioral and cognitive models were predominant forms of treatment, yet there has been a shift back to the relevance and importance of emotion, attachment, relationships, and brain-based theory. The recent parallel interest and research of trauma and neurobiology have been supported by advances in neuroimaging technology and have increased calls for more collaboration between disciplines.

There have been numerous calls for more efficacious treatments for those children who constitute an underserved population (Malchiodi, 2008). Most talk-based therapies require verbal proficiency, insight, and self-reflection, proficiencies that children have not yet developed. Effective therapies for children are developmentally attuned, sensory-rich, encourage movement and play, and occur in a positive, nurturing relational context. Nonverbal, right-brain communication that facilitates creative expression fits well with the dysregulated child. Play, animal-assisted therapies, movement, mind/body, and creative expressive formats such as art, theater, and music are effective modalities for treating the sequelae of trauma (Chapman, 2014; van der Kolk, 2014).

Healing from trauma requires healthy relationships, attunement, acceptance, and an implicit communication system that transmits across the nonconscious pathway from the right brain of the clinician to the right brain of the child. The therapeutic relationship is analogous to a healthy, secure attachment relationship, and a dog is capable of forming interspecies attachment relationships. Dogs provide the child with a sense of safety (Melson & Fine, 2010); aid in the establishment of the therapeutic alliance (Parish-Plass, 2021); provide social and emotional support, and increase the comfort and willingness to share emotions (Bryan et al., 2014).

Incorporating canines into the treatment of trauma exponentially increases options for interventions that address safety, regulation, relationships, emotional, social, and communication skills; all areas that can be impacted by CM, DT, and dysregulation. Working psychotherapy canines offer an ideal solution to this dilemma, as they function as an alternative living being that can participate in attachment, relational, and social realms. The evidence that supports canine mechanisms of change is detailed throughout the book.

The ni-CAP Framework

Neurobiologically infused canine-assisted psychotherapy (ni-CAP) is conceptualized as a therapeutic framework that is developmentally informed, neurobiologically based, and functions as a relational and experiential milieu that is innervated by canine mechanisms of change. Ni-CAP blends psychology and neurobiology to effect positive and enduring change. The polyvagal theory and vagal system are integral to ni-CAP, along with attachment, the oxytocin system, and mirror neurons. This framework is highly flexible and can be integrated with components of other models, particularly play, mindfulness, mind/body, movement-based treatments, and therapeutic education.

The ni-CAP process parallels nature's developmental trajectory that prescribes a sequential and hierarchical pattern of neural development in the child, mining the evolutionarily conserved patterns that have worked for thousands of years. The fulfillment of the child's potential is dependent upon a healthy attachment relationship to maximize the expression of the genetic blueprint. When the quality of the caregiver–infant attachment relationship is altered or disrupted, repair must occur within the context of other healthy relationships.

The neurobiological and developmental focus in treatment has been incorporated into studies and models by Alan Schore (2012), Bruce Perry (2013), and Linda Chapman (2014). Neurodevelopment follows a primitive to complex, inside-out, and bottom-up direction. Primitive structures (such as the brainstem) are formed and organized prior to development of the limbic system, and the prefrontal regions of higher cognition are the last to mature. The advanced maturation of higher structures is dependent upon successful maturation of the lower regions (Perry, 2013).

Psychotherapy processes are capable of promoting plasticity and neurobiological changes through a calculated balance of nurturance and titrated stress (Cozolino, 2017). Ni-CAP and many other therapy modalities can positively impact and change brain circuitry. Young brains are responsive to positive, nurturing, and enriching environments and experiences which are known to increase neuroplasticity and promote neural growth, integration, and organization (Siegel, 2012). Ni-CAP is informed by Kandel's five principles of neuroscience that function as a guide for incorporating neuroscience into psychotherapy (Kandel, 1998). Ni-CAP also taps and integrates elemental mechanisms of nature, synchrony, rhythm, and mimicry into interventions and activities as they function as catalysts for neural growth and organization.

About the Book

The components of this book are drawn from the expertise and pioneering work of multiple scientists, scholars, and clinicians who have studied and advanced the disciplines of psychology, neuroscience, traumatology, and animal sciences that serve children. Their work fueled the author's curiosity, motivation, and desire to learn more about these topics beginning with their early work in the 1990s. Their wisdom, experience, and influence upon the dynamic landscape of human and animal relationships and the neurobiology of development, dysregulation and healing mechanisms were 'front-edge' back then and they continue to lead, advancing the science and clinical fields today. Bruce Perry, Bessel van der Kolk, Alan Schore, Stephen Porges, Louis Cozolino, Eric Kandel, Daniel Siegel, and Sue Carter are notable researchers and clinicians who inspired this work. Additional sources of expertise that also shaped this work include Nancy Parish-Plass, Rise VanFleet, Philip Tedeschi, Meg Olmert, Marc Bekoff, Kate McLaughlin, and Aubrey Fine, among numerous other sources.

The synopsis of neurobiology will hopefully stimulate a deeper interest and exploration into neuroscience for mental health clinicians, professionals, researchers, instructors, and students who are interested in expanding their knowledge base for the treatment of trauma-induced dysregulation and other traditional disorders in children. A large majority of clinicians have not had significant training in the neurosciences as historically it has not been part of the prospectus of most clinical fields. The most enlightening aspect of the expansion of knowledge may be to recognize that what was once conceptualized as 'common' traits of intuition, humanity, compassion, and relational skills has been supported by neurobiological correlates all along.

There are numerous comprehensive educational programs and scholarly sources of scientific information available to clinicians today, and it is predicted that the integration of neuroscience and psychology will continue to advance the field of mental health. The author is also hoping to stimulate increased multidisciplinary collaboration in discussion, programming, treatment applications, and research. Collaborative projects that involve diverse perspectives illuminate, challenge, and exponentially increase the reservoir of knowledge that will improve the lives of humans and animals and our interspecies interactions (HAI).

The neurobiology of early development, maltreatment, dysregulation and developmental trauma (DT) is consolidated in a manner that supports a broader, more comprehensive knowledge of the redirected pathway and its consequences. The information can be translated into a more comprehensive evaluation of the child's needs, more precise, focused targets and increased efficacy in applications for treatment.

An awareness of the influences of the interspecies coevolution on the human–canine relationship enables the professional that works with humans and dogs to develop interventions that not only match needs but are targeted and efficacious. Current and ongoing research is revealing fascinating capabilities of the canine species, information that will be highly useful to clinicians who incorporate dogs, other professionals, *and* those who work and live with dogs and/or children.

Although children and adolescents with dysregulation propagated by maltreatment and developmental trauma are the primary population discussed within this book, neural and multiple domain dysregulation occurs in a wide range of disorders. The principles and mechanisms of neural dysregulation and the therapeutic processes supported by canines, also apply to children identified with autism spectrum disorder (ASD), attention deficit hyperactivity disorder (ADHD), and other disorders that share neural dysregulation and related symptomatology.

The spotlight on canines is due to the recognition that they are the most common animal utilized in psychotherapy and the intention is to highlight the coevolution that is so distinctly relevant to their efficacy. It is recognized that horses also support highly effective models of healing, and their participation in AAIs is expanding through rapidly increasing interest, scientific, study, and programming.

The book is divided into three sections. Part I contains Chapters 1 through 4. The first chapter opens with the story of a child who experiences physical and emotional maltreatment and provides an overview of the primary themes of the book. Case studies are presented throughout the book and are either identity-protected or hybrids of multiple cases. The neurobiology of structures and systems of the brain that are relevant to development, maltreatment, dysregulation, DT, and healing are detailed in the second chapter. The third chapter is a comprehensive look at the crucial role of the attachment process in the development of regulation and resilience. The specific information presented on attachment is significant to designing and implementing treatment for dysregulation and has been augmented with exciting new research. The fourth chapter details how neural dysregulation impacts brain structures, function, connectivity, systems, and networks. Several models are discussed that were developed as explanations of the mechanisms and clinical manifestations of dysregulation.

The second section begins with Chapter 5, a fascinating review of our evolutionary history that brought humans and dogs together. This brief synopsis illuminates the critical factors that seeded and grew the human–canine bond (HCB), and gives a brief summary of the profound changes that resulted from the convergence of our two species. Chapter 6 explains why modern dogs can be efficacious therapeutic agents, detailing their traits, skills, and mechanisms that enable their success. Numerous recent discoveries in canine science have occurred due to advanced neuroimaging technology.

The importance of welfare has risen to the forefront in discussions of animal-assisted interventions (AAI), and should be a primary consideration for all animal-supported therapies (Chapter 7). Consideration of the dog's status as a sentient being, their perception of participation, and their emotional, social, and neurobiological well-being are illuminated and offer a compelling argument for viewing the dog through a more scientific and informed perspective. The incorporation of a canine into therapeutic work must be done with expertise, planning, intention, and a treatment plan. The work requires a synchronous relationship between the clinician and dog that is attuned and authentic. While the framework is flexible and intended to be shaped to the child's needs, the therapeutic relational context does not fit with an additional individual who functions as a dog handler.

The clinician–canine relationship is discussed in detail, listing responsibilities of the clinician, methods of welfare assessment, and the view through the canine lens. The clinician, child, and dog create multiple relationships, and the dog is not simply a soft head to pet, a tool, or 'eye candy.' They are capable of 'working both sides of the room,' attending to each member, and the clinician must also be capable of working on behalf of both the child *and* the dog.

The final section of the book (Part III) demonstrates how a basic knowledge of neurobiological processes can guide clinical work to shape and incorporate canine mechanisms of healing, to restore regulation in the child from the inside out. The dog supports the establishment of an enriched environment, meeting the child in an intersubjective space to support healing and restoration emotionally and socially. Chapter 8 explains the ni-CAP framework, detailing the theory, principles, and components that shape this format.

Chapter 9 shares a template that will guide the clinician in blending neurobiology and psychology to create individualized interventions through the integration of components and mechanisms. This framework is not designed to be standardized into a manual or 'how to' book, as the unique professional experience and personal skills of the clinician are highly influential in the success of the treatment. The power of the relationship with both the child and dog is in its authenticity, implicit communication, and ability to connect.

Conclusion

Supported by evolution-influenced adaptations, relational and social acumen, and neurobiological mechanisms of change, the dog is capable of reaching through the layers of distrust, fear, and distress, to touch the heart of the traumatized child. The beginning chapter will introduce 'Josh,' illuminating the experience of maltreatment viewed through the lens of the child.

References

Beauchaine, T.P. (2015). Future directions in emotion dysregulation and youth psychopathology. *Journal of Clinical Child and Adolescent Psychology*; 44: 875–896. https://doi.org/10.1080/15374416.2015.1038827

Beauchaine, T.P. & Cicchetti, D. (2019). Emotion dysregulation and emerging psychopathology: A transdiagnostic, transdisciplinary perspective. *Development and Psychopathology*; 31(3): 709–804. https://doi.org/10.1017/S0954579419000671

Bryan, J.L. (2014). Pet affinity buffers the negative impact of ambivalence over emotional expression on perceived social support. *Personality and Individual Differences* 68: 23–27.

Chapman, L. (2014). *Neurobiologically Informed Trauma Therapy with Children and Adolescents*. New York, NY: W.W. Norton.

Cole, P.M., Hall, S.E., & Hajal, N. (2017). Emotion dysregulation as a risk factor for psychopathology. In T.P. Beauchaine & S.P. Hinshaw (eds.), *Child and Adolescent Psychopathology* (pp. 265–298). Toronto, Ontario: Wiley & Sons & Sons.

Cozolino, L. (2017). *The Neuroscience of Psychotherapy: Healing the Social Brain* (3rd ed.). New York, NY: W.W. Norton.

Cross, D., Fani, N., Powers, A., & Bradley, B. (2017). Neurobiological development in the context of childhood trauma. *Clinical Psychology* (New York); 24(2): 111–124.

D'Andrea, W., Ford, J., Stolbach, B., Spinazzola, J., & van der Kolk, B. (2012). Understanding interpersonal trauma in children: why we need a developmentally appropriate trauma diagnosis. *The American Journal of Orthopsychiatry*; 82(2): 187–200. https://doi.org/10.1111/j.1939-0025.2012.01154.x

DeBellis, M.D., & Zisk, A. (2014).The biological effects of childhood trauma. *Child and Adolescent Psychiatric Clinics of North America*; 23(2): 182–222.

Dvir, Y., Ford, J.D., Hill, M., & Frazier, J.A. (2014).Childhood maltreatment, emotional dysregulation, and psychiatric comorbidities. *Harvard Review of Psychiatry*; 22(3): 149–161.

Fernandez, K.C., Jazaieri, H., & Gross, J.J. (2016). Emotion Regulation: A Transdiagnostic Perspective on a New RDoC Domain. *Cognitive Therapy and Research*; 40: 426–440. https://doi.org/10.1007/s10608-016.9772-2

Godsil, B.P., Kiss, J.P., Spedding, M., & Jay, T.M. (2013). The hippocampal-prefrontal pathways: The weak link in psychiatric disorders? *European Neuropsychopharmacology*; 23(10): 1165–1181. https://doi.org/10.1016/j.euroneuro.2012.10.018

Grawe, K. (2007). *Neuropsychotherapy: How the neurosciences inform effective psychotherapy*. New York, NY: Psychology Press.

Hebb, D.O. (1949). *The Organization of Behavior*. John Wiley & Sons Inc.

Heim, C., Newport, D.J., Mletzko, T., Miller, A.H., & Nemeroff, C.B. (2008). The link between childhood trauma and depression: Insights from HPA axis studies in humans. *Psychoneuroendocrinology*; 22: 693–710. https://doi.org/10.1016/j.psyneuen.2008.03.008

Jaffee, S.R. (2017). Child maltreatment and risk for psychopathology in childhood and adulthood. *Annual Review of Clinical Psychology*; 8(13): 525–551. https://doi.org/10.1146/annurev-clinpsy-032816-045005

Kandel, E. (1998). A new intellectual framework for psychiatry. *The American Journal of Psychiatry*; 155: 457–469.

Malchiodi, C.A. (2008). *Creative Interventions with Traumatized Children*. 1st ed. Guilford Press.

McCrory, E.J., & Viding, E. (2015). The theory of latent vulnerability: Reconceptualizing the link between childhood maltreatment and psychiatric disorder. *Development and Psychopathology*; 27(2): 493–505. https://doi.org/10.1017/S0954579415000115

McLaughlin, K.A., Sheridan, M.A., Gold, A.L. … & Pine, D.S. (2015).Maltreatment exposure, brain structure, and fear conditioning in children and adolescents. *Neuropsychopharmacology*; 41: 1956–1964.

McLaughlin, K.A., Sheridan, M.A., & Lambert, H.K. (2014).Childhood adversity and neural development: Deprivation and threat as distinct dimensions of early experience. *Neuroscience and Biobehavioral Reviews*; 47: 578–591.

Melson, G. & Fine, A.H. (2010). Animals in the lives of children. In: A.H. Fine (Ed.), *Handbook on animal-assisted therapy: Theoretical foundations and guidelines for practice* (3rd ed.). Cambridge, MA: Elsevier Academic Press.

Parish-Plass, N. (2021). Animal-assisted psychotherapy for developmental trauma through the lens of interpersonal neurobiology of trauma: Creating connection with self and others. *Journal of Psychol Integration*; 31(3): 302–325. https://doi.org/10.1037/int0000253

Perry, B. (2013). The neurosequential model of therapeutics: Application of a developmentally sensitive and neurobiology-informed approach to clinical problem solving in young maltreated children. In K. Brandt, B.D. Perry, S. Seligman, & E. Tronick (Eds.), *Infant & Early Childhood Mental Health: Core Concepts and Clinical Practice* 21–54. Washington, DC: American Psychiatric Publishing.

Perry, B.D. (2000). Traumatized children: How childhood trauma influences brain development. *Ch Trauma Acad*. Retrieved from: https://www.childwelfare.gov

Schore, A.N. (2012). *The science of the art of psychotherapy*. W.W. Norton & Company.

Siegel, D.J. (2012). *The developing mind: How relationships and the brain interact to shape who we are* (2nd ed.). The Guilford Press.

Spinazzola, J., van der Kolk, B., & Ford, J.D. (2018). When nowhere is safe: Interpersonal trauma and attachment adversity as antecedents of posttraumatic stress disorder and developmental trauma disorder. *Journal of Traumatic Stress*; 31: 631–642.

Struck, N., Drug, A., Yuksel, D., Stein, F., Schmitt, S., Meller, T., Brosch, K., Dannlowski, E., Nenadic, I., Kircher, T., Brakemeier, E-L. (2020). Childhood maltreatment and adult mental disorders-the prevalence of different types of maltreatment and associations with age of onset and severity of symptoms. *Psychiatry Research*; 293: 113398. https://doi.org/10.1016/j.psychres.2020.113398

Teicher, M.H., Anderson, C.M., Ohashi, K., & Polcari, A. (2014). Childhood mal-treatment: Altered network centrality of cingulated, precuneus, temporal pole and insula. *Biological Psychiatry*; 76(4): 297–305. https://doi.org/10.1016/j.biopsych.2013.09.016

U.S. Department of Health and Human Services. (2021).Children's Bureau. *Child Maltreatment 2019*. Retrieved from: https://www.acf.hhs.gov/gov/cb/data-research/child-maltreatment

van der Kolk, B. (2003). The neurobiology of childhood trauma and abuse. *Child and Adolescent Psychiatric Clinics of North America*; 12: 293–317.

Van der Kolk, B. (2005). Developmental trauma disorder: Toward a rational diagnosis for children with complex trauma histories. *Psychiatric Annual*; 35(5): 401–408. https://doi.org/10.3928/00485713-20050501-06

van der Kolk, B. (2014). *The Body Keeps the Score*. New York, NY: Penguin.

Zeananah, C.H., & Humphreys, K.L. (2018). Child abuse and neglect. *Journal of the American Academy of Child and Adolescent Psychiatry*; 57(9): 637–644. https://doi.org/10.1016/j.aac.2018.06.007

Part One

Development and Dysregulation of Children through a Neurobiological Lens

Chapter 1   When Bad Things Happen to Good Children

Introduction

Josh felt the threat like a punch in the gut before it even registered in consciousness. The slamming door, foreboding footsteps, and the angry voice were all signals that his father was home. He was drunk, really drunk. Josh's head began to spin. He felt a little sick and his throat had a catch in it. He froze in place and his eyes scanned the room as an image of his mother appeared in his head. She wasn't home, yet a strange sound emerged from his mouth as if he could somehow summon her.

Josh's dad smelled like alcohol and cigarettes and his shirt was dirty and sweat-stained. Josh's head began to pound as his dad stumbled across the room and swung his hand across the face of the small boy. It startled Josh, but he was unaware of any pain. A whimper stumbled out of his mouth. 'Please Dad, I'm sorry.' Josh had nothing to be sorry for, but he knew it did not matter. When his dad turned to set his beer down, Josh felt a surge of adrenaline and turned to run. His dad's deep abrasive voice felt like a hand touching his back and shivers ran down his spine. He ran through the family room to the stairs and bounded up, darting into his room. Josh dove into the closet and shut the door, covering himself with the clothes on the floor.

It was futile and he knew it. He was trapped. His chest felt like he was being pummeled from the inside and he was dizzy with fear. The door flung open and a large hand reached down and plucked the boy from the floor tucking him under his arm. As Josh opened his eyes, he realized they were at the top of the stairs when the front door suddenly opened. Josh's mom looked up and began to yell 'Let him go! Let him go now!' Stomping down the stairs, still gripping the child, the father stopped inches from her face and dropped him at her feet. He then gave her a shove, called her a vile name and stumbled out the door, slamming it behind him.

Josh began to tremble and shake; he realized his pants were wet, and soon sobs overtook his small body. This had happened before, so many times, and Josh felt resigned and hopeless. What had he done to deserve the wrath of his father who was supposed to love and protect him? His mother wrapped her arms around him rocking back and forth, and softly whispered, 'You know you need to stay out of his way when he's like that.' For a brief moment, Josh had felt soothed by the rhythm of the rocking motion and prosody of his mother's voice, but as he processed her words, the soothing moment shattered into little pieces and floated away.

DOI: 10.4324/9781003217534-3

What Happened to Josh's Body?

Throughout evolution, early humans and other mammals have been challenged by threats of danger within their natural environments from predators, unpredictable resources, and even climate change. The primordial goal beneath all challenges is to simply survive (Darwin, 1871). Two primary skills that have been identified as critical to survival are the ability to differentiate safety and threat and the ability to rapidly respond to threats. The competent function of these skills is supported by a complex neurobiological and behavioral response system that is evolutionarily conserved, known as the stress response system (SRS) (Lupien et al., 2016).

The stress response system (SRS) is activated in response to an authentic threat or the *perception* of a threat. The threat is a 'stressor,' and the effects upon the organism are known as 'stress' (Shonkoff & Garner, 2012). The most familiar SRS response is 'fight or flight,' a mobilization response that is generated by the sympathetic nervous system (SNS), a branch of the autonomic nervous system (ANS) (Porges, 2005).

The story of Josh describes an actual threat, and activation of the mobilization response through the lens of a child. Linking emotional and behavioral responses with the neurobiological substrates of the SRS illuminates the complex and critical role that it plays in experiences such as child maltreatment. The SRS is also recognized as a highly relevant system to mental health. This process has been proposed by many scholars as a key component of the pathway that can lead from maltreatment to dysregulation, developmental trauma (DT) and psychopathology (Perry, 2008; van der Kolk, 2005). This pathway is elucidated throughout the book and contributes to the rationale for neurobiologically based treatment

Based on evidence of remarkable similarities between animals and humans who experience threats to safety, Ogden, Minton, and Pain (2006) identified seven stages of the stress response process. The stages begin with a distinct and rapid change in arousal, a heightened orientation to the threat, momentary consideration of attachment and social support, the mobilization strategy, the immobilization strategy, and recuperation, integration, and a return to homeostasis (Ogden et al., 2006).

In the home of this child, the threat was genuine. Josh's body was jolted with a physiological startle before he consciously registered that his father was home. The threat was detected through a process called neuroception, a neural recognition of danger that occurs *prior* to conscious awareness (Porges, 2005). When Josh heard the front door slam, he *felt* an immediate visceral fear as his sensory systems were hit by the smell of whiskey and the low, angry intonation of his father's voice. The SNS rapidly triggers physiological and behavioral changes that prepare the individual with a defense response that prepares them to fight or flee. Fear flooded Josh's lower brain regions that are the locus for the stress response, and his higher cognitive functions shut down. Auditory discrimination devolves away from supportive human voices into a narrow focus on the vocal pitch autonomically associated with the low-frequency sounds of predators. This discriminative bias also tunes into the common high-pitched sounds of other potential victims (Porges, 2005).

A child who is terrified will instinctively *cry out* for aid from the mother or others. That behavior reflects the attachment component and emerges from the vagus nerve as a *primordial scream*. The ability to vocalize, however, can be incapacitated by the survival-based shutdown of the Broca's area (van der Kolk, 2014). Josh felt his mouth open, but no sound emerged. He felt the primal fear of a trapped animal.

Maltreatment is one of the most heinous stressors that can be experienced by a child. While minor stresses play a crucial role in early development, maltreatment often qualifies as toxic stress as it has the power to disrupt the developmental trajectory and dysregulate neural and endocrine systems. These alterations create an increased risk for developing psychopathology, a risk that lasts a lifetime. It should be no surprise that stress-related disorders rank right behind ischemic heart disease in modern health threats (WHO, 2020). An untenable number of children today experience the threat of harm to their emotional and physical integrity, and Josh was one of those children.

The Neurobiology of the Mobilization Response

The mobilization response begins with the activation of the sympathetic-adrenal-medullary (SAM) axis. A signal is sent to the adrenal glands to release epinephrine (adrenaline) and norepinephrine into the bloodstream. These neurotransmitters bind to paired receptors in the brain which activate arousal physiology. Heart rate and blood pressure elevate, oxygen intake increases and sensory functions are sharpened. The individual becomes alert, vigilant, and narrowly focused, ready to fight or flee. Energy required to fuel a capable response to threat is released as glucose and fat from temporary stores, and the body becomes primed for defense. This initial phase is designed to produce a rapid, yet short-term response. After the initial burst of epinephrine subsides, if the threat continues, the second stage is launched.

The hypothalamus-pituitary-adrenal (HPA) axis takes over at this point. This process is slower yet capable of sustained activation. During this phase, the hypothalamus releases the corticotropin-releasing hormone (CRH) which travels to the pituitary gland, releasing the adrenocorticotropic hormone (ACTH) (Frodl & O'Keane, 2013). The ACTH is relayed to the adrenal glands, triggering the production of two glucocorticoids, cortisol and corticosterone. Cortisol is widely known as the 'stress hormone' as it supports the continued physiological and behavioral arousal required for an effective response to a stressor. When the danger has passed, the response is no longer needed so the prefrontal cortex sends an inhibitory command to drop cortisol levels, facilitating activation of the parasympathetic nervous system (PNS), the calming branch of the ANS. When the SNS response shuts down, the process is considered complete or resolved and the body returns to a state of homeostasis.

If Josh's father had quickly stopped his rampage and left the house, Josh's body would have likely returned to a homeostatic state, yet the threat continued. The SRS launched into the second stage involving the HPA axis, sustaining its arousal-supported state. Josh was conditioned to the rough handling of his father, and the internal release of opioids dampened his pain. After the shutdown of response systems, the trauma-triggered and absorbed cache of energy must be released and is necessary for survival (Levine, 1997). In animals, this can be observed in the 'shaking off' behavior after a fear-invoked event, similar to a wet dog shaking water out of its coat. The human rendering of this is the experience of full-body trembling after a terrifying experience. The metabolic cost for a mobilization response is high, and Josh felt a deep consuming fatigue wash over his body. As he lay in his mother's arms, his body began to release his energy through trembling.

If his mother had not returned to interrupt his father's abuse, Josh might have degenerated into a state of immobilization, the most primitive response that is mediated by the parasympathetic branch (PNS). This branch activates when the mobilization response is inadequate to protect the individual. A disconnection occurs between consciousness, body, identity, memory, and thoughts resulting in a continuum of dissociative behaviors ranging from spacing out, fainting, and freezing, to depersonalization and derealization. Heart rate and blood pressure drop, emotions numb, and the body can become unresponsive. The opossum that feigns death is a classic example of dissociation.

It should be considered that the severe and chronic nature of Josh's abuse had possibly already caused aberrations of neural structure, function, and connectivity, compromising multiple areas of function. If the SRS is repeatedly activated, it becomes dysregulated, and the child can become trapped in a survival state. Continued SNS arousal is manifested in hyperarousal, over reactivity, and a hypervigilant state that causes continuous scanning for threat. This pervasive state is metabolically taxing and can dysregulate multiple developmental domains. A child, whose resources are wholly focused upon survival, is unable to attend, learn, academically perform, and engage in meaningful social interaction. In school, Josh might be showing intense, negative emotional reactivity and mood lability, impulsivity, social problems, and academic failure. The most damaging aspect of this behavioral pattern is the fact that often, no one recognizes the source of these problems. Treatment cannot resolve a child's problems if the underlying problem is not identified.

What is Stress?

The National Scientific Council on the Developing Child (2005) produced taxonomy of stress identifying three levels that could be differentiated by their effects upon the stress response system. These categories are positive, tolerable, and toxic. *Positive stress* levels invoke provisional increases in heart rate and mild elevations of stress hormones. This level of stress is related to common life experiences, such as forgetting homework or being late to baseball practice, minor events that are typically mitigated through positive, supportive relationships. Typical or normal experiences of elevated stress and the subsequent successful reduction of that stress are considered healthy experiences as the child learns that stress is temporary, resolvable, and endurable. These experiences trigger neural activation and facilitate the development of a healthy SRS and resilience.

Tolerable stress is evidenced in experiences such as a serious injury or extended separation from a loved one. While this level may be temporally limited, neurobiological disruptions that occur can invoke lasting changes to brain structures and function if they are not buffered by social relationships and support. This level of stress requires a more comprehensive and attentive level of support, yet these events can support the development of adaptive capacity, coping skills, and overall resilience.

Toxic stress is overwhelming to the child and often causes neurobiological alterations in the structures, functions, and connectivity in the brain, leading to dysregulation, clinical impairments, and psychopathology. The effects of severe and chronic maltreatment are intensified if the experiences occur during critical periods of neural plasticity which increase the sensitivity of neural circuitry to environment input.

The ACE Study

The CDC-Kaiser Permanente Adverse Childhood Experiences (ACE) study was one of the largest investigations ever conducted on childhood exposure to and experience of abuse, neglect, family violence, substance abuse, mental illness, divorce, and the incarceration of a family member. The study was conducted from 1995 to 1997, and involved two waves of questionnaires sent to over 17,000 Southern California HMO members, who had received physical exams. The ACE study sought to scrutinize the potential relationship between adverse childhood experiences and the later health status and well-being of those adults. Of the respondents, 30.1% reported physical abuse, 19.9% reported sexual abuse, and 11% reported emotional abuse. Additionally, 23.5% reported exposure to alcohol abuse, 4.9% were exposed to drug abuse, 18.8% reported exposure to mental illness, and 12.5% witnessed domestic violence (Anda et al., 2006).

Study results demonstrated a highly significant relationship between adverse childhood experiences and subsequent depression, suicidal behavior, addiction, interpersonal violence, and sexual promiscuity. Adults with adverse early experiences were also found to be at higher risk for physical health-related illnesses. The ACE study brought the commonality of interpersonal trauma to the forefront of public health.

Child Maltreatment

The maltreatment of children is an environmentally induced, preventable experience that dispenses hardship and devastation to children of all ages, races, and cultures.

Child maltreatment (CM) is defined by the Center for Disease Control (CDC, 2014) as an act (or acts) of commission or omission by a parent or other caregiver that results in harm, the potential for harm, or threat of harm to a child. Acts of commission are characterized as deliberate and intentional, though the consequences may not be intentional. Recognized as physical, sexual, or emotional (psychological) abuse, exposure to domestic violence, or exploitation, these acts can be categorized as events involving threat to the physical and/or mental integrity of the child (McLaughlin et al., 2014).

An act of omission is the failure to provide the basic physical, emotional, or educational needs of a child and also a failure to protect from them from potential or actual harm (Leeb et al., 2011). This form of maltreatment includes the broad range of effects known as neglect or deprivation, and can be defined as the 'absence' of typical and expected environmental experiences (McLaughlin et al., 2014). The World Health Organization defines the perpetrator of CM as one who has 'responsibility, trust, or power' and frames the perpetuated harm as threatening to the child's 'life, health, development and dignity' (WHO, 2020).

Disrupted Attachment as Child Maltreatment

A healthy attachment is considered critical to the safety, coregulation, and healthy neural development of the child. An infant is incredibly vulnerable and completely dependent upon their caregiver. The child of an attuned, nurturing, and responsive caretaker will typically develop a secure style of attachment which instills resilience. The child feels safe, can trust, and will seek social support when needed. When the early caregiver is unresponsive, inconsistent, or rejecting, the child can develop an insecure attachment style. The world, for that child, is perceived as threatening and dangerous, or one of deprivation (Callahan & Tottenham, 2016).

The disruption of the attachment process is an interpersonal betrayal that creates a potentially irresolvable dilemma. When the caregiver is both the source of- *and* the solution to the child's fear, the expected haven of safety and care collapses and the child can be profoundly devastated (Main & Hesse, 1990). It can be suggested that disrupted or impaired attachment can disrupt and alter neural growth, integration, and organization (Siegel, 2015).

During the attachment process 'internal working models' (mental representations) are embedded that reflect the attachment experience. The child is equipped with 'a mobile mother' that functions as an internal guidance system. This internal model shapes the child's expectations of the availability and responsiveness of others (Bowlby, 1982) forming a template for all future relationships and social behaviors. Treatment interventions that target attachment will often consider the integrity of the child's internal working model and can help them develop a contrasting representation of a healthy relationship.

Different neuronal groupings are activated by the specific attachment style, forming what the child experiences as reality (Siegel, 2015). While attachment is believed to be stable across time, studies have shown that attachment style can and does change during psychodynamic treatment. Shifts from less secure to more secure, and also from insecure to secure are supported by research (Diamond et al., 2003). Attachment is also 'relationship-specific.' Children can have one particular style with one caretaker and another with a different individual (Granqvist, et al., 2017). The neural substrates for attachment are also impacted by treatment and help sustain these changes.

A core responsibility of the caregiver during attachment is to regulate the child's affect and arousal. This coregulation supports the infant's homeostasis and promotes the development of their own capacity for regulation. Emotion regulation skills have been associated with the quality of attachment. Deficient coregulation is a key component of early adversity (Lyons-Ruth et al., 2016), and the quality of attachment is believed to be linked to the individual differences in regulatory competency.

The deficiency or lack of an attuned protective relationship magnifies the child's vulnerability and risk for dysregulation and psychopathology (Shonkoff & Garner, 2012). Disrupted attachment processes are considered a causal factor in DT and have been implicated by the National Child Traumatic Stress Network (NCTSN) as one of the earliest forms of maltreatment (Pynoos et al., 2014). Disrupted attachment processes can result in one of three forms of insecure attachment: ambivalent, avoidant, and disorganized.

Ambivalent

Children with an ambivalent attachment style find it difficult to move away from the caregiver to explore new or novel surroundings. They shift between rejection of the parent and dependent and 'clingy' behavior. Children do not seek help from the attachment figure when distressed and are difficult to soothe (Ainsworth, 1979). Attachment anxiety is the unsettling schema that other people are not going to be available or responsive during a vulnerable time. As the child ages, they may exaggerate their emotions to gain the attention of others.

Avoidant

An avoidant attachment style typically results from inconsistency of care. The child cannot predict whether their needs will be met or ignored. They develop a schema that the communication of their needs will not influence the caregiver, thus they try to minimize negative affect as it risks further rejection. The avoidant child appears unusually independent of the caregiver, both emotionally and physically. The child may not seek comfort or support and feels unworthy and inadequate.

The behaviors of these children can be framed as adaptive, as they are trying to appease the caregiver in order to maintain proximity. Children adapt their behavior to adverse environments to cope, yet in a healthier setting, the behaviors are maladaptive and often misunderstood and misinterpreted. A child who forms an avoidant attachment to survive their early environment may be misunderstood in another environment that attempts to nurture and form a close relationship with them.

Disorganized attachment (DA)

Disorganized attachment is often found in the most severely and chronically abused children, and is considered the most virulent form of insecure attachment. It is believed to cause emotional, social, and cognitive impairments, manifesting as interpersonal problems, externalizing disorders, and dysregulation (Pearlman & Courtois, 2005). Studies of DA suggest that it may increase volume in the left amygdala, which contributes to limbic irritability (Lyons-Ruth, et al., 2016).

The child with an insecure attachment is distrustful, suspicious, has difficulty identifying and respecting boundaries, and experiences interpersonal problems. They may have problems with perspective-taking, connecting to others, and can become withdrawn and isolated.

Child Maltreatment and Developmental Trauma

Developmental trauma (DT) is described as neglect and/or abuse inflicted upon a child by an individual, typically a caregiver. Also framed as 'interpersonal trauma,' the devastation from these experiences overwhelms the child's central nervous system as the trauma is beyond their capability to handle the experience. Bessel van der Kolk defines trauma as the embedded footprint of the harm upon the body, 'not the event itself' (van der Kolk, 2014). Childhood maltreatment and trauma are defined by Bruce Perry (2008) as severe and chronic events or experiences that frequently and chronically trigger the SRS, resulting in disruption and dysregulation of multiple other processes.

The recognition and understanding of maltreatment-induced trauma in children is a relatively new field of study. Prior to 2001, no organization existed that dedicated its resources to the study of child trauma. Through an act of Congress, the National Child Traumatic Stress Network (NCTSN) was established, opening 17 centers that were supported by Duke University and UCLA. With this support, Bessel van der Kolk, Joseph Spinazzola, and colleagues began to study the scope of childhood trauma. They quickly discovered a profound dilemma for young victims of maltreatment that no credible diagnostic category existed that fit the sequelae of early trauma. A movement developed and has continued over the past few decades to better meet the needs of these children.

Regulation

One needs to have a reasonable comprehension of what 'regulation' is, in order to conceptualize the construct of 'dysregulation.' Emotion regulation (ER) is a concept that has been well studied and discussed in literature, and is accepted as a relevant construct of mental health. It is considered as the capability to modulate emotion within the context of environmental demands. It is a process that manages the shift out of the comfort zone, or 'window of tolerance' without undue distress (Siegel, 2015).

Emotion regulation is a 'set of processes' that shape emotional experience and expression. These processes include the awareness of emotions, the tolerance and acceptance of feelings, and the use of strategies to manage the experience. While the bulk of literature focuses upon the importance of regulation in *emotion*, 'regulation' in itself can be conceptualized as a system of self-control that crosses neural, emotional, behavioral, cognitive, social, and inter- and intra-personal domains (D'Andrea et al., 2012; van der Kolk, 2005). The brain and body's structures, functions, and systems are integrated, organized, and interdependent, and function as a complex system. This conceptualization of the individual is highly relevant to understanding the broad reach of DT.

Reregulating these complex systems requires a 'whole child, whole system' approach that should not be reduced to components or reliance upon a single model to resolve the problem. There are empirically tested, efficacious treatments that produce positive change, such as behavior therapy or cognitive-behavioral therapy, yet if genuine, enduring change is to occur, *all* components of the system should be addressed, including neurobiology.

Neural Dysregulation

Neural dysregulation may be the most virulent consequence of DT. Early childhood maltreatment that is frequent, severe, and chronic has been shown to alter neurobiology, though mechanisms which direct pathways from maltreatment to dysregulation and psychopathology are difficult to define. The recent advancements in neuroimaging technology that illuminate brain structure, function, and connectivity are supporting the search for answers, yet this information has not been translated into practice (Henderson et al., 2020).

Maltreatment and DT can disrupt, halt, or redirect the developmental trajectory for the immature child in the midst of their developmental ontogeny. Critical periods of neural sensitivity occur during development, which create an increased receptiveness to environmental experiences. Intended to enhance normal neural growth and organization, adverse experiences during these critical periods also heighten negative consequences. Neural dysregulation subsequently impacts developmental domains creating functional impairments in the child (Dvir et al., 2014).

A full 80% of children with maltreatment histories (compared to 37% of controls) showed dysregulation (Maughn & Cicchetti, 2002), and 70% of CM is associated with pervasive neurobiological alterations of brain regions associated with mood regulation (Nemeroff, 2016). All clinical symptomatology is associated with neural correlates, and research is progressing in determining the specific neurobiological alterations involved in dysregulation. Identifying the specific neurobiological substrates that underlie dysregulation from trauma is crucial to understanding the specific mechanisms that impact the child's clinical functioning.

Dysregulation of networks, systems, and processes is often identified through altered patterns of activation and inhibition. Under-modulation and over-modulation are gradations that exist on a continuum, yet trauma effects are not always linear and do not necessarily follow clear principles of science. Dysregulation can have indirect or secondary effects as well. A direct effect of trauma can be dysregulated arousal states which can secondarily compromise the capacity of the child to focus, learn new material, and complete academic tasks.

Emotion dysregulation is the lack of ability to remain within an emotional comfort zone, and it interferes with goal-related functions. A prime example is when unmanageable anxiety (an overwhelming state that shifts a child outside of the comfort zone) disrupts a child's ability to socially engage, though they desperately want to make friends (goal-related behavior).

Dysregulation and Psychopathology

Dysregulation is considered a risk factor for the development of psychopathology in children and adolescents (John & Gross, 2004). Dysregulation has been associated with most of the traditional diagnostic categories including internalizing and externalizing disorders (Beauchaine & Cicchetti, 2019). Emotion dysregulation is a predictor of anxiety, depression, eating disorders, substance abuse, aggression (McLaughlin et al., 2011), and posttraumatic stress disorder (PTSD) (Klaming et al., 2019). Dysregulation has also been associated with childhood disorders such as attention deficit hyperactivity (ADHD), oppositional-defiance (ODD), conduct disorder (CD), and antisocial behavior (Busso and Pollack, 2014).

A 14-year longitudinal study showed a remarkable association between dysregulation in childhood with a broad range of adult psychopathology. Over 2,000 Dutch children were rated with the Child Behavior Checklist/ Dysregulation Profile (CBCL-DP) with findings of severe dysregulation, attention problems, aggression, and anxiety and depression. The study found that these children were at an increased risk for problems in regulation of affect, behavior, and cognition when they reached adulthood (Athoff et al., 2010).

The Diagnostic Dilemma: What about PTSD?

Children with early trauma have an increased risk for being diagnosed with multiple disorders, as the divisions between traditional mental health disorders do not clearly map the complex presentations of these children. Toxic or traumatic stress has traditionally been defined as events outside the normal range of human life, such as war, atomic bombing, transportation accidents, and fire, and weather disasters such as hurricanes, floods, and earthquakes. These types of trauma are what authors had in mind when they drafted the original PTSD diagnosis for DSM-III (APA, 1980). The PTSD diagnosis was highly significant at that time as it was the first acknowledgment of an external etiological agent implicated in clinical pathology.

Relational trauma was not on the radar until the end of the 20th century. During the 1970s and 1980s, interpersonally generated adversities were still considered within the realm of the 'normal' vagaries of life (Friedman, 2019). While PTSD is a respected diagnosis that aligns with adults who experience trauma, studies show that it does not adequately work for traumatized children. A significant percentage of this population does not meet the criteria for PTSD (van der Kolk et al., 2005); and, in fact, may not meet the criteria for *any* diagnosis (D'Andrea et al., 2012). Most ironically, these children have a greater number and severity of functional and psychopathological impairments, compared to controls (D'Andrea et al., 2012).

'Developmental Trauma Disorder' (DTD) was proposed for inclusion in the DSM-V in 2013, to address these problems, but was rejected (van der Kolk, 2014). The movement to include DTD in traditional classification systems continues, and this requires resolution. An accurate clinical description of a child is critical to the determination of treatment. If a child does not meet the criteria for an existing diagnosis, they do not receive any treatment. If they do fit in a category, yet their trauma is not recognized, they may receive treatment that does not meet their needs.

In spite of a lack of recognition by traditional classification systems, 'developmental trauma' is widely accepted and utilized within the literature that discusses children and interpersonal maltreatment. Trauma history should absolutely be part of the initial history and assessment and should include multiple sources of information including self, parent and teacher reports, neuropsychological testing and, if possible, neuroimaging. Recognizing the uniqueness of the child and designing a distinct, personalized treatment plan should be central to all clinical decisions.

Clinical psychology has historically subscribed to a disorder-specific framework in its diagnostic and classification system, research, and treatment. The primary classification system in use today in the United States is the *Diagnostic Statistical Manual* (DSM-5-TR) (APA, 2022). Mental health disorders are currently diagnosed on the basis of identified symptom patterns, and the client either meets the criteria or does not. This system does not capture the dimensionality of psychopathology.

A growing percentage of clinicians believe that the boundaries between categorical disorders do not accurately map the complexity of affected children A significant overlap of symptoms between disorders exists (Cludius et al., 2020; Harrison et al., 2019) which may result from ubiquitous, core symptoms (Krueger, 1999) that cross diagnostic categories. Another substantial issue is the tendency for children to accumulate diagnoses. Known as comorbidity, this pattern has been revealed by epidemiology studies to be extremely common (van der Kolk, 2005).

The Transdiagnostic Solution

Recently, transdiagnostic (TD) models have emerged in response to these issues. Support is rapidly growing for transdiagnostic approaches for diagnosis, treatment, and prevention (Conway, et al., 2018; Lynch et al., 2021). A TD factor is a mechanism that exists across multiple disorders and conveys a risk factor for onset and/or maintenance of disorder symptomatology (Morris, Mansell & McEvoy, 2016). Understanding these mechanisms in the development of multiple mental health disorders holds significant implications for treatment (Buckholtz & Meyer-Lindenberg, 2012).

The transdiagnostic approach is a perspective that re links naturally integrated processes, domains, and functions that are complicit in psychopathology. Emotion and cognition, for example, are recognized as linked, yet traditional diagnoses and past research tended to break down components and domains into increasingly specific entities. The 'decade of the brain' (1990s) brought the perspective of an 'integrated brain composed of interdependent components' back into focus, and neuroimaging research supports this transition. The US Congress approved this initiative to bring scientists from a broad range of disciplines together to improve brain research.

The TD perspective identifies common mechanisms between disorders that can facilitate more functional diagnoses which will drive improved treatment and aid research. Mechanisms can be categories of vulnerability or factors that serve to maintain the symptoms. The National Institutes of Mental Health (NIMH) developed the Research Domain Criteria (RDoC) (2009) initiative to explore the core dimensions of psychopathology (PP) as an alternative to the traditional categorical approach to diagnosis. The initiative seeks to integrate genetics, molecular biology, neurology, cognitive sciences, and other fields to provide an alternative lens through which to examine PP (Suzuki, 2021).

The RDoC has three primary goals: delineate how psychological factors are biologically implemented; explain how neurobiological processes work; and improve the predictability of 'psychopathological phenomena' (Sun et al., 2022). Links between (brain) region-specific circuitry abnormalities and symptomatology are sought to enable neurobiologically targeted treatments.

Dysregulation as a Transdiagnostic Mechanism

Most traditional categories of child psychopathology involve dysregulation as part of their symptomatology. While dysregulation has been long been considered to be a *component* of multiple forms of psychopathology (Aldao & Nolen-Hoeksema, 2010), only within the past two decades, supported by substantial research, has it become established as a potential *mechanism* that *leads* to multiple forms of psychopathology (Dryman & Heimberg, 2018).

The literature primarily focuses on *emotional* regulation, yet early trauma also dysregulates neural structures, functions, and connectivity which may directly or indirectly disrupt multiple developmental domains including emotion, behavior, social, cognitive, and intra- and interpersonal. The return to recognizing the interrelationships between the domains validates the TD approach, and dysregulation may serve as a prototypical mechanism that illuminates a salient path to change.

Further studies will help identify neural mechanisms that correlate with specific forms of psychopathology. It is necessary to identify both psychological and neural mechanisms that underlie the dimensions of psychopathology that seem to cut across diagnoses. There are multiple transdiagnostic mechanisms that are currently being studied for integration into mental health processes, diagnosis, and treatment, and the model can be predicted to evolve as collaborative research continues.

Over the next year, Josh began to act out in school. He became defiant with teachers, refused to complete work, and his grades dropped. When he escalated to physical aggression, he was placed in a day-treatment therapeutic school. The program was founded on a stringent behavioral program with rewards for compliance and consequences for noncompliance. Josh struggled to adjust as he once again found himself 'at the mercy' (his words) of another. One morning a few weeks later, Josh refused to go to school.

His mom called the school principal who told her to 'just get him in the car and bring him to the door of the school' with the assurance that staff would take it from there. Josh's father intervened and shoved the pajama-clad child into the car and his mother drove the screaming child to the school. Some behaviorally based programs have 'hands-on' policies to 'ensure the safety of the child and others' thus; three staff met the car and tried to safely extract Josh from the car.

Josh avoided capture for a few minutes by hopping back and forth across the seats, but they soon secured him, wrapped him in a blanket and carried him into the school. Josh was still screaming as he was set down on the floor of a clinician's office. He was in such a state of distress that he vomited on the carpet. The child then seemed to shift from a state of angry defiance to one of resignation, hopelessness, and dissociation. Josh scooted as far back into a corner as he could, retreated into a fetal position, and hid under the blanket. The boy's screams were now sobs which shook his entire body. The empathetic clinician tried to soothe the child, employing multiple techniques to help him calm down, yet nothing seemed to work. The clinician decided to ask her supervisor for support, and he simply said, 'Let's get Lilly.'

Lilly was a familiar presence in the school and was frequently called upon to help calm children, assist transitions, and improve the well-being of the students. When she was 'off duty', she napped in a quiet office in an adjacent building. Lilly was a dog that worked hard, played hard, and napped hard in between gigs. One of the core principles of incorporating dogs into therapy situations is to maintain safety. A clinician must not put the dog (or child) into a situation that might cause harm to them. As Josh had not yet spoken, the clinician was uncertain of his potential risk to the dog. She asked Josh if it was ok to bring her in, asking if he would 'keep her safe?' He nodded and clearly said, 'Yes.'

The door opened, and Lilly confidently trotted right across the room, discreetly side-stepping the liquid on the carpet. Though her nose twitched ever so briefly as she recognized the odor, she quickly hopped onto Josh's lap and presented herself to him. The blanket slowly slid off of Josh as he wrapped his arms around her. The dog leaned into his shoulder and buried her nose into his neck. The boy's breathing slowed, his body softened, and the trembling slowly dissipated. After ten minutes, Josh got dressed and Lilly escorted him into his classroom.

After that incident, Lilly became the 'go-to' girl to help children transition from their cars or the parking lot into the school. She would get the call when a child would 'be stuck' in the car and would eagerly join them in their space. In the five years that she held her job, no physical carries were required to bring a child into the school. While physical control of a child is preferable to dangerous, unsafe behavior, for the physically or sexually abused child the contact required for a hold can be a trigger. The tenet of 'do no harm' is supposed to govern all clinical and medical interventions, and the principles of this intervention should continue to be studied.

Lilly, as a competent working therapy dog, succeeded in calming and engaging a child who was overwhelmed with emotion and physical arousal. She succeeded while professionals were struggling, and did it with intuition and intention. She provided Josh with a sense of safety, nurturance, and coregulation, shepherding him to a place where he could reconnect with himself and the other humans trying to help him.

Conclusion

Child maltreatment remains a critical threat to young children, and when perpetuated by a caregiver, engenders a severe interpersonal betrayal that can overwhelm the child's resources. A 'destabilization' occurs, and the child who lacks resilience and social buffering is unable to recover without help. Their developmental trajectory can become disrupted, delayed, or even halted. Severe and chronic maltreatment is capable of causing neurobiological alterations in the structures, function, connectivity, systems, and networks which is defined as 'dysregulation.' Neural dysregulation can disrupt multiple or even all functional domains of the child, which include emotion, behavior, cognition, somatic/physiology, social, and intrapersonal (the self) and interpersonal (relationships). Dysregulation is proposed as a mechanistic link between CM and psychopathology and serves as a transdiagnostic target.

Imagine how beneficial a fundamental comprehension of the neurobiological processes in children could be in their treatment. This awareness could create a functional roadmap and guide to designing a treatment that would be capable of restoring and reregulating the dysregulated child.

References

Ainsworth, M.S. (1979). Infant-mother attachment. *American Psychologist*, 34(10), 932–937. https://doi.org/10.1037/0003-66X.34.10.932

Aldao, A. & Nolen-Hoeksema, S. (2010). Specificity of cognitive emotion regulation strategies: A transdiagnostic examination. *Behavior Research and Therapy*; 48(10): 974–983. https://doi.org/10.1016/brat.2010.06.002

Anda, R.F., Felitti, V., Bremner, J.D., Walker, J.D., Whitfield, C., Perry, B.D., Dube, S.R., & Giles, W.H. (2006). The enduring effects of abuse and related adverse experiences in childhood. *European Archives of Psychiatry and Clinical Neuroscience*; 256(3): 174–186. https://doi.org/10.1007/s00406-005-0624-4

APA. (1980). *Diagnostic and Statistical Manual of Mental Disorders* (3rd Ed.). Washington DC: American Psychiatric Publishing.

APA (2022). *Diagnostic and Statistical Manual of Mental Disorders (5th Edition-TR)*. Washington DC: American Psychiatric Publishing.

Athoff, R.R., Verhulst, F., Rettew, D.C., Hudziak, J.J., & van der Ende, J. (2010). Adult outcomes of childhood dysregulation: A 14-year follow-up study. *Journal of the American Academy of Child and Adolescent Psychiatry*; 49 (11): 1105–1116. https://doi.org/10.1016/j.jaac.2010.08.006

Beauchaine, T.P., & Cicchetti, D. (2019). Emotion dysregulation and emerging psychopathology: A transdiagnostic, transdisciplinary perspective. *Development and Psychopathology*; 31: 799–804. https://doi.org/10.1017/S0954579419000671

Bowlby, J. (1982). Attachment and loss: Retrospect and prospect. *The American Journal of Orthopsychiatry*; 52(4): 664–678. https://doi.org/10.1111/j.1939-0025

Buckholtz, J.W. & Meyer-Lindenberg, A. (2012). Psychopathology and the human connectome: toward a transdiagnostic model of risk for mental illness. *Neuron*; 74(6): 990–1004. https://doi.org/10.1016/j.neuron.2012.06.002

Busso, D.S., & Pollack, C. (2014). No brain left behind: Consequences of neuroscience discourse for education. *Learning, Media and Technology*. https://doi.org/10.1080/1743988.2014.908908

Callahan, B.L. & Tottenham, N. (2016). The stress acceleration hypothesis: Effects of early-life adversity on emotion circuits and behavior. *Current Opinion in Behavioral Sciences*; 7: 78–81. https://doi.org/10.1016/j.cobeha.2015.11.018

Center for Disease Control (CDC) (2014). Understanding Child Maltreatment-Fact Sheet 2014. Retrieved from https://www.cdc.gov

Cludius, B., Ehring, T., & Mennin, D. (2020). Emotion regulation as a transdiagnostic process. *Emotion*; 20(1): 37–42. https://doi.org/10.1037/emo0000646

Conway, CC., Raposa, E.B., Hammen, C., & Brennan, P.A. (2018). Transdiagnostic pathways from early social stress to psychopathology: A 20-year prospective study. *Journal of Child Psychology and Psychiatry*; 59(8): 855–862. https://doi.org/10.1111/jcpp.12862

D'Andrea, W., Ford, J., Stolbach, B., Spinazzola, J., & van der Kolk, B.A. (2012). Understanding interpersonal trauma in children: why we need a developmentally appropriate trauma diagnosis. *The American Journal of Orthopsychiatry*; 82(2): 187–200. https://doi.org/10.1111/j.1939-0025.2012.01154.x

Darwin, C. (1871). *The Descent of Man and Selection in Relationship to Sex*. London: J Murray.

Diamond, D., Clarkin, J.F., Stovall-McClough, C., & Levy, K. (2003). Patient-therapist attachment in the treatment of borderline personality disorder. *Bulletin of the Menninger Clinic*; 67(3): 227–259. https://doi.org/10.1521/bumc.67.3.227.23433

Dryman, M.T., & Heimberg, R.G. (2018). Emotion regulation in social anxiety and depression: A systematic review of expressive suppression and cognitive reappraisal. *Clinical Psychology Review*; 65: 17–42. https://doi.org/10.1016/j.cpr.2018.07.004

Dvir, Y., Ford, J.D., Hill, M., & Frazier, J.A. (2014). Childhood maltreatment, emotional dysregulation, and psychiatric comorbidities. *Harvard Review of Psychiatry*; 22(3): 149–161. https://doi.org/10.1097/HRP.0000000000000014

Friedman, M.J. (2019). PTSD: History and overview. Retrieved from http://www.ptsd.va.gov

Frodl, T., & O'Keane, V. (2013). How does the brain deal with cumulative stress? A review with focus on developmental stress, HPA axis function and hippocampal structure in humans. *Neurobiology of Disease*; 52: 24–37. https://doi.org/10.1016/j.nbd.2012.03.012

Grandvist, P., Sroufe, L.A., Dozier, M., Hesse, E., ... & Duschinsky, R. (2017). Disorganized attachment in infancy: A review of the phenomenon and its implications for clinicians and policymakers. *Attachment & Human Development*; 19(6): 534–558. https://doi.org/10.1080/14616734.2017.1354040

Harrison, L.A., Kats, A., Williams, M.E., & Aziz-Zadeh, L. (2019). The importance of sensory processing in mental health: A proposed addition to the research domain criteria (RDoC) and suggestions for RDoC 2.0. *Frontiers in Psychology*. https://doi.org.10.3389/fpsyg.2019.00103

Henderson, T.A., van Lierop, M.J., McLean, M., Uszler, J.M., Thornton, J.F., Siow, Y-H., Pavel, D.G., Cardaci, J., & Cohen, P. (2020). Functional neuroimaging in psychiatry-aiding in diagnosis and guiding treatment. What the American psychiatric association does not know. *Frontiers in Psychiatry*; 11: 276. https://doi.org/10.3389/fpsyt.2020.00276

John, O.P., & Gross, J.J. (2004). Healthy and unhealthy emotion regulation: Personality processes, individual differences, and life span development. *Journal of Personality*; 72: 1301–1334.

Klaming, R., Spadoni, A.D., Veltman, D.J., & Simmons, A.N. (2019). Expansion of hippocampal and amygdala shape in posttraumatic stress and early life stress. *Neuroimage Clinical*; 24: 101982. https://doi.org/10.1016/j.nicl.2019.101982

Krueger, R.F. (1999). The structure of common mental disorders. *Archives of General Psychiatry*; 56(10): 921–926. https://doi.org/10.1001/archpsyc.56.10.921

Leeb, R., Lewis, T., & Zolotor, A. (2011). A review of physical and mental health consequences of child abuse and negelct and implications for practice. *American Journal of Lifestyle Medicine*; 5(5): 454–468. https://doi.org/10.1177/1559 827611410266

Levine, P.A. (1997). *Waking the Tiger: Healing Trauma: The Innate Capacity to Transform overwhelming Experiences*. Berkeley, CA: North Atlantic Books. ISBN 155643233X 9781556432330

Lupien, S.J., Quellet-Morin, I., Herba, C.M., Juster, R., & McEwen, B.S. (2016). From vulnerability to neurotoxicity; A developmental approach to the effects of stress on the brain and behavior. Abstract Retrieved May 1, 2022 https://doi.org/10.1017/978-3-319-24493-8-1

Lynch, S.J., Sunderland, M., Newton, N.C. & Chapman, C. (2021). A systematic review of transdiagnostic risk and protective factors for general and specific psychopathology in young people. *Clinical Psychology Review*. https://doi.org/10.1016/j.cpr.2021.102036

Lyons-Ruth, K., Pechtel, P., Yoon, S.A., Anderson, C.M., & Teicher, M.H. (2016). Disorganized attachment in infancy predicts greater amygdala volume in adulthood. *Behavioural Brain Research*; 308: 83–93. https://doi.org/10.1016/j.bbr.2016.03.050

Main, M., & Hesse, E. (1990). Parents' unresolved traumatic experiences are related to infant disorganized attachment status: Is frightened and/or frightening parental behavior the linking mechanism? In M.T. Greenberg, D. Cicchetti, & E. Cummings (Eds.), *Attachment in the Preschool Years: Theory, Research, and Intervention* (161–182). Chicago, IL: U. of Chicago.

Maughn, A. & Cicchetti, D. (2002). Impact of child maltreatment and interadult violence on children's emotion regulation abilities and socioemotional adjustment. *Child Development*; 73(5): 1525–1542. https://doi.org/10.1111/1467-8624.00488

McLaughlin, K.A., Sheridan, M.A., & Lambert, H.K. (2014). Childhood adversity and neural development: Deprivation and threat as distinct dimensions of early experience. *Neuroscience and Biobehavioral Reviews*; 47: 578–591.

McLaughlin, K.A., Hatzenbuehler, M.L., Mennin, D.S., & Nolen-Hoeksema, S. (2011). Emotion dysregulation and adolescent psychopathology: a prospective study. *Behaviour Research and Therapy*; 49: 544–554. https://doi.org/10.1016/j.brat.2011.06.003

Morris, L., Mansell, W., & McEvoy, P. (2016). The take control course: Conceptual rationale for the development of a transdiagnostic group for common mental health problems. *Frontiers in Psychology*. https://doi.org/10.3389/fpsyg.2016.00099

National Institute of Mental Health (2009). Research Domain Criteria (RDoC). Retrieved March 25, 2022, from https://www.nimh.nih-gov/research-priorities/rdoc/index.shtml

National Scientific Council on the Developing Child (2005). *Excessive Stress Disrupts the Architecture of the Developing Brain* (Working paper 3). Harvard University: Author.

Nemeroff, C.B. (2016). Paradise lost: The neurobiological and clinical consequences of child abuse and neglect. *Neuron*; 82(5): 892–909. https://doi.org/10.1016/j.neuron.2016.01.019

Ogden, P., Minton, K., Pain, C., & Siegel, D. (2006). *Trauma and the Body: A Sensorimotor Approach to Psychotherapy*. New York N.Y.: W.W. Norton & Co.

Pearlman, L.A. & Courtois, C.A. (2005). Clinical applications of the attachment framework: Relational treatment of complex trauma. *Journal of Traumatic Stress*; 18(5): 449–459. https://doi.org/10.1002/jts.20052

Perry, B. (2008). Child maltreatment: A neurodevelopmental perspective on the role of trauma and neglect in psychopathology. In Chapter 4 T.P., Beauchaine & S.P. Hinshaw (Eds.), *Child and Adolescent Psychopathology*. Hoboken, N.J.: Wiley.

Porges, S. (2003). Social engagement and attachment: A phylogenetic perspective. *Annals of the New York Academy of Sciences*; 1008: 31–47.

Porges, S. (2005). The role of social engagement in attachment and bonding: A phylogenetic perspective. In C.S. Carter (Ed.), *Attachment and Bonding: A New Synthesis* 33–54). Cambridge, MA: Boston Review.

Pynoos, R.S., Steinberg, A.M., Layne, C.M., Liang, L-J., Vivrette, R.L., Briggs, E.C., Kisiel, C., Habib, M., Belin, T.R., & Fairbank, J.A. (2014). Modeling constellations of trauma history in the national child traumatic stress network core data set. *Psychological Trauma Theory Research Practice and Policy*; 6(1): S9–S17.

Shonkoff, J.P. & Garner, A.S. (2012). The lifelong effects of early childhood adversity and toxic stress. *Pediatrics*; 129(1): e232–e246. https://doi.org/10.1542/peds.2011-2663

Siegel, D. (2015). *The Developing Mind: How Relationships and the Brain Interact to Shape Who We Are*. New York: Guilford Press.

Sun, M., Vinograd, M., Miller, G.A., & Craske, M.G. (2022). Research Domain Criteria (RDoC) and emotion regulation. https://doi.org/10.1093/med:psych/9780198765844.003.0005

Suzuki, T. (2021). The transdiagnostic dimensional approach: Another way of understanding mental illness. *NAMI*.

van der Kolk, (2014). *The Body Keeps the Score*. New York: Penguin Books.

van der Kolk, B. (2005). Developmental trauma Disorder: Toward a rational diagnosis for children with complex trauma histories. *Psychiatric Annals*; 35(5): 401–408. https://doi.org/10.3928/00485713-20050501-06

World Health Organization (2020). Retrieved from https://www.who.int

Chapter 2   Growing the Baby Brain

Introduction

This chapter provides a concise synopsis of the central nervous system and brain that is relevant to understanding the neurobiology of early development, child maltreatment, dysregulation, developmental trauma, and psychopathology in a child. The presented information will support the clinician in designing and applying remedial interventions that draw from a blending of neurobiology and psychology.

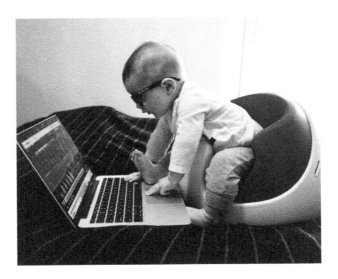

The Dynamic Science of the Brain

The 1990s were designated as the 'Decade of the Brain' as part of an interagency initiative that sought to highlight the importance of brain research (Tandon, 2000). The initiative was successful in increasing scientific study of the brain and succeeded in bringing scientists together, educating the public, and drawing international collaboration. The decade also produced

DOI: 10.4324/9781003217534-4

a number of paradigm-changing discoveries regarding the relationship between the brain and development, dysfunction, and treatment. Three of these discoveries are distinctly relevant to the content of this book.

Prior to the run-up to the new millennium, most scientists believed that the brain was not malleable past early development. More recently, however, scientists found that the brain *does* remain receptive to environmental stimuli into adulthood and neural connectivity can occur rapidly. Called 'neuroplasticity' this phenomenon is highly relevant to understanding development, dysregulation, and treatment mechanisms. Scientific knowledge of 'critical periods' of neural growth and development was also elucidated. These time-limited periods of heightened sensitivity to the environment help explain how positive and negative experiences, relationships, and environmental factors impact neural growth. The third and possibly most prolific breakthrough during this decade was the development of the functional magnetic resonance neuroimaging (fMRI).

This technological advance allowed researchers to look inside the brain in real time and identify structures, function, connectivity, and processes in normal and atypical behavior. Previous research was focused on discrete, narrow targets, and neuroimaging opened the door to viewing the entire brain as a complex system. Studies could now view circuits, networks, and connectivity as potential culprits in dysfunction and dysregulation. Research in the upcoming years is predicted to substantially increase the reservoir of brain knowledge as neuroimaging is producing massive amounts of raw data. While this data shows activation patterns, collaboration of brain regions, and abnormalities, it is the accurate analysis of this data that will provide critical interpretation, conclusions, and direction for useful applications (Sui et al., 2014).

Prior to this period, the study of psychopathology was centered on treatments that remediated symptoms. Our traditional diagnostic system, the *Diagnostic and Statistical Manual of Mental Disorders* is based on symptom criteria. Throughout the past century, scientists and clinicians have developed treatments (primarily pharmaceutical and behavioral), for most mental health disorders, yet little was understood about the brain mechanisms that were complicit in psychopathology. TR Insel (2010), director of the National Institute of Mental Health, shared how scientists are now beginning to identify the brain mechanisms that are instrumental in development, dysfunction, and psychopathology.

All of this leads to the recognition that the integration of neuroscience and psychology is predictably the catalyst for propelling this field forward. All behavior has neurobiological correlates, and viewing the child as a complex system of interrelated components mandates inclusion of all domains of function. While this is exciting and sounds futuristic, it should be remembered that pioneers such as William James and Sigmund Freud suggested similar theorems over a century ago (Cozolino, 2017).

Sharing the momentum of this recent research, the neurosciences have experienced other models of study that will further impact this field. One significant change is the transition from a 'one brain' to a 'two brain' model of study (Hasson et al., 2012; Redcay & Schilbach, 2019). Studies using a single brain model fail to capture the reciprocity and social processes that occur *between* dyads, particularly how the brain reacts, adjusts, and responds to other brains. Our brains are designed to interact with other brains, and humans require interpersonal interactions which, along with the environment, interface with the genome to form a template for development and function throughout life. These concepts are relevant to treatment that restores regulation, as repairing the consequences of developmental trauma requires a context of nurturing and coregulating relationships. Identifying mechanisms that shape and power relationships will improve the healing and restoration of the disconnected, dysregulated child.

This more practical model also opens the door to understanding 'brain-to-stimuli coupling' and 'brain-to-brain coupling.' The individual brain couples with physical stimuli (or objects) in the environment, as a way of actively perceiving the environment. Information is transmitted to the brain through chemical, mechanical, and electromagnetic signals that are converted to electrical impulses in the brain, called oscillations, the language of the brain (Hasson et al., 2012).

Brain-to-brain coupling is the same concept yet occurs between two brains, which has been characterized as a 'wireless connection.' Another difference between the two coupling models is that linking brain-to-brain requires a similarity between organisms and taps emotions and various sensations to enable coupling. EEG-based hyper-scanning is a neuroimaging technique that facilitates the study of neural relationships between two brains. This tool permits scientists to observe social interaction through a neurological lens, illuminating real-time modifications of oscillations and interbrain synchronization (Valencia & Forese, 2020). The University of California, Los Angeles (UCLA) recently conducted studies on social synchrony between mice and were first to document interbrain synchrony in this species on a cellular level. Interbrain coupling supports engagement in reciprocal complex social interactions, and was observed in mice to predict future behavior and to aid in the establishment of a hierarchy (Kingsbury et al., 2019).

Within the attachment relationship, brain coupling joins the right hemisphere (RH) of the caregiver and that of the infant; an implicit channel of communication that both creates synchrony and is enhanced by it. Right brain-to-right brain coupling of the clinician and child is also a powerful mechanism of the therapeutic relationship that facilitates connection, synchrony, and coregulation (Schore, 2000). *Interspecies* brain-to-brain coupling has recently begun to emerge as a research topic of interest as a result of case studies. While in training for equine-assisted therapy several years ago, the author was able to experience a coupling with an unrestrained unfamiliar horse that upon joining followed her around a large paddock. The connection was achieved through the calm establishment of proximity, visualizing the horse (and nothing else) in the mind, and clearly avoiding any gestures or language that might insinuate an attempt to control the animal. Being totally 'present' is a mind, body, and spiritual commitment to the moment and conveys the message to the animal that we are there for them. These implicit mechanisms of communication are elements of the language of the animal. If we are quiet and listen with all of our being, they can hear us, and perhaps we can hear them. These types of experiences will likely open up exciting new avenues for cross-species relationships, and it is predicted that research will establish interspecies coupling as an empirically valid concept.

The Role of Neuroplasticity in Brain Development

The amazing development of neural circuitry is accentuated by time-limited states of neuroplasticity, called *critical periods*. Critical periods denote a heightened receptiveness to external stimuli and subsidize rapid, prolific growth and change. The term emerged as a concept from Spanish neuroanatomist Santiago Ramon y Cajal who, in the late 19th century identified the neuron as the primary component of the central nervous system (Mateos-Aparicio, 2019).

While critical periods have typically been associated with sensory systems, such as visual and auditory, animal studies have also revealed the relevance of these periods for emotional and social development (as in anxiety and stress) (Yang et al., 2012). Each brain structure and region matures by an individual timetable and has distinct periods of receptivity. This implies that the timing of child maltreatment is a mediator of outcomes.

Neural change happens when synaptic strength is enhanced through repeated excitation between cells. When prolonged, the experience creates synchronized firing patterns and promotes the organization of neural networks (Hebb, 1949). Most of us are familiar with the saying, 'Neurons that fire together wire together.' The process of repeated neural excitation activates the transcription of RNA, causing protein synthesis that is necessary for neuronal growth.

Plasticity cuts both ways, however, and the same neural capacity for growth and expansion also incurs a susceptibility to the detrimental effects of adverse environmental experiences (Shonkoff & Philips, 2000). The child who experiences chronic maltreatment is highly vulnerable to neurobiological alterations and dysregulation of their still-maturing brain. These alterations can create dysfunction and dysregulation in existing neural circuitry, and impair developmental growth, organization, and connectivity that are emerging or yet to develop.

As neuroplasticity is now understood to extend far beyond early childhood, new learning and experiences are now believed to contribute to the continuous processes of shaping and organizing neural networks, as they continue to be instrumental in growth and change (Voss et al., 2017). This principle is also central to therapeutic change. Treatment intended to reduce symptoms, and restore and re-regulate the brain requires new learning and experiences that affect neural change. Clinicians can advantage treatment with awareness of the principles of plasticity. Lasting change from treatment requires a supportive neural substrate, and neural change requires plasticity which can be activated and extended by patterned input and enriched environments and experiences (Cozolino, 2017).

It's not Nature *or* Nurture. It's Nature *and* Nurture

The developmental trajectory of the child is now understood to be directed and shaped by an elaborate interface between the genome and the environment (Perry et al., 1995). The primary architecture of the brain is developed during the initial six months of gestation, and is guided by the genomic blueprint. The instructions within DNA provide the *template* for this early growth which is predominantly free from environmental influence. Genes, as templates, provide the basic anatomical architecture of the brain. *Experience-expectant stimuli* are species-typical experiences that are common to most members of a species. An example of this is the visual cortex that genetically *expects* the experience of exposure to patterns of light. The deprivation of these specific sensory experiences is known to compromise neural organization within specific sensory systems.

From the last trimester forward, environmental factors and experiences become critical inputs that influence the further development of the infant human brain (McGowan & Roth, 2015). Multiple factors determine how the *template (genotype)* is expressed as a *genetic transcription (phenotype)* and how protein synthesis becomes manifested in physical and behavioral features (Kandel, 1998; Siegel, 2015). Transcription genes are associated with neuroplasticity, the ability for adaptation and change, and are considered *experience-dependent*. The clinician can advantage therapeutic change with an enriching environment and experiences that promote plasticity and change. The age-old question of 'Is it nature or nurture?' can be put to rest as the exquisite development of the human brain is actualized within the space between nature and nurture.

Adaptations Promote Survival

Adaptation is a primary principle of evolution, a process that living organisms employ to improve their fitness (reproductive success) and survival. Adaptations are adjustments or changes in the organism to the dynamic environment, and can be behavioral, anatomical, or physiological. These changes can lead to alterations in genetic expression, and become herita-ble and transmittable across generations. The human brain continuously interacts with the environment, and its ability to adapt to change within their world is central to species survival. Adaptations may solve one prob-lem yet create another, and they may become maladaptive in a different environment.

Adaptation is a relevant concept to understanding maltreated children. The biological nature of children is to adjust their behavior to ensure sur-vival in an environment that is threatening or neglectful. A child who is sexually abused while young may experience a precocious puberty. This is a physiological adaptation that likely formed during early evolution to en-sure the ability to reproduce as the victim's survival was threatened. In modern times, however, this can be maladaptive, as accelerated cellular aging is associated with negative physical and mental health outcomes (Colich et al., 2020).

Epigenetics

Childhood maltreatment, dysregulation, and developmental trauma con-stitute an environmentally precipitated perturbation (experience) that can alter gene expression. This could be considered *experience-unexpected*, as it represents an environmental experience that procures powerful adverse consequences that can derail normal development. Any action that alters gene function without altering the DNA sequence is known as epigenetics. Genes can be turned on or off, most commonly by a chemical process called DNA methylation. These changes can become heritable and helps explains how specific family patterns are transmitted between generations. Some of these changes can also be reversible, however, which is good news for treatment interventions.

The Developmental Trajectory of the Human Brain

This brief summary of the ontogeny of the brain will serve the clinician whose treatment is based upon a multidisciplinary foundation of psychol-ogy and neuroscience. Awareness of these processes supports a perspective of the individual as a complex multidimensional system. The ontogeny of the brain begins with a mass of immature and undifferentiated neural cells that grow, organize, and differentiate, at an exponential tempo. The human brain in a four-week-old embryo comprises a set of microscopic lumps at the end of a neural tube. It is the auspicious beginning of a complex and protracted process that continues into early adulthood. The genomic design dictates the sequence of development which involves billions of interactions across multiple micro (e.g., the neuron) and macro domains (e.g., maternal–child interactions). The most defining attribute of neurons is their ability to respond to external cues and influences by altering themselves (Perry et al.,

1995). These neural processes culminate in an exquisite expression of a child's genetic potential, creating a unique individual.

Dramatic and detrimental aberrations in neural development can occur if 'experience-dependent' cues are absent, such as a lack of critical sensory stimulation (as in neglect), or are atypical, extreme experiences (such as physical maltreatment) which confer abnormal neural activation (Perry et al., 1995). The immature child is substantially more vulnerable to adverse experiences, as their neural development is incomplete and can be disrupted, dysregulated, or even halted.

The ontogeny of the brain unfolds in a sequential and hierarchical pattern and can also be conceptualized in vertical integration and organization (Tucker, 2000). Growth progresses from the bottom up, beginning with the most primitive components and processes and progressively developing into complex circuitry and networks (Perry, 2000). *Neurogenesis* is the intense and rapid proliferation of neural cells, micro units that subsidize the grand scheme of the brain. A massive amount of neurons are produced; around 100 billion that are later reduced during sorting and assignment of final roles. Neurons travel along with glial cells (neuron supports) to predetermined regions of the brain, in a radial migration that travels from the inside of the brain to the outside. After migrating to their assigned locations, neurons then differentiate and become a sensory neuron, a motor neuron, or an interneuron. Neurons connect with each other, building circuitry and forming networks and systems that collaborate to produce specific functions. Around 40–60% of these relocated neurons mature and differentiate. The rest are deemed redundant and suffer a predetermined fate called apoptosis.

Synaptogenesis is the formation of connections between neurons, called synapses. Serving as conduits of signaling, the synapse is composed of an opposed duet, the presynaptic terminal, and the postsynaptic target, separated by a gap or cleft (Hong & Park, 2016). Regulation of these processes is critical for the success of these sequences as this delicate construction requires precision and timing.

After this process peaks, which temporally varies between regions, a *pruning* occurs, eliminating weak, ineffective synapses. The neural connections are created and pruned in a prescribed order, beginning with simple structures, and progressing to high-level, more complex systems. This process optimizes circuitry and network processes which support functions such as learning. The timing of peak synapse production is related to the plasticity of that region and each structure and region have their own timeline of maturation. Some regions mature early, such as the amygdala and hippocampus, while others, such as the prefrontal cortex (PFC), have a protracted development that extends into early adulthood (Nelson & Guyer, 2011). Pruning of the cortical regions associated with visual and auditory processes is complete when the child reaches 4–6 years of age, whereas circuits serving regulation, including inhibitory controls, are not pruned until young adulthood.

Neural Communication

Proficient communication between components of complex systems as intricate as the brain is essential for efficient, productive function. From micro units (neurons) to complex networks, the channels of information-sharing must be in good working order and need to perform with regulatory competence. Neurons must communicate with each other to complete their function and they rely upon *neurotransmitters* which perform a critical chemical process essential in the transmission of signals. The neuron can be visualized as a tree with three sections: the cell body, an axon, and dendrites. Using this analogy, the cell body is the trunk; the axon is the root, and the dendrites are formed as branches (Ludwig, 2017). The cell body stores DNA within its nucleus and houses the mechanisms that produce neurotransmitters. Dendrites serve as a reception point for signals, and their growth patterns appear to be shaped by both intrinsic and extrinsic determinants.

The axon carries information as an electrical impulse (action potential) through itself to its end (a terminal). The synaptic gap sits between this terminal and a dendrite extending from another neuron. A neurotransmitter, emitted by the cell body, is secreted into the gap, filling it, and bridging across into a receptor that sits on the receiving dendrite. Neurotransmitters can be imagined as a unique key that will fit into a specific lock. This action either stimulates or inhibits the next neuron, similar to a light that is switched on or off. This form of messaging is analogous to an electrical wire and the transmission takes around 100 milliseconds. While there are about 100 neurotransmitters, norepinephrine, epinephrine, dopamine, and serotonin are highlighted due to their relevance to development, dysregulation, and psychopathology.

Myelination

Myelination, the final process of this sequence, is the protective wrapping of the neural pathways that facilitate communication. A sheath of fatty tissue (white matter) encapsulates and insulates the nerves, ensuring smooth and rapid transmission of information between structures and networks. These communication highways permit disparate regions to collaborate to produce specific functions (Stiles & Jernigan, 2010). Myelination typically begins during the period from late gestation into the early postnatal period, but continues into early adulthood in the prefrontal regions of the brain (Giedd, 2004). Protracted completion of prefrontal myelination accounts for the difficulty in children and teens to employ executive functions which support regulation, inhibition, decision-making, and judgment.

Recent studies have investigated the potential of myelination to be influenced by learning and experiences, generating enthusiasm for the possibility that neural modifications of brain structure and function can be forged throughout life. Most previous studies of neuroplasticity have targeted neuronal synapses, and though precise mechanisms require further study, these processes are still relevant and applicable to treatment (Bonetto et al., 2020). Animal and human studies have shown structural modifications in white matter that result from cognitive functions (Schlegel et al., 2012), motor learning (Xiao et al., 2016), sensory experience (Hill et al., 2018), and social behavior (Liu et al., 2016).

Neural Oscillations

Oscillations or brain waves are rhythmic and synchronized 'frequency patterns' reflecting neural activation in the central nervous system (Cebolla & Cheron, 2019). The organism's emotions, thoughts, and behavior are communicated through these electrical pulses at different frequencies. Known as delta, theta, alpha, beta, and gamma waves, they serve as indicators of neurological processes such as memory, sleep, consciousness, perception, information processing, and neural abnormalities. Electroencephalograms (EEG) are used to measure oscillatory patterns and use units of Hertz (Hz) which indicate one cycle per second.

The Endocrine System

The endocrine system represents a complex network of glands that regulate most processes in the body including metabolism, growth and development, and stress, emotions, mood, and sleep. This system is also tasked with cardiovascular regulation prior to being replaced during evolution by the unmyelinated vagus and ultimately the myelinated vagal system. The glands manufacture and release hormones that carry messages through the bloodstream to skin, tissue, muscles, and organs to perform specific functions that may take minutes or days to be triggered.

Three neural structures that are particularly relevant to the themes of this book are the hypothalamus, the pituitary, and the adrenal glands. These form the hypothalamic-pituitary-adrenal (HPA) axis, a primary regulator of the stress response system (SRS). The hypothalamus, located within the brain, processes information from the central nervous system to inform its regulatory role in multiple processes in the body. The pituitary is a pea-sized gland located at the base of the brain. It secretes hormones and regulates production in other glands. The two adrenals, located on top of the kidneys, regulate blood pressure, metabolism, sexual development, and the stress response.

Three of the hormones which are also pertinent to multiple critical functions include cortisol, oxytocin (OT), and vasopressin (AVP). Cortisol, produced by the adrenals, is known as 'the stress hormone' and regulates the stress response, metabolism, inflammation, blood pressure, and blood sugar. Measurable by blood, urine, and saliva, cortisol levels peak during early morning and are at their lowest in the evening. Oxytocin and AVP are hormones that function as neuropeptides, as they are released into fluids and diffuse to multiple locations, near and far from their point of release (Kovacs, 2004). They are considered an adaptive integrative system and support homeostasis, reproduction, social behavior, and function under conditions of safety and threat.

The Nervous System

The nervous system of the body has two divisions, the central nervous system (CNS) and the peripheral nervous system, which collaborate to regulate all functions. The CNS contains the brain and spinal cord, and the peripheral system consists of nerves and ganglia which connect organs and limbs of the body to the CNS. The brain comprises roughly 2% of body weight, yet consumes 20% of the energy reserves in its functions as the control center for the organism. MacLean characterized the human brain as 'three brains in one.' Though criticized for its simplicity, the model is widely used and reflects the evolutionary hierarchical blueprint for growth and complexity. The brainstem (reptilian) is most primitive, home to the nervous system, and serves autonomic, life-preserving functions. The limbic system (paleomammalian), known as the emotion center, includes cortical, and subcortical structures that serve emotional processes, memory, attachment, reward systems, and threat detection. The prefrontal cortex (PFC) (neomammalian) was the last area to evolve and is also the last brain region to mature during development. The center of higher cognition, this area is the source for problem solving, reasoning, personality, and social cognition (MacLean, 1985).

The most significant responsibility of the CNS is to sense, process, and respond to environmental input. All human experience is received through the sensory systems which include visual (sight), auditory (hearing), olfactory (smell), gustatory (taste), tactile (touch), proprioception (sensations from muscles and physical orientation to space), and vestibular (sense of head movement in space). Sensory input tracks through the brain from the bottom up, adding increasingly complex processing to the initial visceral perception. The nature of sensory, frequency, intensity, and visceral response influences the regulation, connectivity, and organization of the brain (Gaskill & Perry, 2014).

The peripheral nervous system is divided into the autonomic nervous system (ANS) and the somatic nervous system. The somatic system innervates skin, muscles, and joints. The ANS, situated in the brainstem, is tasked with visceral regulation, or homeostasis. Its function is autonomic and non-conscious, and provides regulation of heart rate (HR), respiration, digestion, and metabolism (Kreibig, 2010). The ANS supports growth, healing, and restoration in the individual and also serves as a neural platform for physiological and behavioral responses to threat.

The components of the mammalian nervous system are specifically designed to support survival, safety, and homeostasis.

The Role of the Vagus Nerve in ANS Functions

Stephen Porges outlined the polyvagal theory to conceptualize the role of the nervous system in the regulation of body, emotional, and behavioral states, and ascribed the evolutionary path that coupled the ANS to emotional experience, expression, and contingent social engagement (Porges, 2007).

The vagus, the tenth cranial nerve, is a fibrous bundle that serves as a communication highway to facilitate a bidirectional flow of information between the brain and internal organs (the viscera). This neurobiological 'feedback loop' consists of *afferent* messages sent from the organs to the brain (sensory information) and *efferent* transmissions (regulating data) sent from the brain to the organs. The connections between the brain and the viscera enable the organs to adapt or adjust to the environment of the individual. The vagus comprises two pathways that are structurally and functionally distinct: the dorsal vagus and the ventral vagus. The dorsal vagus, the oldest and predominantly unmyelinated component of the ANS, originates in the dorsal nucleus; and the ventral vagus, the most recently evolved, consists of primarily myelinated fibers and emerges from the nucleus ambiguous. Both fibrous bundles exit the brainstem and travel to their respective territories of responsibility. The ventral vagus serves the supradiaphragmatic region above the diaphragm, while the dorsal vagus attends to the organs below, in the subdiaphragmatic region (Dana, 2018).

The ANS consists of two familiar branches, the parasympathetic nervous system (PNS) and the sympathetic nervous system (SNS), along with a third, the enteric nervous system that serves the brain-gut connection. The PNS, along with the vagus nerve and SNS, provides the neural substrate for three subsystems that are phylogenetically ordered and produce the physiological and behavioral responses to threats or challenges (stress responses). These subsystems have emerged over time and include the immobilization response (behaviors such as fainting, feigning death, and system shutdown), served by the PNS and unmyelinated vagus; the mobilization response (fight or flight behaviors) served by the SNS; and the social engagement system (social communication such as facial expressions, voice, and optimized hearing) which is served by the PNS and myelinated vagus. The function of these three circuits is to adaptively respond to conditions of safety, danger, and threat to life (Porges, 2009).

As the brain evolves and adapts, newer circuitry, and functions are added, but the older circuits are not eliminated. The older two systems continue to exist and function following Jackson's principle of dissolution

(Jackson, 1882). Younger circuits inhibit the older circuits unless they become contextually inadequate. At that point, the older circuits become available for recruitment.

The Parasympathetic Nervous System (PNS)

The dorsal vagus fuels the most primitive response to danger, is reflected in a continuum of immobilization behaviors, gradations of metabolic shutdown, intended to preserve resources. When activated, it moves the individual away from connection and into a state of protection. Coming online about 500 million years ago, the dorsal vagus, responsible for the immobilization response, is shared by reptiles and mammals, and is activated in the face of extreme danger, such as a threat to physical integrity or life (Porges, 2001). In early vertebrates, the unmyelinated vagus was critical in the neural regulation of the entire body. Animals that do not require much oxygen could handle the significant metabolic drop of an immobilization response.

Deb Dana links the responsibility of the dorsal vagus for the area of the body below the diaphragm with the types of trauma that involve that region, such as sexual and physical abuse, medical treatments, and injuries, citing the dorsal response as a common reaction to those forms of trauma (Dana, 2018). Victims of sexual abuse speak of dissociating during the assault as an effective mechanism of survival.

The Sympathetic Nervous System (SNS)

Emerging 400 million years ago, the SNS, situated in the middle region of the spinal cord was responsible for the mobilization (fight or flight) response that Josh experienced. The SNS functions as a 'gas pedal' that accelerates the metabolic processes that equip the individual to stand their ground or flee the scene. When the gas pedal is depressed, systems accelerate; heart rate and blood pressure are elevated and blood flow is prioritized to skeletal musculature. Attention increases and focus narrows, as breathing becomes more rapid, increasing oxygen. The systems that support mobilization divert resources from daily homeostatic functions, such as gastrointestinal function, growth and healing, and tasks that require higher cognition. Intended as a short-term solution, the mobilization response becomes metabolically and emotionally taxing, if extended.

When the child experiences a pervasive state of pervasive sympathetic arousal, cortical regions that support decision-making, judgment, and logic go offline. Brainstem and limbic regions become dominant, and the child appears emotionally reactive, hyperactive, and vigilant. Fearful and distressed, they lose their ability to accurately decipher facial expressions and will misinterpret other social cues. As the child is distrustful, resistant, and defensive, they are unable to access social support. The child develops an attention bias toward threat and focuses their energy on scanning the environment for threats, leaving minimal resources to attend, engage, and learn.

The Social Engagement System (SES)

As mammals phylogenetically diverged from reptiles, the ANS underwent a substantial neuroanatomical and neurophysiological adaptation in response to the increased mammalian sociality. This adaptation was conceptualized by Porges in his polyvagal theory as 'the social engagement system' (SES), which provided a third neural platform that rendered social connection into a mechanism to reduce fear and stress (Porges, 2003).

The neural pathways that travel to the face and head became integrated with the ventral vagus creating a 'face-heart' connection. This connection subsidized emotional expression and communication with others. This neural linkage enabled the use of facial, eye, and middle ear muscles; laryngeal and pharyngeal muscles; and directional head movements to both express safety and differentiate safety and threat in others.

An example of the SES influence can be observed as two dogs engage in a game of chase. During normal intraspecific canine play, the line between play and threat can become blurred. If the pursuing dog nips the hind end of the other, the pursued dog will look back to view the other's face for information that clarifies their intent. Depending on the interpretation, play will either continue (if cues signal safety) or turn aggressive (if threat is signaled).

Relevant to canines and humans, the SES promotes calm and restorative states and promotes connection, as it dampens SNS activation and the HPA axis (Porges, 2009). The SES components also interact with oxytocin and vasopressin and the immune system (Porges, 2001). The child who can access the SES becomes able to attend, engage, be social, and learn, as the mobilization and immobilization circuits are inhibited by this state. Coregulation by others becomes a viable option, as a child who feels safe and part of a nurturing relationship is able to socially engage.

The Vagal Brake

In order to coexist, these two neurobiological states (SNS and PNS) required the capacity to rapidly and adaptively switch from a defensive stance to a social state, and back again, an important responsibility for the vagus (Porges & Furman, 2011). A homeostatic state and social behavior are incompatible with the defensive responses.

When the vagal tone is high, the vagus is functioning as a brake, inhibiting the heart rate and relaxing the individual. When the tone is low, the brake is released and heart rate elevates. Without a functional vagal break, individuals are compromised for bonding, relationship formation, and social learning.

Vagal Tone

'Vagal tone,' a measure of vagal activity, is an index of functional and regulatory efficiency and can be predictive of psychological, social, and physiological health (Kok & Fredrickson, 2010). High vagal tone is associated with reduced anxiety, improved mood, efficient digestion, and the ability to recover quickly from stress or exercise. Vagal tone is measurable through an index called heart rate variability (HRV). Heart rate variability is the difference between the heart rate upon breath inhalation (which raises HR) and exhalation (which lowers HR). Existing biomarkers of physiological processes that accurately measure functional efficiency have already benefited research and the recent development of user-friendly mobile index systems holds significant promise for assessment purposes in future treatment.

The Gut Microbiome

The gut microbiome is technically the third branch of the ANS along with the sympathetic and parasympathetic branches. While it does not receive the amount of attention as the SNS and PNS, it is relevant to mental health and produces substantial sensory information to the brain. Around 90% of signaling via the vagus nerve is afferent, traveling from the gut to the brain. The gastrointestinal system (the gut) is lined with a network of neurons, nerves, and neurotransmitters that extend from the esophagus all the way through the digestive tract to the anus. The gut produces more than 30 distinct neurotransmitters, including 95% of serotonin. As the ENS contains the same neural structures as the brain, some call it the 'second brain.'

The gut provides regulatory functions for brain chemistry, influencing neural, and endocrine systems associated with the SRS, memory, and anxiety (Breit et al., 2018). The CNS also dysregulates gut microbe composition during psychological stress conditions via endocrine release. Gut dysregulation is also associated with risk for physical disease. While it has been suggested that the gut is impacted as a result of depression and anxiety, scientists are beginning to look at the possibility that the gut can be a causal mechanism in affective disturbances.

Brain Structures

The architecture of a child's brain is formed through a 'bottom-up' process, creating the components and structures that support all functional processes of the organism. The brain has three primary sections: the cerebral cortex, the limbic system, and the brainstem. Following the hierarchical direction, growth begins in the primitive section of the brainstem and culminates in the cognitive functions of the cerebral cortex. The integrity and organization of the lower regions support development of the higher areas. It is useful to employ the perspective that higher, more complex regions govern the lower; and they do, yet it is far more complicated. All of the areas function in an interdependent, coordinated, and collaborative dance, and the communication between these regions is critical.

The *brainstem*, the most primitive region of the brain, is influenced by genetics and is fully functional at birth. Comprising three sections, the brainstem regulates the autonomic processes that are critical to life itself: heart rate, breathing, hunger, and sleep. The brainstem is also responsible for the regulation of the CNS and provisions the primary motor and sensory nerve supply to the face and neck.

The *limbic system* includes cortical and subcortical structures that subserve emotional processes, attachment, reward systems, and threat detection. It also performs roles in memory, motivation, and learning. The limbic system regulates autonomic neural and endocrine processes involved with the organism's responses to emotional and sensory stimuli, including the stress response system (SRS). The limbic system connects the sensory networks with the action organization networks and serves as a link between the unconscious, autonomic functions of the brainstem and the consciousness and intellect of the cerebral cortex. Its dense connectivity with these regions supports the necessary communication for collaboration needed to produce specific functions. The system's most well-known structures include the amygdala, hippocampus, hypothalamus, and thalamus.

The *amygdala* is a small, almond-shaped structure that is a key component of multiple networks that serve sensory, emotional, and complex cognitive processes. Involved in emotion (particularly fear and anxiety), attachment, early memory and fear, one of its roles is to attach emotional significance to encoded memories which factors into the strength of that memory. Experiences and events associated with intense emotion tend to be encoded more easily, with less repetition required. A significant portion of the US population clearly remembers where they were, and what they were doing on September 11, 2001. The amygdala is evolutionarily conserved and functions as a threat detector for the stress response system (SES).

The *hippocampus* is anatomically linked with structures that serve emotion and, along with the amygdala; it matures early, yet has extended neuroplasticity and is sensitive to trauma. The *hippocampus* is considered the memory center of the brain and encodes episodic memory paired with sensory stimuli, such as encrypting a specific odor with a specific event. It is also involved in spatial memory, memory consolidation, and transfer.

The *thalamus and hypothalamus* are both associated with emotional reactivity. The thalamus connects the limbic structures to the other sections of the brain and sorts sensory information (from sight, sound, taste, and touch systems) prior to relaying it to the cerebral cortex. The hypothalamus sits at the intersection of the nervous system, which communicates with electrical impulses, and the endocrine systems that use hormones (chemicals) as a signaling mechanism. The hypothalamus functions as a monitor, often first to detect critical changes within the body. The monitor becomes a responder and sets the messaging systems in motion. This organ also serves as a translator turning emotion into a physical response. When an external or internal threat triggers fear, the hypothalamus signals the ANS and pituitary gland, beginning a cascade of physiological changes to prepare the body for defense (the stress response system). When dysregulated, the HPA axis can purvey significant disruption to neural, psychological, and behavioral function.

The cerebral cortex is the outer layer of the brain and is responsible for higher level processes such as thought, consciousness, language, memory, personality, and emotion. It is subdivided into four lobes: the frontal, temporal, occipital, and parietal, each of which have specific functions. Contrasting with the brainstem, the development of the cerebral cortex is heavily influenced by its environment.

The *prefrontal cortex (PFC)*, the most complex and recently evolved brain region is the last neural area to mature and constitutes about 30% of the cerebral cortex. The PFC serves as a regulatory system and is densely connected with multiple other structures, including the brainstem, amygdala, hippocampus, and other limbic regions. This connectivity allows the PFC to access emotional states, sensory information, and multiple systems, such as the stress response system.

The PFC is able to create and maintain representations of knowledge that regulate emotion, thoughts, and actions. The PFC regions can meld and compare the past with the future, form complex associations that involve multiple modes of information, and incorporate temporal aspects. This center of higher cognition is a primary source of regulation for other brain regions and exerts its control through mechanisms of inhibition and goal-directed actions.

The PFC is the source of executive functions, attention, and memory. Executive functions include the ability to problem solve, plan and make decisions, analyze, form judgments, and self-monitor. Working memory, task initiation, organization, emotional control, and flexible thinking are also functions of the executive system.

Attention properties include alertness, spatial attention and sustained attention, and the ability to control interference or distraction. Attention components are believed to reach maturity at about 12 years of age. Neuroimaging studies reveal the role of the PFC for developing episodic memory and actions that promote the formation and retrieval of memory. The PFC is divided into several regions based on function.

The *dorsolateral prefrontal cortex (dlPFC)* is responsible for working memory, cognitive flexibility and planning, problem solving, and sustained attention. Approach and avoidance behaviors are lateralized in the left and right hemispheres of the dlPFC.

The *orbitofrontal cortex (OFC)* is associated with emotion regulation, attachment and relationship processes, and social cognition. The OFC, the amygdala, anterior cingulate, and the front sections of the temporal lobes are the neural components of the social brain. This group of structures formed a network in response to the dramatic increase in sociality during evolution. As a result of its proximity to subcortical regions, the OFC incorporates emotion and sensory information to interpret complex social situations. The OFC functions as a point of convergence, as it consolidates information from multiple sources to integrate the internal and external world.

The ventromedial prefrontal cortex's (vmPFC) duties overlap somewhat with the responsibilities of the OFC, as it is also well connected and receives information from the amygdala, thalamus, temporal lobe, ventral tegmental area, and olfactory system. These regions of higher cognition contribute their executive knowledge and regulatory competence to the emotional and sensory data which substantially support multiple social and interpersonal functions. The vmPFC is credited with producing compassion, courage, shame, and guilt (Siddiqui et al., 2008).

The cortex has two hemispheres, the right, and the left, which have lateralized functions. The left brain is more verbal and analytical than the right, and is designed for reading, writing, and mathematics. The right brain is tasked with more abstract thinking, nonverbal communication, imagination, and intuition. The two sides work together, communicating via the corpus callosum (CC), a large bundle of 200 million nerve fibers (McGilchrist, 2009). The CC permits information to cross over to the other hemisphere allowing integration of information for more complex processing.

Functional Connectivity

The brain may contain 100 billion neurons, but it creates 100 trillion connections. It was believed for some time that specific functions were generated by singular brain structures and regions. Recent investigations using advanced neuroimaging technology now show that collaboration occurs between multiple, often geographically disparate regions to produce specific functions. Communication pathways composed of bundled white matter connect brain regions, providing an efficient mechanism for sharing information and collaborating to produce a specific function. Known as *functional connectivity (FC)*, the strength and integrity of this system is critical to regulatory functions. Disrupted FC has been implicated in multiple forms of dysregulation and psychopathology.

While higher cognitive systems regulate lower, subcortical regions, lower systems also confer regulatory action upon higher, more complex systems. Within the past few decades, research investigations have produced a substantial fund of evidence that highlights the critical importance of genome-environment interaction in neurobiological development of the young brain (Perry et al., 1995). Maltreatment is now recognized as potentially toxic and traumatic, with the power to alter and dysregulate the brain. These adverse experiences are exacerbated by critical periods of neural plasticity which increase receptivity of the brain to the environment.

Conclusion

This brief fundamental explanation of basic neural development components and processes is highly relevant to understanding normal development and neural and functional disruption, dysregulation, and psychopathology. The interdependence and connectedness of the brain components make it easy to understand the cascade of consequences of dysregulation, as change in one region leads to changes in another.

Dysregulation of structures, function, connectivity, and systems and networks are detailed in Chapter 4. This knowledge can enhance and support diagnosis and treatment design and application. Use this chapter as a reference as these concepts are revisited and further integrated throughout the book. The attachment relationship is widely believed to be the most influential environmental experience upon brain growth and organization. A secure attachment is synonymous with regulation and resilience, and that relationship is detailed in the following chapter.

References

Bonetto, G., Kamen, Y., Evans, K.A., & Karadottir, R.T. (2020). Unraveling myelin plasticity. *Frontiers in Cellular Neuroscience* https://doi.org/10.3389/fncel.2020.00156

Breit, S., Kupferberg, A., Rogler, G., & Hasler, G. (2018). Vagus nerve as modulator of the brain-gut axis in psychiatric and inflammatory disorders. *Frontiers in Psychiatry*; 13. https://doi.org/10.3389/fpsyt.2018.00044

Cebolla, A.M., & Cheron, G. (2019). Understanding neural oscillations in the human brain: From movement to consciousness and vice versa. *Frontiers in Psychology*, 10(1930): 1–6. https://doi.org/10.3389/fpsyg.2019.01930

Colich, N.L., Rosen, M.L., Williams, E.S., & McLaughlin, K.A. (2020). Biological aging in childhood and adolescence following experiences of threat and deprivation: A systematic review and meta-analysis. *Psychological Bulletin* 146(9): 721–764. https://doi.org/10.1037/bul0000270

Cozolino, L. (2017). *The Neuroscience of Psychotherapy*. New York, NY: W.W. Norton & Co.

Dana, D. (2018). *The Polyvagal Theory in Therapy: Engaging the Rhythm of Regulation*. New York: WW Norton & Co.

Gaskill, R.L. & Perry, B.D. (2014). The neurobiological power of play: Using the neurosequential model of therapeutics to guide play in the healing process. In *Creative Arts and Play Therapy for Attachment Problems*. C.A. Malchiodi & D.A. Crenshaw, Eds. (pp. 174–194). New York: Guildford Press.

Giedd, J.N. (2004). Structural magnetic resonance imaging of the adolescent brain. *Annals of the New York Academy of Sciences*; 1021: 77–85.

Hasson, U., Ghazanfar, A.A., Galantucci, B., Garrod, S., & Keysers, C. (2012). Brain-to-brain coupling: A mechanism for creating and sharing a social world. *Trends in Cognitive Sciences* 16(2): 114–121. https://doi.org/10.1016/j.tics.2011.12.007

Hebb, D.O. (1949). *The organization of behavior: A neuropsychological theory*. New Jersey: Lawrence Erlbaum Associates, Inc.

Hill, R.A. Li, A.M., & Grutzendler, J. (2018). Lifelong cortical myelin plasticity and age-related degeneration in the live mammalian brain. *Nature Neuroscience* 21: 683–695. https://doi.org/10.1038/s41593-018-0120-6

Hong, J-H. & Park, M. (2016). Understanding synaptogenesis and functional connectome in C. elegans by imaging technology. *Frontiers in Synaptic Neuroscience*. https://doi.org/10.3389/fnsyn.2016.00018

Insel, T.R. (2010). Understanding mental disorders as circuit disorders. In: A Decade after the Decade of the Brain. *Cerebrum*. Dana Foundation. Retrieved from dana.org

Jackson, J.H. (1882). On some implications of dissolution of the nervous system. *Medical Press and Circular*; 2: 411–414.

Kandel, E. (1998). A new intellectual framework for psychiatry. *The American Journal of Psychiatry*. https://doi.org/10.1176/ajp.155.4.457

Kingsbury, L., Huang, S., Wang, J., Golshani, P., Wu, Y.E. & Hong, W. (2019). Correlated neural activity and encoding of behavior across brains of social interacting animals. *Cell*; 178(2): 429–446. https://doi.org/10.1016/j.cell.2019.05.022

Kok, B.E. & Fredrickson, B.L. (2010). Upward spirals of the heart: Autonomic flexibility, as indexed by vagal tone, Reciprocally and prospectively predicts positive emotions and social connectedness. *Biological Psychology*; 117: 240. https://doi.org/10.1016/j.biopsycho.2010.09.005

Kovacs, G.L. (2004). The endocrine brain: Pathophysiological role of neuropeptide-neurotransmitter interactions. *EJIFCC*; 15(3): 107–112.

Krebig, S.D. (2010). Autonomic nervous system activity in emotion: A review. *Biological Psychology*; 84(3): 394–421. https://doi.org/10.1016/j.biopsycho.2010.03,010

Liu, J.,Kupree, J.L., Frawley, R., Sikder, T., & Naik, P., et al. (2016). Clemastine enhances myelination in the prefrontal cortex and rescues behavioral changes in socially isolated mice. *The Journal of Neuroscience*; 36: 957–962. https://doi.org/10.1523/JNEUROSCI.3608-15.2016

Ludwig, M. (2017). How your brain cells talk to each other-whispered secrets and public announcements. *Frontiers for Young Minds*; 5: 39. https://doi.org/10.3389/frym.2017.00039

MacLean, P.D. (1985). Evolutionary psychiatry and the triune brain. *Psychological Medicine*; 15(2): 219–221. https://doi.org/120.1017/s0033291700023485

Mateos-Aparicio, P. & Rodriguez-Moreno, A. (2019). The impact of studying brain plasticity. *Frontiers in Cellular Neuroscience* https://doi.org/10.3389/fncel.2019.00066

McGilchrist. (2009).*The Master and His Emissary: The Divided Brain and the Making of the Western World*. New Haven and London H: Yale University Press.

McGowan, P.O., & Roth, T.L. (2015). Epigenetic pathways through which experiences become linked with biology. *Development and Psychopathology* 27 (2): 637–648. https://doi.org/10.1017/S0954579415000206

Nelson, E.E. & Guyer, A.E. (2011). The development of the ventral prefrontal cortex and social flexibility. https://doi.org/10.1016/j.dcn.2011.01.002

Perry, B.D., Pollard, R.A., Blaicley, T.L., Baker, W.L., & Vigilante, D. (1995). Childhood trauma, the neurobiology of adaptation, and "use-dependent" development of the brain: How "states" become "traits". *Infant Mental Health Journal*; 16(4): 274.

Perry, B.D. (2000). The neuroarcheology of childhood maltreatment: The neurodevelopmental costs of adverse childhood events. *Child Trauma Academy*. Retrieved from https://www.aaets.org/article196.htm

Porges, S.W. (2001). The polyvagal theory: Phylogenetic substrates of a social nervous system. *International Journal of Psychophysiology*; 42(2): 123–146. https://doi.org/10.1016/S0167-8760(01)00162-3

Porges, S.W. (2003). The polyvagal theory: Phylogenetic contributions to social behavior. *Physiology & Behavior*; 79: 503–513. Por 03 https://doi.org/10.1016/S0031-9384(03)00156-2

Porges, S.W. (2007). The polyvagal perspective. *Biological Psychology*; 74(2): 116–143. https://doi.org/10.1016/j.biopsycho.2006.06.009

Porges, S.W. (2009). The polyvagal theory: New insights into adaptive reactions of the autonomic nervous system. *Cleveland Clinic Journal of Medicine*; 76(2): S86–S90. https://doi.org/10.3949/ccjm.76.s2.17

Porges, S.W. & Furman, S. (2011). The early development of the autonomic nervous system provides a neural platform for social behavior: A polyvagal perspective. *Infant and Child Development*; 20(1): 106–118. https://doi.org/10.1002/icd.688

Redcay, E., & Schilbach, L. (2019).Using second-person neuroscience to elucidate mechanisms of social interaction. *Nature Reviews. Neuroscience*; 20(8): 495–505. https://doi.org/10.1038/s41583-019-0179-4

Schlegel, A.A., Rudelson, J.J., & Tse, P.U. (2012). White matter structure changes as adults learn a second language. *Journal of Cognitive Neuroscience*; 24: 166401670. https://doi.org/10.1162/jocn_a_00240

Schore, A.N. (2000). Attachment and the regulation of the right brain. *Attachment & Human Development*; 2: 23–47

Shonkoff, J.P., & Philips, D.A. (2000). *From Neurons to Neighborhoods: The Science of Early Childhood Development*. Washington, D.C.: National Academy Press.

Siddiqui, S.V., Chatterjee, U., Kumar, D., Siddiqui, A., & Goyal, N. (2008). Neuropsychology of prefrontal cortex. *Indian Journal of Psychiatry*; 50(3): 202–208.

Siegel, D. (2015). *The Developing Mind*. New York: Guilford Press.

Stiles, J. & Jernigan, T.L. (2010). The basics of brain development. *Neuropsychology Review*; 20: 327–348. https://doi.org/10.1007/s11065-010-9148-4

Sui, J., Huster, R., Yu, Q., Segall, J.M., & Calhoun, V.D. (2014). Function-structure associations of the brain: Evidence from multimodal connectivity and covariance studies. *NeuroImage*; 102(1): 11–23. https://doi.org/10.1016/j.neuroimage.2013.09.044

Tandon, P.N. (2000). The decade of the brain: A brief review. *Neurology India*; 48: 199–207.

Tucker, D.M. (2000). Anatomy and physiology of human emotion: Vertical integration of brainstem, limbic, and cortical systems. In: J. Borod (Ed.), *Handbook of the Neuropsychology of Emotion*. New York: Oxford.

Valencia, A.L., & Forese, T. (2020). What binds us? Inter-brain neural synchronization and its implications for theories of human consciousness. *Neurosci Consciousness*; 2020(1): niaa010. https://doi.org/10.1093/nc/niaa010

Voss, P., Thomas, M.E., Cisneros-Franco, J.M., & de Villers-Sidani, E. (2017). Dynamic brains and the changing rules of neuroplasticity: Implications for learning and recovery. *Frontiers in Psychology* https://doi.org/10.3389/fpsyg.2017.01657

Xiao, L., Ohayon, K., McKenzie, I.A., Sinclair-Wilson, A., Wright, J.L., Fudge, A.D., Emery, B., Huiliang, L., & Richardson, W. (2016). Rapid production of new oligodendrocytes is required in the earliest stages of motor-skill learning. *Nature Neuroscience*: 19: 1210–1217. https://doi.org/10.1038/nn.4351

Yang, E-J., Lin, E.W., & Hensch, T.K. (2012). Critical period for acoustic preference in mice. *PNAS*; 109(supplement_2): 17213–17220. https://doi.org/10.1073/pnas.1200705109

Chapter 3   Attachment Provisions Regulation and Resilience

The Importance of Attachment

Rooted in developmental evolution, the attachment relationship is a distinguishing feature of mammals and represents one of the most critical tasks of childhood. The increasingly complex human brain evolved to be implicitly linked at birth with an adult brain that would provision the immature brain with the resources it needs (Siegel, 2015). Citing the pioneering work of Colwyn Trevarthen on the intersubjectivity of the infant–caregiver relationship, Schore reiterates that the infant's brain development requires the neural synchronization or coupling with another that is actualized through the mechanisms of implicit nonverbal communication. The resonant coupling provisions the dyad with coregulation and shared emotion in an unconscious dialog between the right brain of the caregiver and the right brain of the infant (Schore, 2021; Trevarthan, 1993).

Significant research endorses the caregiver–infant relationship as a prototype and perhaps the most significant influence upon the neurobiological maturation of the young brain, particularly the affective, social, and stress response system (SRS) (Rincon-Cortes & Sullivan, 2014).

British psychologist John Bowlby (1969, 1973) along with Mary Ainsworth, transformed thinking about the role of the attachment relationship as they developed one of the most prominent theories of modern time. The attachment theory explains how the attachment relationship sculpts the development of the self and influences social relationships throughout life (Banai et al., 2005).

Bowlby proposed that infants are born with an innate biological drive to seek proximity with another to attain the protection, nurturance, emotional support, and care necessary for its survival and development. The attachment relationship functions as an implicit regulation system that is critical to the homeostasis of the helpless infant. The relationship itself is designed to be rewarding to both the infant and caregiver (Mikulincer & Shaver, 2007). When the child feels safe, loved, and their needs are met, a secure attachment will be established.

DOI: 10.4324/9781003217534-5

Bowlby identified four fundamental attributes of the attachment relationship that distinguish it from other affectionate affiliations: safe haven, secure base, proximity maintenance, and separation distress (Bowlby, 1969). Close proximity between children and their caregivers is essential for protection, communication, touch, and play, and the absence of propinquity is associated with profound consequences (Barnett, et al., 2022). The physically immature infant is not capable of ambulating toward or away from positive or negative events or relationships, inferring a profound vulnerability. They have few resources of their own, yet are born with a functional system of striated musculature of the face, head, and neck, served by corticobulbar pathways. This musculature supports vocalization, facial expressions, gazing, smiling, and even scowls. These are mechanisms of expression that solicit positive maternal attention and response (Schore, 1994). When the tiny infant responds to the caregiver's soft voice with excited vocalizations, they are engaging their potential for reciprocity, and demonstrating their capacity for connection.

The Caregiver and Child

The psychobiological attunement of the caregiver to the infant is central to the successful establishment of a secure attachment. The proficient caregiver creates a milieu of synchronicity and intersubjectivity and is available, responsive, and compassionate. The internal, autonomic arousal states of the infant are recognized, appraised, and addressed through a symbiotic synchronicity that is soothing and nurturing. Reciprocal body-based messaging is conveyed through facial expression, voice prosody and tone, posture and gestures, and variances of arousal (Schore, 2021), The right hemispheres of both brains are the locus of communication and the site of key structures, systems, and processes during early attachment. Through this bidirectional communication beneath conscious awareness, the infant is nurtured and regulated.

The Clinician and Child

Nonverbal communication promotes a nonconscious relational connection, and as it is central to the caregiver–infant relationship, so is it to efficacious treatment. The clinician who works with the dysregulated child must connect with the child in a format that allows them to sync with the child. The clinician must be present, attuned, and mirror the child, joining them 'where they are.' The presence of a dog enhances the child's perception of the clinician. When the child witnesses the compassion, kindness, and affection of the clinician (toward the dog), they witness a healthy relationship model and can begin to consider that they can be valued and loved as well.

Secure Attachment

The experience of a healthy relationship establishes a secure attachment and has been associated with regulatory competence (Bretherton & Mun-holland, 2008), resilience, and the development of a cohesive self (Basso, et al., 2021; Schore, 2003). A secure attachment procures an advantageous developmental trajectory, optimizing brain development and equipping the child with resources and resilience that promote mental and physical health (Lahousen, 2019). The child develops an enduring sense of security, the ability to trust, the capability to be empathic and intimate, and the ability to interpret the intentions, emotions, and thoughts of another. Secure children are optimistic, take risks, and will seek relational and social support to solve problems.

Primary Provisions of Attachment

The attachment process unfolds through the psychological, social, and neural resources of caregiver behavior that are evolutionarily shaped to provide safety, coregulation of arousal and affect, and resources that guide and optimize brain development. These three primary provisions of a secure attachment promote resilience in the child; the ability to recover from challenges and adversity. As the attachment process is believed to be critical in the development of self and all future behavior, it follows that a poor attachment experience has been predicted to be one of the most profound stressors in the infant (Bick & Nelson, 2016; Rincon-Cortes & Sullivan, 2014). Impairments in the early attachment relationship are suggested to infer a heightened vulnerability to future onset of psychopathology (Lima et al., 2010).

Safety and Protection

The provision of safety is a biological requisite for the maintenance of homeostasis, for social engagement, learning, and survival itself. The synchrony of the attachment relationship maintains a relational and physiological homeostasis. When proximity and protection are maintained during threat, physiological and emotional arousal in the infant can be regulated by physical contact (George and Solomon, 2008). Skin-to-skin contact has been shown to support the maturation of the autonomic system, improves state regulation, and supports neurodevelopment (Feldman & Eidelman, 2003).

While the concept of protection is central to attachment for actual survival, the notion of 'safety' can be thought of in terms of 'felt' emotion (Gendlin, 1978). *Feeling safe* is a powerful component and requisite of well-being, relational and social interest and engagement, and learning. Homeostasis, balance, and equilibrium are terms that reflect regulation and invoke sensations of safety.

Coregulation

The central nervous system (CNS) of the infant is equipped to function in a safe environment where gradations of arousal are monitored and stabilized through coregulation. The caregiver shields the child from overwhelming stress and reregulates the physiology and emotion of the child with nurturing responsiveness. Coregulation of these states supports synchrony in the pair, and in a context of attuned reciprocity, synchrony more effectively maintains homeostasis in the infant (Busuito, et al., 2019). The quality of early care is unequivocally correlated with this early experience of coregulation and is directly associated with the emergence of the child's own regulatory system Bretherton & Munholland, 2008). The maturity of the child's regulatory competence is reflected in their emotional and physiological response to threat (George & Solomon, 2008; Mikulincer & Shaver, 2007).

Regulatory competence is served by neurobiological substrates that are formed during early caregiving (Tottenham, 2015). This neural circuitry supports regulation, an essential component of all functional domains, including emotion, behavioral, cognition, social, and physiological. Deficient attachment experiences can inhibit development of the regulatory frontolimbic circuits that are experience-dependent, causing dysregulation in these functional domains.

Optimized Brain Development

The infant brain experiences a major growth spurt that is predominantly postnatal, continuing to about 24 months of age. The enormous neural activity in the little brain is strongly influenced by the child's environment, particularly the social and emotional aspects (Schore, 1994).

The right hemisphere (RH) matures ahead of the left analytical side, thus is central to attachment functions, coregulation, stress response, and the processing of emotional and social information. The RH is densely interconnected with the autonomic nervous system (ANS), neurochemical systems, and subcortical limbic circuits. Through the coregulation of affect and arousal, the attachment process shapes and balances the stress response system (SRS). Increasingly, research is finding links between attachment insecurity and distinct physiological response patterns to threat and stress events. Primary components of the SRS, the HPA axis (Gunnar et al., 1989), SAM, and immune systems (Doom & Gunnar, 2013; Padgett & Glaser, 2003) have been identified as systems that become dysregulated in children with maltreatment and developmental trauma.

Secure attachment reflects a homeostatic balance between the sympathetic (SNS) and parasympathetic nervous systems (PNS), the two branches that serve the SRS. Shaped by early experiences, an imbalance (manifested as arousal or withdrawal) can become a pervasive pattern of dysregulation. Dysregulation and persistent dominance of either the SNS or PNS are believed to infer a vulnerability to psychopathology.

The attachment period functions as a growth-inducing environment, and the integrity of functional connectivity in the cortical and limbic networks reflect the environment during development. The attachment experience plays a substantial role in limbic circuitry, and neural organization, integration, and connectivity become compromised by poor attachment experiences (Cozolino, 2017). Emotional and physiological synchrony in the duo also directly shapes the neural circuitry of the orbital prefrontal cortex (OFC), a site of regulatory systems. The PFC regions register and appraise sensory input from all of the senses, along with facial expressions, as higher cognition interprets and formulates responses to these signals.

Resilience

Resilience can be conceptualized as the ability to cope with threats, challenges, and destabilizing events. Many assume that resilient children do not suffer the negative effects of trauma, that they are somehow protected from suffering. While some experts believe resilience is genetic and innate, others believe that thoughts and behaviors can be learned that foster the ability to recover from adversity. Resilient children are indeed, impacted by trauma, yet they actively draw from a multitude of resources that support adaptive change and recovery.

Eric Nestler, MD, PhD, frames resilience as an issue with plasticity. In a study of mice exposed to severe stress, many appeared defeated, yet one-third showed the potential to recover. The difference was that the mice with resilience showed adaptive changes *after* the initial consequences of stress. Plasticity for them seemed to endure (Patoine, 2019).

Ming-Hu Han, PhD, and team looked at resilience from a genetic perspective and also found significant differences in gene expression between two groups of mice in a social-defeat model. Resilient mice showed three times the amount of activated genes as the defeated group. They were not immune to stress consequences, yet they utilized resources to adapt on a molecular level (Patoine, 2019). Scientists and clinicians agree that mechanisms of resilience should be robustly studied.

Studies have shown that adults maltreated as young children, *without* psychological disorders, have remarkably similar neurobiological alterations as maltreated adults *with* psychopathology (McCrory & Viding, 2015; Teicher et al., 2016). Resilience is the protective mechanism that prevents individuals from a redirected pathway. These results highlight the importance of preventive programming and early intervention. These types of studies also infuse hope that effective treatment will identify the factors that diverted the child's pathway, build resilience, restore regulation, and successfully redirect them to an optimal outcome. Current treatment designs that strive to increase resilience use relational and social scaffolding as primary resources. Specific interventions also utilize learning and skill development, movement and exercise, social skills, and mindfulness. Canine-assisted models are capable of incorporating all of these modalities and enhance their effectiveness.

The extreme climate and habitat changes during the Pleistocene Epoch drove many species to extinction yet it brought humans and wolves, two distant species, into a relationship that bound them. Each had factors of resilience that were species-specific, yet their collaborative relationship increased adaptation and survival in both. Humans and dogs supported each other, cooperated with each other, and learned from each other. Perhaps one of the most enduring lessons they absorbed was the power of affiliations and relationships to mitigate stress. Our social species require a social context to thrive, and the ability to access the support of others is a major key to regulatory competence, mental health, and even survival. Individuals who have been harmed by interpersonal betrayal have great difficulty accessing and accepting human support. This is another argument for the profound relational capability of dogs to provide an alternative, yet authentic and trustworthy mechanism of resilience.

The social engagement system (SES), conceptualized in the polyvagal theory (Porges, 2007), evolved to support these principles as a powerful adaptation that supports the increased sociality of humans and other mammals. Accessing the SES during ni-CAP provides an acceptable safe alternative for social support, attachment benefits, and the necessary co-regulation that supports healing.

Stress Training and Resilience

Childhood mastery of minor levels of adversity is requisite in the development of functional resilience that equips the individual with resources to combat future challenges. The capability of maltreated children to develop and employ mechanisms of resilience, however, is negatively impacted by the toxic quality and quantity of early adversity. A longitudinal study of young adults with histories of maltreatment revealed that only 22% developed functional resilience. (McGloin & Widom, 2001) Lacking a functional level of resilience leaves the child with a significant vulnerability and risk for future mental and physical health disorders.

Studies show that mild to moderate stress experience promotes coping and emotion regulation. The developmental experience of periodic, mild stress serves as a mechanism that 'trains the brain' through repetitive episodes of 'rupture and repair.' Human caregivers are by nature, 'human'. Dyadic *misattunement* episodes are typical in any relationship, and these moments create a minor *rupture* in the bond that is then *repaired* (remediated) by the attuned caregiver. Attachment is predicated on the process of *synchrony*. If stress can be classified as *asynchrony*, then the movement of an infant from synchrony to asynchrony and back to synchrony builds resilience. If the relationship is *not* repaired, however, the child endures highly stressful periods of frightening arousal.

These experiences provide building blocks for regulatory capacity which instills resilience in the child. Positive reciprocal exchanges of emotion trigger the dopaminergic and opioid systems which not only enhance brain development; they increase the child's tolerance of higher levels of emotion and arousal. This represents coregulation and stress training which encodes as part of the 'internalized mother' or 'internal working model' (Bowlby, 1969). The attachment relationship becomes a *template to-go* providing guidance as the child becomes autonomous.

The Role of the Oxytocin System

Meg Olmert (2009) illuminated the importance of oxytocin when she coupled the evolution of humans and animals with neuroscience. Oxytocin (OT) is a neuropeptide signaling molecule that evolved over 700 million years and is present in all vertebrates. It functions as a hormone and neurotransmitter through two release mechanisms to permit adaptations in an organism to the ever-changing environment. Oxytocin has supported multiple mammalian processes, including reproduction and birthing, metabolism, and homeostasis. These neurobiological changes account for the emotional, cognitive, and executive priming that prepares for the birth of the infant. Oxytocin calms the sympathetic nervous system of the mother after birth, lowering heart rate and blood pressure to inhibit stress reactivity. Olmert suggests that the oxytocin-fueled intense fascination and focus that occurs in the new mother is analogous to early humans who were captivated by the animals they observed. Both processes are served by visual and attention systems.

Oxytocin plays a significant role in the attachment process and enhances the positive neurobiological effects. Both OT and dopamine are associated with parenting and bonding. Breastfeeding, mutual eye gazing, and skin-to-skin contact increase maternal OT levels and also decrease blood pressure and cortisol levels. While OT functions as an acute relatively short-term effect, repetitive behaviors can extend their effects (Handlin et al., 2012). Oxytocin levels of parents and the infant become synchronized after birth, and OT is also believed to synchronize with the activation of reward circuits during mother–infant interaction. This hormonal influence increases the attunement and commitment of parents to the infant (Chambers, 2017; Olmert, 2009). Infants produce OT prior to birth and postnatal relational experiences such as skin-to-skin contact increase their plasma levels (Vittner et al., 2018).

Oxytocin also serves as a regulator for stress states and overall wellbeing. It can be triggered through sensory signals such as gentle tactile stimulation of the skin, positive touch activity such as nursing, stroking, grooming, and skin-to-skin contact. These behaviors that are believed to reduce stress and anxiety in the child are known as 'soothing mechanisms' (Unväs-Moberg et al., 2014). The capability of the mother to produce nutrition from her body is an evolutionarily conserved function specific to mammals. Supported by the collaboration of OT with dopamine release, regulation of serotoninergic and cortisol levels, and its influence upon the sympathetic and parasympathetic nervous systems (SNS and PNS), nursing provides a powerful mechanism for regulation (Unväs-Moberg et al., 2014; Schore, 2003). When maternal chemistry and behavior (as in oxytocin release and soothing techniques) confer a reduction in elevated cortisol levels in the infant, plasticity is enhanced, and resilience is increased (Vela, 2014).

The caregiver, whose infant is premature or has neurodevelopment or medical issues, faces an increased challenge to coregulate their baby. Parents have preconceived expectations about their new arrival, and unexpected complications can be devastating. Parents of today lack the familial and community support of earlier times, compounding the stress and pressure. Social programs that offer services such as accessible and no-cost nursing/medical advice, parent support groups, counseling, and respite could potentially mitigate long-term issues that arise from early challenges.

Oxytocin also mediates social behavior and stress regulation, and plays a role in the use of social relationships to mediate stress (Yirmiya et al., 2020). While the OT system gets the most credit, it often collaborates with vasopressin (AVP) and other endocrine components (dopamine, serotonin, and opioids) to serve functions in both kinship and non-kinship relationships (Cozolino, 2017).

Studies have shown links between OT and both empathy and theory of mind; trust and generosity (Zak et al., 2007); social synchrony (Levy et al., 2017); and face recognition and memory (Savaskan et al., 2008). The OT system also increases the duration of mutual gaze (Guastella, et al., 2008), promotes attention and attunement to emotional cues (Ma et al., 2016), and underlies the ability to recognize emotions in others (Jiang & Platt, 2018). For a long time, humans and other primates were considered the only species to be capable of attributing a mental state to others (theory of mind) yet canines have been shown to 'read' human emotion and predict behavior.

Ma and colleagues provided the first neural evidence showing that oxytocin reduced negative affect in humans, a result that has been replicated. Using intranasal methods, amygdala activity was reduced in response to states of fearful, angry, and sad faces. Intranasal OT also reduced amygdala activity in conditions involving social trust betrayal and social threats (Ma et al., 2016). Securely attached individuals typically have higher levels of oxytocin which increase during episodes of stress and play. Secure attachment is correlated with elevated OT and also a reduction of subjective distress during stressful events.

The Role of Opioids

Animal research suggests that the activation of the opioid systems of mother and child supports and regulates the attachment process (Cozolino, 2017). Endogenous opioids promote a sense of safety and increase feelings of well-being in the infant. This chemistry is shaped through the collaboration of environmental experience and internal physiological processes.

The mechanism of coregulation is evident in the behavior of the mother who mitigates infant distress and discomfort through nursing. Molecules within breast milk trigger receptors linked to opioids which produce a physical and emotional calming effect. This familiar attachment behavior supports the reciprocal activation of the duo's endogenous opiate systems and also regulates the dopamine levels in the infant.

The reward system consists of neural circuitry that is dichotomously split into the *familiarity* system and the *novelty seeking* system (Tops et al., 2014). Both of these systems are associated with attachment. The dorsal striatal pathway serves the implicit rewards of familiarity and comfort, while the ventral striatal pathway serves the seeking of novelty as a reward. The infant initially seeks the mother's face as novel, then, as she becomes categorized as familiar, her face is sought as a source of comfort. When the healthy development of these pathways is disrupted, implicit attachment can result. The deficient maturation of the familiarity circuitry diminishes its salience and the individual becomes focused on novelty. Unfortunately, further study showed a diminished response to the novel reward system as well for individuals with early child maltreatment (Teicher et al., 2016). Bonding, relationships, and prosocial behaviors can become compromised, robbing the child of the joy, comfort, and resilience that others enjoy. When the reward system is dysregulated, other, often maladaptive, forms of stimulation may be sought, such as drugs and high-risk behavior.

Elemental Mechanisms of Attachment (Synchrony, Rhythm, and Mimicry)

Organisms are programmed for rhythms and cycles, and nature provides us with numerous prompts that support synchrony. The sun rises and sets each day; the tides come in and out, and the seasons change throughout year. Our hearts beat with a rhythm that aligns with the inhalation and exhalation of breath, and we wake and sleep in a circadian cycle.

Synchrony has been framed as a temporal organization of sensory and physiological messaging into patterns that nurture the relationship (Feldman, 2007). Biobehavioral synchrony occurs between the brains of the attachment dyad, involves autonomic processes, hormones, and behavior, and supports long-term mental health, regulation, empathy, and stress management. Synchrony can result from a shared environment or cooperative task and is more common in familiar dyads. Significant research of this construct has been conducted in the context of the caregiver–infant relationship as it is considered the prototypical social relationship.

Autonomic synchrony is reflected in the simultaneous release of oxytocin, heart and breathing rhythms, and pupil dilation, and is associated with improved immune function and higher respiratory sinus arrhythmia (Feldman et al., 2011). Emotions, gaze, vocalizations, and touch can also sync in dyads. Emotional synchrony develops as the mother shapes and regulates the infant's affective states through nuanced and implicit visual signals and other nonverbal cues.

Synchrony within the attachment process readies the infant's social brain for future relationships and social functioning. Feldman and team also found that synchrony at three and nine months could predict the level of self-regulation in children at two, four, and six years. Follow-ups found early synchronous patterns were associated with healthy attachment, reduced behavior problems, self-regulation, and empathic behavior at later ages (Feldman, 2007). These examples of synchronicity between caregiver and infant are measurable using several tools. One example currently used in attachment research, is magnetoencephalography (MEG), a technology that measures brain oscillations involved in synchrony (Hari & Kujala, 2009).

Categorized as alpha, beta, delta, gamma, and theta waves, oscillations encode information and create the experience of consciousness (Cebolla & Cheron, 2019). Brain-to-brain coupling occurs with synchronized alpha and gamma oscillation rhythms (Levy et al., 2017). This phenomenon is considered a valid index of bidirectional information flow. Oscillations subserve motor movement and movement conversely stimulates cortical spindle oscillations (Basso et al., 2021). Movement stimulates neural plasticity, facilitates neural network communication, and optimizes brain functionality (Headley & Pare, 2017). Oscillations also support the development of cognitive skills, language, and social and emotional learning (Cirelli et al., 2018).

The phenomenon of mimicry was positively selected through evolution for its benefits to the social development of humans and mammals. Traits that increase the survival potential of a species are continued throughout time, and mimicry and social competency were, and still are, essential for healthy function among species. The presence of this ability in human and mammal infants speaks to the adaptive evolutionary value (Palagi & Scopus, 2017).

The discovery of *mirror neurons* in the 1990s was a significant contribution to learning and communication theories. With advanced neuroimaging, a single neuron can be identified as firing in an observer of another organism as the other performs a task. The firing neuron in the observer is comparable to the neuron in the one performing the task. (Rizzolatti & Craighero, 2004).

Humans automatically and unconsciously mimic the facial expressions of others, a form of embodied emotion. With the help of mirror neurons, individuals activate the specific facial musculature of observed facial expressions of their emotion. For instance, when someone is smiling or laughing, the *zygomaticus major* in the observer is activated (cheek musculature). Mimicry accentuates emotional engagement and, in a bidirectional loop, emotional engagement increases mimicry. Pleasurable emotional interactions increase familiarity, bonds, and synchronization, and this process may serve emotional bridges between humans and other animals (Palagi and Scopa, 2017).

The process of repeated reinforcement of this early developmental mimicry then leads to more complex components of social interaction. Mimicry is believed to be related to the skill of recognizing and interpreting nonverbal social cues which supports healthy reciprocal interaction.

Rhythm, synchrony, and mimicry each support the attachment process and are key components of social development. A newborn infant has the reflexes to automatically mimic facial gestures such as tongue protrusion and open mouth (Meltzoff & Moore, 1983), and this ability supports and increases face-to-face interactions, strengthening a platform for early communication. Humans can mimic facial expressions and motor activity, but mimicry also synchronizes heart rate, pupil diameter (Kret & De Dreu, 2017), and hormonal levels (Saxbe et al., 2014). Blushing, crying, and the well-known yawning contagion are other examples that demonstrate this mechanism which is considered the precursor of emotion contagion (Kret, 2015).

Elemental mechanisms of nature, including synchrony, mimicry, and rhythm can be found throughout life processes. These mechanisms facilitate healthy growth and development and have a regulating effect on neurobiological processes that will support a restoration of multiple domains of function.

Modes of Communication in Attachment

Right-Brain Coupling

The right hemisphere (RH) matures prior to the analytic left, and is thus dominant in the very young child. This discovery was confirmed by a single photon emission computed tomography (SPECT) scan less than 25 years ago (Chiron et al., 1997). The right brain is often referred to as the 'emotional brain,' as it is involved in emotion, stress, self-awareness, and body perception. Highly receptive to relational experiences, the internalized attachment model and relational knowledge are stored within the right brain.

The RH of the infant becomes coupled with the regulated and regulating caregiver RH, which supports emotional attunement, reciprocity, and coregulation (Tronick et al., 1977). The coupling provides the pair with a direct channel of implicit and nonverbal messaging that operates beneath the level of consciousness. The communication of emotion is expressed in the facial musculature, tone and prosody of voice, gestures and posture. The flow of energy between the pair is choreographed with a rhythm that taps into neural circuitry (Basso et al., 2021). The RH processes the implicit modes of communication and builds a neural substrate for perception and processing of faces, voices, and gestures (Schore, 2003).

The implicit awareness of the relevance of the RH to attachment led scientists to conceptualize a state of experience-expectancy in the infant brain that requires maternal input transmitted by the mother's right hemisphere. More recently, it has been recognized that a 'right brain-to-right brain' coupling occurs between infant and caregiver that provides the unconscious channel of implicit communication. This process that underlies bonding, security, coregulation, and critical learning that is time-sensitive makes sense, as the physiology and cognition of the infant are precariously immature. The RH is now believed to be a core component of the attachment process.

Implicit processing is automatic and supports rapid categorization and decision-making (Lyons-Ruth & Jacobvitz, 1999). Along with its essential role in emotional attachment, the RH supports the ability to grasp reality as a whole and is involved in the integration of affect, behavior, and autonomic activity (Schore, 2003). Empathy, self-awareness, identification with others, and other intersubjective processes are also largely dependent upon right-brain resources.

The RH also mediates basic physiological and endocrinological functions whose primary control centers are located in subcortical areas of the brain. Along with these functions, the RH has dense connectivity with the limbic and autonomic nervous system, making it a key player in emotional, social, and stress response systems (SRS). These factors support the relevance of the RH in stress response, and particularly in adversity involving interpersonal betrayal and disrupted attachment. Preverbal memories of early maltreatment and trauma tend to be encoded in the RH as images, sounds, smells, and other sensory forms which are viscerally experienced. Without a paired verbal narrative, these memories are difficult to put into context or process.

Consider the potential influences these modes of communication have in a relationship-based therapeutic context. They are instrumental in creating safety and coregulation, and also optimize brain development, primary attributes of a healthy attachment relationship. The clinician and canine are also capable of coupling with the RH of the child; connecting, communicating, and recreating or strengthening the essential attachment relationship. The coupling of brains fosters an implicit, body-based intersubjectivity that funds a powerful connection. A healthy attachment relationship can be formed creating a new, alternative template. The niCAP framework integrates many of these processes of the attachment experience to reregulate the child with dysregulation.

Crossing Eyes and Brains

The RH is thought to have become dominant for rapid response to threats during human and canine evolution (Bonati et al., 2013). Dogs also share this lateralization bias (Guo et al., 2009). Both visual and auditory cues associated with a threat trigger RH activation.

A left visual preference fits with the tendency of humans to access the RH for processing of emotional and social information. Circuitry correlated with the interpretation of facial expressions is also RH positioned. Interestingly, the lateralization of the brain implicitly informs maternal instinct for this mode of communication, and it is recognized at work in her behavior. The mother cradles the child on the left side of her body lining up visual connections that feed messaging of relational and social messaging between the two right brains. From that vantage position, the infant faces the 'more expressive' left profile of the mother (Lindell, 2018). This lateralization bias is believed to be gender-specific for females, be subject to multiple variables, and is potentially related to biases for the left ear and left side of the body. A diminished preference for left-cradling was found to be inversely related with psychological health, as in maternal separation and mental health conditions (Malatesta et al., 2019). It has been suggested that hemispheric specialization of functions may have been a precursor for more complex cognitive and social behavior (Forrester et al., 2018a).

Program developer, director, and art therapist, Linda Chapman's treatment model incorporates neurobiological principles that are active during attachment and early development that strengthen intervention effectiveness. Working with art mediums, she shares how she uses her left eye to look into the left eye of the child, a process that supports joining of her right brain with the child's right brain (Chapman, 2014). Right-brain coupling is a powerful mechanism for reaching the child and is further detailed in later chapters.

The Visual System

The occipital cortex develops in the infant around two months of age resulting in a significant expansion of emotional and social capacity. Eye contact and mutual gaze are powerful mechanisms of expression and shared synchronous states. The occipital cortex is both a benefactor (facilitator) *and* a beneficiary of attachment.

The SES that developed through evolutionary changes to the ANS finetuned these mechanisms. Human expression of emotion was accentuated by neural changes providing enhanced regulation of eyelids and facial musculature. The eyes are a primary mode of communicating feelings in humans, and are becoming so for dogs, as well. An adaptation to the increasing interdependence and sociality of dogs and humans was the anatomical change to a tiny muscle above the eye (Kaminski et al., 2019). Multiple species of modern dogs can raise a single eyebrow which substantially increases their capability for emotional and social facial expression. Dogs today seem capable of soliciting human attention through this expanded repertoire of eye movement.

The face is a dynamic social tool of communication that is used for the expression, transmission, and interpretation of information (such as emotion, thoughts, and motivation). While body gestures, touch, and vocalizations also provide information, in early development, it is the face that is central in communication. As the infant matures, they begin to identify particular reference points on the caregiver's face which leads to an ability to interpret the nuances of specific micro-movements. Most humans develop a repertoire of these expressions and this allows familiarity to be established relatively quickly. The face reflects an individual's emotions, thoughts, and motivations, thus mutual gaze is a primary component of interpersonal relationships and communication.

Affective Touch Is Direct Messaging to the Child

Affective pleasant touch by the caregiver is perceived and processed through somatosensory channels and is an important mechanism of communication. This form of touch regulates the physiology of the infant and promotes calming, encourages emotional closeness, and increases engagement of the infant (Fairhurst et al., 2014). Affective touch is gentle positive tactile stimulation that is believed to be critical for emotional, social, neurobiological, and neurocognitive growth in mammals (Cascio et al., 2016). Parents have not always had the benefit of scientifically sound advice. In 1894, Dr Luther E. Holt, a renowned US pediatrician, wrote a parenting book that remained the gold standard for 50 years. Holt advocated 'hands off' parenting and discouraged holding, cuddling, and playing with children (Holt, 1894). His advice was apparently based on opinion and lacked supportive research.

Rene Spitz, an Austrian psychoanalyst found mortality rates in orphanages in the 1940s and 1950s to be as high as 70%. He proposed it was due to a lack of touch and performed the first systematic research, yet his hypothesis was not readily accepted (Spitz, 1945). Fellow scientist Harry Harlow then tested Spitz's theory with Rhesus monkeys that were deprived of maternal touch and nurturance. His results endorsed the theory (Harlow & Zimmerman, 1958) and the two studies are among the most well known in child development fields. Mammals and human children can be profoundly stunted across all domains when deprived of touch.

Positive touch is an ancient mechanism of healing in Asian societies, practiced for over 2,000 years (Xiong et al., 2015). Western experts today are currently encouraging parents to be nurturing and abundant with gentle touch of their children. Physical contact between caregiver and infant is capable of producing cardiac and respiratory coupling. This physiological synchrony has also been shown to regulate vagal tone and cortisol activity (Feldman, et al., 2011).

C-Tactile (CT) fibers are peripheral nerves within the skin, activated during slow, gentle touch (McGlone et al., 2014). This type of touch has been shown to increase activation of the parasympathetic nervous system which reduces heart rate and calms physiological arousal (Tanaka et al.,

2021). CT fibers are considered mediators for oxytocin release and endogenous opioids (Uvnas-Moberg et al., 2014). Gentle and pleasant touch can elicit a state of calm relaxation and urge to connect through the release of oxytocin and endorphins.

It should be noted that infants with sensory integration dysfunction may show touch aversion and avoidance (Kilroy et al., 2019). This sensitivity increases the challenge for caregivers to establish healthy attachment, as the sensory impairment may appear like rejection or infer an inferior quality of care. Similar challenges occur for parents of children with autism (Cascio et al., 2016), eating disorders (Feldman et al., 2004), pain, or premature birth. An interesting consideration is that early defensiveness to touch likely reduces their experiences which in itself may alter development of the social brain. Further exploration will hopefully reveal information that can be used for the benefit of these children. Notably, the palm of the hand is not innervated with CT fibers, which may partially explain the willingness of defensive children to stroke a dog.

Jack, diagnosed with Asperger Syndrome, appeared to his parents and teachers as highly touch-aversive. His mother complained that he refused to hug her throughout his 13 years. During his second appointment, however, Jack lay down on the floor and at arm's length, vigorously petted Bentley with both hands for most of the session. Stretched out side by side, the two were equal in height, though the large Newfoundland outweighed the teen. Bentley seemed to respect Jack's space, perhaps interpreting the gentle bracing of his arms. He never attempted to move closer. When Jack began to approach the dog from above, Bentley demonstrated the skill called self-handicapping, by remaining on his back. This behavior continued over the course of several weeks and gradually Jack began to lay next to the dog with his sleeve-covered arm across his back. Jack did continue to resist human-to-human hugging, though he did state, 'I haven't ruled it out yet!'

Animal studies have shown significant differences in neural connectivity between children given 'high' amounts of touch vs. 'low' levels (Seelke et al., 2015). Humans were found to employ touch during 65% of face-to-face communications resulting in immediate reductions in both dysregulated behavior and physiology. The paradox for clinicians and other professionals who provide services for children is that while we now recognize the importance of touch for the development, health, and well-being of children, it has been highly discouraged. This dilemma, fortunately, can be mitigated through the incorporation of dogs into treatment. Dogs are natural and authentic in their affection for children and do not trigger similar liability concerns. Children need positive and affective touch for both development *and* healing, thus the dog can fulfill this crucial role with minimal issues.

Voice/Auditory

The instinctive orienting of the infant to the caregiver's voice increases mutual eye gaze and stimulates the networks of attachment and neural growth (Schore 1994). When a child hears the mother's voice, emotional processing areas (the amygdala and orbito-frontal cortex) are activated (Dehaene-Lambertz, et al., 2010). Research has shown that soothing speech triggers the release of oxytocin and reduces salivary cortisol, a chemical formula that reduces stress reactions (Seltzer et al., 2012). The prosody and tonal cues are believed to confer these responses, not linguistic content. Characterized as *motherese*, the melodic prosody of the caregiver is suggested to regulate infant affect and arousal, calming heart and breathing rates (Fancourt & Perkins, 2018).

Researchers have investigated the influence that singing (music) has upon bonding, prosocial behavior, shared attention, motivation, and increased well-being, and results support its power to effect positive change. Oxytocin and endogenous opioids are biochemical mechanisms that support these effects (Weinstein et al., 2016). Parents who sing to their young create an experience of interpersonal intimacy that can evoke an emotional and physiological response. Interpersonal relations that source music draw from mechanisms such as synchrony and rhythm, which evoke perceptions of emotional closeness.

The modern day phenomenon of texting as a substitute for in-person social interaction presents a potential risk for emotional and social development of youth today. The lack of sufficient exposure to prosodic, auditory cues may deprive children of valuable hormonal influences. Parental voices, even for teens, are a critical source of nurturing, support, and co-regulation. Texting also deprives the child of the entire repertoire of non-verbal communication. Healthy development relies on the multitude of signals that face-to-face communication provides.

Sharing Saliva: A Recently Proposed Mechanism of Communication

Most individuals consider the body fluids of others as distasteful and even unhealthy, yet fortunately parents still universally accept the drool and saliva of their infants as a tolerable occupational hazard (Fawcett, 2022). Scientists are unsure if the 'shared saliva' behavior is innate or learned, yet researchers have identified shared saliva as an implicit cue of a primordial intimate relationship. Thomas and colleagues at Harvard and MIT tested their hypothesis through multiple studies, each time expanding subject diversity for increased rigor. Their conclusion was that saliva sharing serves as an informative cue that signals the quality of relationship and also shapes infant expectations about adult response and care (Thomas, et al., 2022).

Evolutionary theory shows that individuals benefit from kinship relationships, and children possess a biological encoding for identifying kin that is activated very early. Infants develop an attribution bias for familiarity due to their extreme reliance upon another human for survival. After birth, they are able to quickly identify their caretaker, and gradually they acquire insight into the formation of in- and out-group membership and schema, expanding their circle as they age.

The discovery of this potential additional cue that communicates and enhances the attachment relationship is suggested to be a biological mechanism that also might serve the human–canine bond. Children tend to interpret the licking behavior of a dog as 'friendly' and will attribute the action as a sign that 'he likes me!' The human–canine interspecies relationship mirrors multiple elements of the attachment process, factors that are discussed throughout the book. These similarities lend themselves to investigation of their potential relevance and the therapeutic effect of dogs in the healing of children.

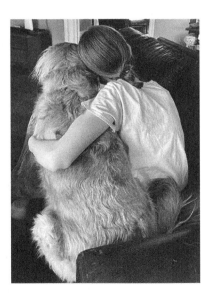

The Child and Dog Relationship

Human–animal bonds (HABs) have been rigorously studied within the past two decades and the infant–caregiver relationship has provided a salient template for comparison. Humans do envision their relationships with dogs as 'attachments,' and they seem to fulfill the requisites of infant–caregiver pairs (Kurdek, 2008; Wanser et al. 2019). Literature discusses the role of the clinician in establishing an attachment relationship to provide the client with a figure of trust, safety, and coregulation. While this component of treatment is part of an effective modality, forming this level of relationship may be very difficult for a maltreated child. The experience of being harmed, neglected, and betrayed by another human creates distrust, fear, and dysregulated physiology which can lead to attrition or poor outcomes in treatment. Now, imagine the working therapy dog.

Dogs are exceedingly interested and attentive to humans, and one way to frame their unique ability with children is that they are not compromised by language. There are no biases, attitudes, or judgment in their communication. They are not constrained by tone, intensity, rhythm, intonation, and prosody. The dog meets the child in their intersubjective space and can reach inside the child in a manner that bypasses the obstacles of human relationships.

Studies show that an individual can form secure relationships with dogs in spite of existing insecure attachments with humans (Beetz, et al., 2012). As the clinician–dog bond models a healthy relationship to the child, a child–dog relationship affords the actual *experience* of a strong bond. In a study of children in abusive home environments, they were found to be four times more likely to have formed a secure attachment to an animal in the home than to their caregiver (Wanser et al., 2019).

The working therapy dog also serves as a bridge for the child to form a strong therapeutic alliance with the clinician. As the child witnesses the clinician–canine relationship, they recognize this human is safe and can be trusted. The canine-assisted therapeutic milieu offers a synchronous and attuned relational, attachment, and social support permitting the child's neural systems to be accessed and reedited. The secure base felt in the presence of a canine companion enables the child to feel safe and more comfortable to explore their internal world (Zilcha-Mano et al., 2012). Once the child feels safe, is engaged in a positive therapeutic alliance, and has a bond with the canine, work can begin on identified targets.

Conclusion

The attachment relationship is crucial to optimizing early development. With the coregulation of the caregiver, the child develops the ability to self-sooth, to manage unpleasant emotions and situations, and acquires resilience. All humans experience challenges and stress; the difference between individuals is the ability to recover, to 'bounce back.' Regaining homeostasis is a primary neurobiological goal and when dysregulated, the state of equilibrium is difficult to regain.

Interventions that are designed to incorporate canine mechanisms of change can positively promote attachment needs, safety, and neural regulation. The recalibration of neural dysregulation is a tall order, however. Chapter 4 describes how neural dysregulation impacts brain structures, function, connectivity, and networks and how those aberrations manifest clinically in the child.

References

Banai, E., Mikulincer, M., & Shaver, P. (2005). 'Selfobject' Needs in Kohut's Self Psychology: Links with attachment, self-cohesion, affect regulation, and adjustment. *Psychoanalytic Psychology*; 22(2): 224–260. https://doi.org/10.1037/0736-9735.22.2.224

Barnett, W., Hansen, C.L., Bailes, L.G., & Humphreys, K.L. (2022). Caregiver-child proximity as a dimension of early experience. In *Development and Psychopathology, First View* (pp. 1–19). Cambridge University Press. https://doi.org/10.1017/S0954579421001644

Basso, J.C., Satyal, M.K., Rugh, R. (2021). Dance on the brain: Enhancing intra- and inter-brain synchrony. *Frontiers in Human Neuroscience.* https://doi.org/10.3389/fnhum.2020.584312

Beetz, A., Julius, H., Turner, D., & Kotrschal, K. (2012). Effects of social support by a dog on stress modulation in children with insecure attachment. *Frontiers in Psychology*; 3: 352.

Bick, J., & Nelson, C.A. (2016). Early adverse experiences and the developing brain. *Neuropsychopharmacology*; 41(1): 177–196. https://doi.org/1038/npp.2015.252

Bonati, B., Csermely, D., & Sovrano, V.A. (2013). Looking at a predator with the left or right eye: Asymmetry of response in lizards. *Laterality*; 18(3): 329–339. https://dx.doi.org/10.2307/4012563

Bowlby. J. (1969). *Attachment and Loss: Vol. 1. Attachment.* New York: Basic Books.

Bowlby, J. (1973). *Attachment and Loss: Vol. 2. Separation: Anxiety and Anger.* New York: Basic Books.

Bretherton, I., & Munholland, K.A. (2008). Internal working models in attachment relationships: Elaborating a central construct in attachment theory. In J. Cassidy, & P.R. Shaver (Eds.), *Handbook of attachment: Theory, research, and clinical applications* (pp. 102–127). New York: Guildford Press.

Busuito, A., Quigley, K.M., Moore, G.A., Voegtline, K.M., & DiPietro, J.A. (2019). In sync: Physiological correlates of behavioral synchrony in infants and mothers. *Developmental Psychology*; 55(5): 1034–1045. https://doi.org/10.1037/dev0000689

Cascio, C.J., Woynaroski, T., Baranek, G.T., & Wallace, M.T. (2016). Toward an interdisciplinary approach to understanding sensory function in autism spectrum disorder. *Autism Research*; 9(9): 920–925. https://doi.org/10.1002/aur.1612.

Cebolla, A.M., & Cheron, G. (2019). Understanding neural oscillations in the human brain: From movement to consciousness and vice versa. *Frontiers in Psychology*; 10: 1930. 1–6. https://doi.org/10.3389/fpsyg.2019.01930

Chambers, J. (2017). The neurobiology of attachment: From infancy to clinical outcomes. *Psychodynamic Psychiatry*; 45(4): 542–563. https://doi.org/10.1521.4.542.

Chapman, L. (2014). *Neurobiologically Informed Trauma Therapy with Children and Adolescents: Understanding Mechanisms of Change.* New York: W.W. Norton.

Chiron, C., Jambaque, I., Nabbout, R., Lounes, R., Syrota, A. & Dulac, L. (1997). The right hemisphere is dominant in human infants. *Brain: Journal of Neurology*; 120(6): 1057–1065. https://doi.org/10.1093/brain/120.6.1057

Cirelli, L., Trehub, S., & Trainor, L. (2018). Rhythm and melody as social signals for infants. *Annals of the New York Academy of Sciences*; 1423: 66–72. https://doi.org/10.1177/2059204318761622

Cozolino, L. (2017). *The Neuroscience of Psychotherapy. Healing the Social Brain* (3rd ed.). New York: W.W. Norton & Co.

Dehaene-Lambertz, et al. (2010). Language or music, mother or Mozart? Structural and environmental influences on infants' language networks. *Brain and Language*; 114(2): 53–65. https://doi.org/10.1016/j.bandl.2009.09.003

Doom, J.R., & Gunnar, M.R. (2013). Stress physiology and developmental psychopathology: Past, present and future. *Development and Psychopathology*; 25(4). https://doi.org/10.1017/S095457941300066

Fairhurst, M.T., Loken, L., & Grossmann, T. (2014). Physiological and behavioral responses reveal 9-month-old infants' sensitivity to pleasant touch. *Psychological Science* https://doi.org/10.1177/0956797614527114

Fancourt, D. & Perkins, R. (2018). The effects of mother-infant singing on emotional closeness, affect, anxiety, and stress hormones. https://doi.org/10.1177/2059204317745746

Fawcett, C. (2022). Kids attend to saliva sharing to infer social relationships. *Developmental Psychology*; 375 (6578). https://doi.org/10.1126/science.abn5157

Feldman, R. (2007). Parent-infant synchrony: Biological foundations and developmental outcomes. *Current Directions in Psychological Science* 16(6): 300–345.

Feldman, R., & Eidelman, A.I. (2003). Skin-to-skin contact (Kangaroo Care) accelerates autonomic and neurobehavioural maturation in preterm infants. *Dev Med & Ch Neuro*; 45: 274–281.

Feldman, R., Keren, M., & Gross-Rozval, M et al. (2004). Mother-child touch patterns in feeding disorders: Relation to maternal, child, and environmental factors. *Journal of the American Academy of Child and Adolescent Psychiatry*; 43: 1089–1097.

Feldman, R., Magori-Cohen, R., Galili, G., Singer, M, & Louzoun, Y. (2011). Mother and infant coordinate heart rhythms through episodes of interaction synchrony. *Infant Behavior and Development*; 34(4): 569–577. https://doi.org/10.1016/j.infbeh.2011.06.008

Gendlin, E.T. (1978). *Focusing*. Everest House.

George, C., & Solomon, J. (2008). The measure of attachment security and related constructs in infancy and early childhood. In J. Cassidy and P.R. Shaver (Eds.), *Handbook of Attachment-Theory, Research and Clinical Applications* (3rd ed.: 366–398). New York, NY: Guildford Press.

Guastella, A.J., Mitchell, P.B., & Dadds, M.R. (2008). Oxytocin increases gaze to the eye region of human faces. *Biological Psychiatry*; 63(1): 3–5.

Gunnar, M.R., Mangelsdorf, S., Larson, M., & Hertsgaard, L. (1989). Attachment, temperament, and adrenocortical activity in infancy: A study of psychoendocrine regulation. *Developmental Psychology*; 25: 355–363.

Guo, K., Meints, K., Hall, C., Hall, S., & Mills, D. (2009). Left gaze bias in humans, rhesus monkeys and domestic dogs. *Animal Cognition*; 12(3): 409–418. https://doi.org/10.1007/s10071-008-0199-3

Handlin, L., Nilsson, A., Ejdeback, E., Hydbring-Sandberg, E., & Uvnas-Moberg, K. (2012). Associations between the psychological characteristics of the human-dog relationship and oxytocin and cortisol levels. *Anthrozoös*; 25(2): 215–228.

Hari, R., & Kujala, M.V. (2009). Brain basis of human social interaction: From concepts to brain imaging. *Physiological Reviews*; 89: 453–479. https://doi.org/10.1152/physrev.00041.2007

Harlow, H. & Zimmerman, R. (1958). Affectional responses in the infant monkey. *Science*130: 421–432.

Headley, D.B., & Pare, D. (2017). Common oscillatory mechanisms across multiple memory systems. *NPJ Science of Learning*; 2(1). https://doi.org/10.1038/s41539-016-0001-2

Holt, L.E. (1894). '*The Care and Feeding of Children*' *A Catechism for the use of Mothers and Children's Nurses*. New York and London: D. Appleton & Co.

Jiang, Y. & Platt, M.L. (2018). Oxytocin and vasopressin flatten dominance hierarchy and enhance behavioral synchrony in part via anterior cingulate cortex. *Scientific Reports*, 8(8201). https://doi.org/10.1038/s41598-018-25607-1

Kaminski, J., Waller, B.M., Diogo, R., Hartstone-Rose, A., & Burrows, A.M., et al. (2019). Evolution of facial muscle anatomy in dogs. *PNAS*, 116929). https://doi.org/10.1073/pnas.1820653116

Kilroy, E., Aziz-Zadeh, L., & Cermak, S. Ayres. (2019). Theories of autism and sensory integration revisited: What contemporary neuroscience has to say. *Brain Sciences* 9(3): 68. https://doi.org/10.3390/brainsci9030068

Kret, M.E. (2015). Emotional expressions beyond facial muscle actions. A call for studying autonomic signals and their impact on social perception. *Frontiers in Psychology*; 6(711). https://doi.org/10.3389/fpsyg.2015.00711

Kret, M.E., & De Dreu, C.K.W. (2017). Pupil-mimicry conditions trust in exchange partners: Moderation by oxytocin and group membership. *Royal Society B-Biological Sciences*; 284(1850): 20162554.

Kurdek, L.A. (2008). Pet dogs as attachment figures. *Journal of Social and Personal Relationships*; 25: 247–266.

Lahousen, T. (2019). Psychobiology of attachment and trauma-some general remarks. *Frontiers in Psychiatry*; 10: 914.

Levy, J., Goldstein, A., & Feldman, R. (2017). Perception of social synchrony induces mother-child gamma coupling in the social brain. *Social Cognitive and Affective Neuroscience*; 12(7): 1036–1046. https://doi.org/10.1093/scan/nsx032

Lima, A.R., Mellow, M., & Mari, J. (2010).The role of early parental bonding in the development of psychiatric symptoms in adulthood. *Current Opinion in Psychiatry* https://doi.org/10.1097/YCO.0b013e32833a51ce

Lindell, A. (2018). Lateralization of the expression of facial emotion in humans. *Progress in Brain Research*. 238: 249–270. https://doi.org/10.1016/bs.pbt.2018.06.005

Lyons-Ruth, K., & Jacobvitz, D. (1999). Attachment disorganization: Unresolved loss, relational violence, and lapses in behavioral and attentional strategies. In J. Cassidy & P.R. Shaver (Eds.), *Handbook of Attachment: Theory, Research and Clinical Applications* (520–554). The Guildford Press.

Ma, U., Shamay-Tsoory, S., Han, S., & Zink, C.F. (2016). Oxytocin and social adaptation: Insights from neuroimaging studies. *Trends in Cognitive Sciences*; 20(2): 133–145. https://dx.doi.org/10.1016/j.tics.2015.10.009

Malatesta, G., Marzoli, D., Rapino, M., & Tommasi, L. (2019). The left-cradling bias and its relationship with empathy and depression. *Scientific Reports*; 9(6141).

McCrory, E.J., & Viding, E. (2015). The theory of latent vulnerability: Reconceptualizing the link between childhood maltreatment and psychiatric disorder. *Development and Psychopathology*; 27(2): 493–505. https://doi.org/10.1017/S0954579415000115

McGloin, J.M., & Widom, C.S. (2001). Resilience among abused and neglected children grown up. *Development and Psychopathology*; 13(4): 1021–1038.

McGlone, F., Wessberg, J., Olausson, H. (2014). Discriminative and affective touch: Sensing and feeling. *ScienceDirect*; 82(4): 735–755. https://doi.org/10.1016/j.neuron.2014.05.001

McLaughlin, K.A., et al. (2015). Causal effects of the early caregiving environment on development of stress response systems in children. *Proceedings of the National Academy of Sciences of the United States of America*; 112(18), 5637–5642. https://doi.org/10.1073/pnas.1423363112

Meltzoff, A.N., & Moore, M.K. (1983). Newborn infants imitate adult facial gestures. *Child Development*; 54: 702–709.

Mikulincer, M., & Shaver, P.R. (2007). *Attachment in Adulthood: Structure, Dynamics, and Change*. New York: Guildford Press.

Olmert, M.D. (2009). *Made for Each Other*. Cambridge, MA: Da Capo Press.

Padgett, DA & Glaser, R. (2003). How stress influences the immune response. *Trends in Immunology*; 24(8): 444–448. https://doi.org/10.1016/s1471-4906(03)00173-x

Palagi, E. & Scopa, C. (2017). Integrating Tinbergen's inquiries: Mimicry and play in humans and other social mammals. *Learning & Behavior*; 45: 378–389.

Patoine, B. (2019). The resilient brain. *Dana Foundation*. https://dana.org/article/the-neurobiology-of-resilience/.

Porges, S.W. (2003). Social engagement and attachment: A phylogenetic perspective. *Annals of the New York Academy of Sciences*; 1008: 31–47. https://doi.org/10.1196/annals.1301004

Porges, S.W. (2007). The polyvagal perspective. *Biological Psychology*; 74(2): 116–143. https://doi.org/10.1016/j.biopsycho.2006.06.009

Rincon-Cortes, M., & Sullivan, R.M. (2014). Early life trauma and attachment: Immediate and enduring effects on neurobehavioral and stress axis development. *Frontiers in Endocrinology*; 5: 33. https://doi.org/10.3389/fendo.2014.00033

Rizzolatti, G., & Craighero, L. (2004). The mirror-neuron system. *Annual Review of Neuroscience*;27:169–192.https://doi.org/10.1146/annurev.neuro.27.070203.144230

Savastan, E. Ehrhardt, R., Schulz, A., Walter, M., Schachinger, H. (2008). Post-learning intranasal oxytocin modulates human memory for facial identify. *Psychoneuroendocrinology*; 33(3): 368–374. https://doi.org/10.1016/j.psyneuen.2007.12.004

Saxbe, D.E., Margolin, G., Spies Shapiro, L., Ramos, M., Rodriguez, A., & Iturralde, E. (2014). Relative influences: Patterns of HPA axis concordance during triadic family interaction. *Health Psychology*; 33(3): 273–281. https://doi.org/10.1037/a0033509

Schore, A.N. (1994). *Affect Regulation and the Origin of the Self*. Mahwah, NJ: Lawrence Erlbaum Associates.

Schore, A.N. (2003). *Affect Regulation and the Repair of the Self*. New York: W.W. Norton & Co.

Schore, A.N. (2021). The Interpersonal Neurobiology of Intersubjectivity. *Frontiers in Psychology*; 12: 648616. https://doi.org.10.3389/fpsyg.2021.648616

Seelke, A.M.H., Perkeybile, A.M., Grunewald, R., Bales, K.L., & Krubitzer, L.A. (2015). Individual differences in cortical connections of somatosensory cortex are associated with parental rearing style in prairie voles (Microtus ochrogaster). *The Journal of Comparative Neurology*; 524(3): 564–577. https://doi.org/10.1002/cne.23837

Seltzer, L.J., Prosoki, A.R., Ziegler, T.E., & Pollak, S.D. (2012). Instant messages vs. speech: hormones and why we still need to hear each other. *Evolution and Human Behavior*; 33(1): 42–45. https://doi.org/10.1016/j.evolhumbehav.2011.05.004

Siegel, D.J. (2015). *The Developing Mind: How Relationships and the Brain Interact to Shape Who We Are*. (2nd ed.). New York: The Guilford Press.

Spitz, R.A. (1945). Hospitalism: An inquiry into the genesis of psychiatric conditions in early childhood. *Psychoanalytic Study of the Child*; 1: 53–74.

Tanaka, Y, Kanakogi, & Myowa, M. (2021). Social touch in mother-infant interaction affects infants' subsequent social engagement and object exploration. Humanities and *Social Sciences Communications*; 8(32). https://doi.org/10.1057/s41599-020-00642-4

Teicher, M.H., Samson, J.A., Anderson, C.M., & Ohashi, K. (2016). The effects of childhood maltreatment on brain structure, function, and connectivity. *Nature Reviews. Neuroscience*; 17(10): 652–666. https://doi.org/10.1038/nrn.2016.111

Thomas, A.J., Woo, B., Nettle, D., Spelke, E., & Saxe, R. (2022). Early concepts of intimacy: Young humans use saliva sharing to infer close relationships. *Science*; 375 (6578). https://doi.org/10.1126/science.abh1054

Tops, M., Koole, S.L., Ijzerman, H. & Buisman-Pijlman, F.T.A. (2014). Why social attachment and oxytocin protect against addiction and stress: Insights from the dynamics between ventral and dorsal corticostriatal systems. *Pharmacology, Biochemistry, and Behavior* 119: 39–48. https://doi.org/10.1016/j.pbb.2013.07.015

Tottenham, N. (2015). Social scaffolding of human amygdala-mPFCircuit development. *Social Neuroscience*; 10: 489–499.

Trevarthon, C. (1993). The self born in intersubjectivity: The psychology of an infant communicating. *Psychology*. https://doi.org/10.1017/CBO9780511664007.009

Tronick, E.D., Als, H., & Brazelton, T.B. (1977). Mutuality in mother-infant interaction. *The Journal of Communication*; 27(2): 74–79. https://doi.org/10.1111/j.1460-2466.1977.tb01829x

Unväs-Moberg, K., Handlin, L., & Peterson, M. (2014). Self-soothing behavior with particular reference to oxytocin release induced by non-noxious sensory stimulation. *Frontiers in Psychology*; 5: 1529.

Vela, R.M. (2014). The effect of severe stress on early brain development, attachment, and emotions. *Psychiatric clinics of North America*; 37: 519–534. https://doi.org/10.1016/j.psc.2014.08.005

Vittner, D. et al. (2018). Increase in oxytocin from skin-to skin contact enhances development of parent-infant relationship. *Biological Research for Nursing*; 20(1): 54–62.

Wanser, S.H., Vitale, K.R., Thielke, L.E., Brubaker, L., & Udell, M.A.R. (2019). Spotlight on the psychological basis of childhood pet attachment and its implications. *Psychology Research and Behavior Management*; 12: 469–479. https://doi.org/10.2147/PRBM.S158998

Weinstein, D., Launay, J. Pearce, E., Dunbar, R.I.M., & Stewart, L. (2016). Singing and social bonding: Changes in connectivity and pain threshold as a function of group size. *Evolution and Human Behavior*; 37: 152–158. https://doi.org/10.1016/evolhumbehav.2015.10.002

Xiong, X.J., Li, S.J., & Zhang, Y.Q. (2015). Massage therapy for essential hypertension: A systematic review. *Journal of Human Hypertension*; 29: 143–151.

Yirmiya, K., Motsan, S., Zagoory-Sharon, O., & Feldman, R. (2020). Human attachment triggers different social buffering mechanisms under high and low early life stress rearing. *International Journal of Psychophysiology*; 152:72–80. https://doi.org/10.1016/j.ipsycho.2020.04.001

Zak, P.J., Stanton, A.A., & Ahmadi, S. (2007). Oxytocin Increases Generosity in Humans. *PLoS One* https://doi.org/10.1371/journal.pone.0001128

Zilcha-Mano, S., Mikulincer, M., & Shaver, P.R. (2012). Pets as safe havens and secure bases: The moderating role of pet attachment orientations. *Journal of Research in Personality*; 46(5): 571–580.

Chapter 4   The Neurobiological Dysregulation of Early Trauma

Introduction

The brain is highly vulnerable in a young child in the midst of development, as neural receptivity to the environment is heightened during critical periods of plasticity. Growth is genetically programmed yet also reliant upon specific healthy relationships and experiences to fulfill its potential. When the brain incurs significant deprivation or chronic assault, neurobiological alterations to this sensitive organ are evidenced by dysregulation and impairment of developmental domains. Incessant violation of a vulnerable child can result in a reorganization of their brain, body, and perception of the self and the surrounding world.

This chapter provides a brief synthesis of literature and research that illuminate neurobiological alterations and dysregulation of the brain that may occur as a result of maltreatment-induced developmental trauma, leading to psychopathology. Brain structures are intricately connected, and detangling their complex interactions presents a significant challenge to scientists in their attempt to separate and delineate processes and pathways. Most studies target and study a specific suspected pathway from maltreatment to psychopathology, yet experts agree that a multitude of factors, along with their temporal sequence, interface to produce the heterogeneous outcomes that are noted in individuals. The commonality between proposed trajectory models is that they involve dysregulation.

Homeostasis

One of the primary responsibilities of the brain is to maintain homeostasis within the neural structures, networks, systems, and processes of the body. When equilibrium is disrupted by intense and chronic environmental events, such as maltreatment, the brain seeks to 'right the ship' and reestablish its baseline of function. The brain is always changing through continuous interaction with the environment, and when regulatory processes are successful, homeostasis is sustained and life is good.

Maltreatment experiences are toxic, however, and can leave a deep imprint upon the brain and body of a child. The complex and interdependent

DOI: 10.4324/9781003217534-6

nature of the brain produces an amazing range of functions, yet that same design also renders a vulnerability to disruption. Dysregulation occurs when the child's systems are overwhelmed and unable to restore a homeostatic state. Dysregulation can occur at molecular and cellular levels up through circuitry and networks, increasing vulnerability and compromising regulatory, cognitive, and emotional systems (Teicher et al., 2016).

Brief Overview of Theoretical Models of Trauma-Induced Neural Alterations

There are several models that propose specific pathways that lead from maltreatment to psychopathology. The following section briefly details the most recognized pathways, though this is not an exhaustive list. These models are based upon neurobiological aberrations of structures and function, the stress response system (SRS); the frontolimbic bi-nodal network, large-scale networks and, possibly the most plausible, functional connectivity (FC). While various models represent differing theories, there is relative conceptual concordance. It is suggested that these (maltreatment-induced) neurobiological alterations can be conceptualized as *neural dysregulation* which serves as a linking mechanism between maltreatment/DT and psychopathology.

As stated earlier, well-controlled studies have shown a direct correlation between early child maltreatment and neurobiological alterations in structures and functions of the brain (Agorastos, et al., 2019; DeBellis & Zisk, 2014). Along with anatomical alterations, the connectivity *between* these structures and regions is also susceptible to trauma resulting in potentially profound consequences. Functional connectivity (FC) is the integrity of communication that transmits crucial information between structures and regions. Efficient communication is clearly critical to productive function.

Scientific thinking has shifted from viewing the brain as a modular structure to a perspective of distributed networks. Individual brain structures are separate entities yet do not operate in isolation. They fill numerous roles and participate in multiple networks. Specific functions were previously believed to be served by localized regions, but neuroimaging research has demonstrated that collaborations of multiple structures and regions are involved in specific functions.

Networks can be geographically disparate, yet are enabled by a scaffold of global connectivity that supports communication and collaboration. The basal ganglia and thalamus have been suggested to support this long-distance integration, functioning beyond mere association structures, fulfilling a more critical need than previously thought (Bell & Shine, 2015).

Functional Connectivity (FC)

Bundles of fibrous white matter serve as conduits of communication or 'messaging highways' to subsidize functional connectivity (FC). The integrity of connectivity is directly correlated with the degree of functional competence as it facilitates communication and collaboration between regionally disparate structures (Uddin, et al., 2019). Typical brain maturation is reflected in the strengthening of connectivity, increased localized specialization, and experience-dependent plasticity. Developmentally, top-down regulation (demonstrating appraisal and other cognitive regulation strategies) is supported by this maturation along with sufficient connectivity between the PFC and subcortical structures (Casey et al., 2014).

Through the process of neural maturation, structures and networks follow organizational network dynamics of segregation and integration processes relevant to distinct and collaborative functional integrity. A synchronized balance between the two is crucial in the transmission of neural communication, both locally and globally (Shine, 2019; Wang et al., 2021).

Connectivity within and between multiple networks and structures is shown to be highly sensitive to environmental conditions, particularly the prefrontal cortices and limbic structures. Emerging empirical evidence suggests that perturbations in FC occur from early adversity (Herzberg & Gunnar, 2020) and are associated with increased risk for psychopathology (Herringa et al., 2013). Studies of individuals with trauma history showed a more global pattern of diminished connectivity, involving multiple regions (Uddin et al., 2019). Vulnerability of these specific structures is believed to be a byproduct of developmental timing (Lupien et al., 2009) and the density of glucocorticoid receptors. Children with developmental trauma, neural alterations, and dysregulation often cannot utilize top-down strategies, due to the diminished integrity of FC, particularly in the frontolimbic regions. Bottom-up interventions that address lower, more primitive brain regions, such as sensory-motor systems, are more practical and developmentally appropriate.

The Human Connectome Project (HCP) launched in 2009 with the purpose of mapping connectivity or neural pathways in the brain using neuroimaging (Van Essen & Barch, 2015). Producing a map of the 'wiring' of the brain would profoundly illuminate our understanding of the relationship between structures and functions, yet, to date, the only completed connectome map is of a version of the roundworm C. *elegans*, a tiny organism with a neural network of 300 neurons and 7,000 connections. Human brains have 90 billion neurons and 150 trillion connections (Van Essen & Barch, 2015). The task is clearly daunting, yet the project has already had a transformative impact upon the field, with more to come.

Another well-known study was the Adolescent Brain Cognitive Development (ABCD) study, a longitudinal investigation that measured resting-state functional connectivity (rs-FC) to investigate the clinical and neurobiological consequences of early adversity (Brieant et al., 2021). Using a large population, multiple sites, and repetitive neuroimaging technology, this study has highlighted the role of connectivity between circuits in dysfunction and dysregulation. Aberrations in connectivity have been implicated in deviations from normal developmental trajectories. Both accelerated (Callahan & Tottenham, 2016) *and* delayed (Rakesh et al., 2020) neural maturation have been found in children with early trauma, conditions believed to increase risk for internalizing symptoms and externalizing behaviors. These contrasting patterns reflect adaptations by the brain to its current environment yet only provide short-term resilience.

As the brain continuously attempts to maintain homeostasis, correct imbalances, and dysregulation, changes are considered adaptations. The evolutionarily designed core intent of adaptations was to ensure survival. For example, a precocious puberty supports the individual under threat of a shortened life with the ability to reproduce, passing on their heritage. When adaptations occur, however, they can trigger further adaptations that may not be complementary, or may persist, becoming maladaptive in later timeframes or changing circumstances.

Disrupted functional connectivity has been linked with stress disorder symptoms and deficits in multiple domains. FC can disrupt memory consolidation and the fear and arousal circuitry, including the amygdala, hippocampus (limbic structures), and sgACC (subgenual anterior cingulate cortex), a component of the vmPFC (ventromedial PFC). The sgACC activates in response to threat and plays a role in the nonconscious (autonomic) regulation of negative emotion (Herringa et al., 2013). Disrupted or impaired FC has also been implicated in multiple mental health disorders, disrupted fear extinction, and deficient emotion regulation (Ross & Cisler, 2020).

The Stress Response System (SRS)

Disruption of the SRS has long been considered one of the primary mechanisms that cause dysregulation in children (Hart and Rubia, 2012). This pathway of dysregulation begins with a normal activation of the SRS in response to maltreatment that should return to baseline if the event is short term and not overwhelming. When maltreatment is chronic and severe, however, the SRS may become dysregulated and can become chronically activated.

The SRS is mediated by an infrastructure composed of molecular, cellular, and endocrine constituents that, when dysregulated, impact physiological and behavioral changes. These can be transient or permanent (Godoy et al., 2018). The conceptualization of a dysregulated SRS system implies susceptibility to the specific constituent structures and processes of that system, as well. Dysregulation of the hypothalamus-pituitary-adrenal (HPA) axis and the endocrine system, two prominent components of the SRS, have also specifically been linked to impaired function and psychopathology (Nemeroff, 2016), as the HPA axis is considered a primary system in the transcription of environmental experiences into internal function (Hibel et al., 2019). Numerous animal studies show that trauma effects on the HPA axis also confer dysregulation in hormones and neurotransmitters (such as cortisol, norepinephrine, and epinephrine).The HPA axis mediates the dynamic interaction of the central nervous system and the endocrine system (Doom & Gunnar, 2013), through its regulation of glucocorticoids (cortisol), the hormonal end product of the HPA process. Metabolic, cardiovascular, and immune systems are also mediated by this relationship.

Chronic repetitive HPA axis activation results in prolonged elevation of circulating cortisol levels. Dysregulated levels of cortisol can confer damage to neural processes and structures, reducing neurogenesis and synaptogenesis; causing atrophy and reducing the volume of structures (McEwen, 2012). Cortisol inflicts damage to the hippocampus, as it has abundant sensitive glucocorticoid receptors, by causing an excitotoxic effect that also reduces connectivity (Bremner, 2006). Repetitive activation of the stress response, including chronic activation of the HPA axis causes neural and physiological dysregulation (Shonkoff, 2016).

The functional capability of the HPA axis is related to the quality of the attachment experience (Schuder & Lyons-Ruth, 2004), and attunement is crucial to the child's ability to manage stress and participate in social relationships. Coregulation of the infant by the caregiver dampens the SRS, HPA axis, and endocrine system (Gunnar & Donzella, 2002). One of the first studies to investigate the actual transmission of physiology between the mother and child suggests that attunement may be critical in mediating this regulation. Attunement is the sensitivity, synchrony, and responsiveness that support physiological, behavioral, and neural organization of the child. Researchers found that non-maltreating mothers are able to recognize their child's stress physiology yet do not transmit their own stress physiology to the child (Hibel et al., 2019).

The maltreatment group of mother–child pairs showed little emotional and physiological synchrony with their children and had distorted perceptions of the child's signals. They were also shown to transmit substantial levels of cortisol to the child. Dysregulated caregiver physiology is suggested to predict dysregulation in the child, reflected in transmission of cortisol. Researchers concurred with Cicchetti and Tucker (1994) that transmission of stress physiology may contribute to dysregulated physiology and behavior in children, increasing the risk for psychopathology through life. When the SRS is dysregulated, neural and endocrine paths which support communication are compromised which can affect interoception. Interoception is brain-body bidirectional communication supports the sensing and processing of visceral signals produced by the central nervous system which leads to a conscious perception of bodily processes and states. When the HPA axis becomes dysregulated, the individual becomes vulnerable to psychopathology as well as maladaptive responses to future stress.

Neural Brain Structures

Three primary structures that are particularly susceptible to childhood maltreatment and developmental trauma are the prefrontal cortex, amygdala, and hippocampus. Their interdependent collaborations are central in multiple key functions, including the aforementioned SRS, and emotional and cognitive functions (executive, memory, and attention) (Cancel et al., 2019). Additional structures also suggested to suffer trauma-induced aberrations include the corpus callosum, the insula and cingulate gyrus (Teicher et al., 2016), and anterior cingulate cortex (ACC) (Hart & Rubia, 2012). When integration and connectivity between these regions is impaired, memory formation is impacted and information flow is disrupted.

Specific anomalies are evidenced in deviations of volume, cortical thickness, and myelination (Jeong et al., 2021). Diminished cerebral volumes and larger cortical and prefrontal cortical cerebrospinal fluid (CSF) volumes have been found in children with trauma histories. Degradation and cellular death that reduce volume may occur in primary regions of the prefrontal cortices, amygdala, hippocampus, and corpus callosum (CC) along with trauma-induced neuronal atrophy (Herringa et al., 2013). Reduced hippocampal volume is one of the most notable neurological effects of trauma (Sapolsky, 2021). Studies of hippocampal alterations from childhood trauma, however, have been mixed, as the effects of trauma do not always reveal themselves until adulthood.

Both cortical thickness and myelination that undergo significant maturational changes during normal development are susceptible to environmental experiences, and have been implicated in various mental health disorders that emerge during development (Nelson and Gabard-Duram, 2020).

The Prefrontal Cortex

The prefrontal cortex (PFC) constitutes one-third of the cerebral cortex and contributes to emotion, learning, and memory systems. This regulatory system is the source of higher cognition and provides the complex processes necessary for regulation, such as attention, response inhibition, working memory, planning, and decision-making. These along with other higher cognitive processes are known as the executive functions.

The positioning of the PFC permits a convergence of multiple cortical and subcortical regions subsidized by dense reciprocal connectivity. Most regulatory actions involve either activation (neural excitation) or inhibition (dampening of neural activity), and though the PFC is often simplified as 'the regulator' of the emotional limbic system, the signaling between the cognitive and emotional regions is bidirectional. The PFC and dorsal anterior cingulate (dACC), along with the amygdala are suspected in dysregulated emotion and fear learning (Phelps, 2004).

The PFC plays a critical role in the stress response by shutting down the process when the threat is over, restoring homeostasis. Diminished FC hinders the PFC from this inhibitory role contributing to dysregulation of the SRS, as it is unable to effectively communicate the relevant neural information to the HPA axis.

Children with histories of trauma have been found to suffer from emotional, cognitive, and neuropsychological dysregulation in substantial numbers. Recent research has delved into the more nuanced aspects of the executive system, looking into the role·of relationships in brain development (Op den Kelder et al., 2018). Dysregulation and dysfunction that result from unsuccessful attachment experience are known to impair executive functions including attention, memory, abstract thinking, and memory (DeBellis & Van Dillen, 2005). Early interpersonal trauma may also decrease emotional attunement to self and others, diminish empathic ability, and impair development of theory of mind. Emotion regulation and cognitive flexibility, both negatively affected by interpersonal trauma, are prerequisites for effective problem solving which is a critical skill of healthy functioning. Dysregulation of PFC regions also clinically manifest as impulsivity, inappropriate social behaviors, increased motor activity, and sexual disinhibition.

Several neural systems overlap due to connectivity, location, and multiple roles, as well as a kinship of sorts that exists between attachment, emotion regulation, and fear systems. These functions serve as a foundation for development of self-identity that is shaped by early caregiving experiences (DeBellis & Zisk, 2014).

Limbic Structures

The limbic system, comprising the amygdala, hippocampus, thalamus, hypothalamus, and basal ganglia, is commonly referred to as the emotional center of the brain. Positioned above the brainstem and just below the cerebral cortex in the cerebrum, the limbic system is highly connected to the endocrine and autonomic nervous system (ANS). The early maturation of the amygdala and hippocampus and their distinct sensitivity to endocrine activation create a vulnerability to early experiences and attachment processes.

The limbic system, an essential component of the stress response, is also well known for its responsibilities for emotion processing and regulation. The limbic system mediates stress regulation through complex and integrated neural messaging with other specific regions related to sensory processing, fear response, and cognitive oversight. The amygdala is involved in emotion perception, generation, processing, and expression. This tiny structure is also involved in the assessment of threat stimuli, behavioral regulation, attachment, and the assignment of valence to memories encoded in the hippocampus. The proximally situated structures are presumably an evolutionary design that enhances survival by linking threat experiences with negative emotion, which promotes life-preserving adaptive behavior. The perception of danger paired with fear often results in avoidant behavior.

The healthy child is capable of detection of suspicious eye movement, posture, and behavior and their neuroceptive ability informs them with somatic responses to the presence of a potential threat. As the amygdala is

a core component of the social brain in humans, alteration of this structure, occurring as a result of chronic trauma, can impair social judgment
and communication. Damage is manifested in the inability to read faces
(recognize emotion in facial expressions), predict behavior, and moderate
approach and avoidance choices. These functions are critical to safety and
survival, as they support the child in recognition and assessment of the
nuanced visual signs that signal safety or threat.

One consequence of a dysregulated SRS is a kindling of the amygdala
that results in a heightened oversensitivity to perceived threat. 'Kindling'
occurs as a result of repetitive, intermittent, and unpredictable neuronal
stimulation and is a persistent hypersensitivity to that stimulus, a form of
dysregulation. This electrical dysregulation is identified in studies as *limbic
irritability*, a state that is similar to epilepsy. These neural disruptions are
also associated with alterations of the hippocampus.

Neural dysregulation results in a deficient ability to accurately differentiate between safety and threat. Called a *threat bias*, the child begins to see
threat in objectively less threatening, benign, or generalized conditions,
and can become *stuck* in a survival mode. This entrapment disables the
capability to participate emotionally, socially, and academically, as survival is metabolically consuming. Directing energy and resources to survival leaves little available for social interaction and learning.

Alterations in the amygdala can result in persistent irritability, aggression, deficient recognition of emotion, and dysregulation of emotional experience and expression. Studies show differences in the amygdala between
controls and individuals with PTSD and mood disorders. Early trauma
can disrupt the sufficient ascription of salience to emotional cues, create
deficits in reality testing, and impair short-term memory.

The Hippocampus

Shaped like a seahorse, the hippocampus is associated with memory, spatial learning, and behavioral regulation. The hippocampus stores memories and accompanying sensory experience that can be conscious and
described in words. These memories are called declarative or explicit and
can be shared in a verbal narrative. Memories associated with intense emotion are strongly encoded; fear learning can occur with minimal repetitions
of fear-provoking events.

Primitive, nonverbal, nonconscious, and visceral memories are stored in
the amygdala. Trauma occurring prior to the acquisition of language and
maturity of memory systems may be encoded as visual or sensory representations in the amygdala which stores all implicit memory (Parish-Plass,
2022). Neuroanatomical mapping has produced data that also suggests
some early memories may be encoded into areas that have few pathways to
the frontal cortex. Trauma has been shown to disrupt the encoding and
integration of memory thus; fear-laden memories may be inefficiently

encoded, fragmented, or even lost (van der Kolk, 2005). These fragments of sensory and emotional experiences are distressing and confusing, and often the individual will create an inaccurate or false memory to make sense of them. Trauma experiences have been shown through neuroimaging to increase the activation and reactivity of both the amygdala and hippocampus (Jeong et al., 2021) and damage the FC between these structures.

Limbic and FC damage is associated with emotion dysregulation including anxiety, anger, agitation, memory impairments, altered biological rhythms, and abnormal sexual behavior. Early trauma can disrupt the normal developmental trajectory, disrupting maturation of limbic circuitry. These neural alterations can lead to impairments in cognition and behavior, learning, social functioning, and an array of emotional disturbances, such as PTSD, bipolar, anxiety, and depression.

Corpus Callosum

The CC consists of a bundle of white matter fibers and functions as a liaison between the left and right hemispheres. Integrity of the CC is critical to maintain necessary communication and integration of these lateral brain regions. Myelination of this fibrous structure is a crucial step in development, as it supports efficacious transmission of information between the hemispheres. Excessive stress hormones can interfere with normal myelination and pruning. Decreases in volume and integrity of white matter are one of the more consistent observations found in imaging studies of trauma victims (Teicher et al., 2016).

Electrophysiological Abnormalities

A study conducted by Ito and colleagues in 1993 investigated the relationship between a history of abuse and neurological abnormalities in 115 consecutive admissions to a child and adolescent psychiatric inpatient unit. Fifty-four percent of patients with histories of abuse were found to have electrophysiological abnormalities primarily in the left side of the frontal, temporal, or anterior regions, compared to 26.9% of non-abused patients. Results support the hypothesis that early childhood maltreatment alters brain development. (DeBellis & Zisk, 2014).

In subsequent research, Teicher and colleagues identified a constellation of brain abnormalities in children victimized by abuse and trauma. Using electroencephalogram (EEG) imaging, evidence of disrupted brain wave patterns were found that are similar to temporal lobe epilepsy (TLE). Individuals with TLE experience a wide array of symptoms including headaches, numbness, dizziness/vertigo, tingling sensations, and illusions within any of the sensory systems, such as an unpleasant taste or smell, ringing of the ears, and visual distortions (Ito et al., 1993). In a study of adults served by a mental health clinic, more than half of the patients reported physical and/or sexual abuse. All patients were administered the limbic system checklist (LSCL-33) which measures TLE symptom history; individuals with both abuse forms averaged scores that were 113% higher than controls (Teicher et al., 1993). In a subsequent study that investigated the relationship between abuse and atypical neurobiology, patients with early trauma had twice the rate of abnormal EEGs (Teicher, et al., 1993).

The Frontolimbic Network

The frontolimbic network, consisting of the prefrontal cortex and amygdala, has served as the 'classic' model of stress-impacted neural circuitry for several decades (Kebets et al., 2021). This region serves a vast number of functions, including regulation. While this model has been criticized for being overly simplified, it provides a useful model of dysregulated circuitry that can inform clinicians in the identification of treatment targets and design of applications.

Regulatory competence is associated with maturation of these regions and stress-related systems, and that maturation is shaped by healthy early relational and environmental experiences. Altered FC within this bi-nodal system has also been implicated in attention deficit disorder, borderline personality disorder, and bipolar disorder. Both genetics and childhood trauma are implicated in these disorders, adding credence to conceptualizing trauma-induced dysregulation as a transdiagnostic construct (Moukhtarian, et al., 2018).

Considered vulnerable to trauma experiences, aberrations of this network impact the function and collaborative competency of both structures. The amygdala becomes over activated and highly reactive, concurrent with diminished inhibitory conveyance of the PFC. Emotion is over-produced and under-regulated (Hart & Rubia, 2012). The neural circuitry of the PFC with its protracted development continues to mature structurally and functionally through the late 20s (Rakesh et al., 2020). Comparatively, the subcortical regions of the brain mature earlier, creating a maturational disparity and possibly conferring an age-related difficulty employing cognitive controls to regulate emotion. While this developmental factor may not be a strong causal factor in childhood psychopathology, it could be considered highly relevant to the design of treatment for children. Psychotherapy should strive to match or 'fit' the child's developmental age and stage, and it must also be considered that maturity may substantially vary between domains (Perry, 2009).

Dysregulation of the frontolimbic network is suggested to cause widespread impairment across multiple domains, compromising emotion awareness and social cognition which support regulation, and manifesting as chronic irritability, hyperarousal, heightened reactivity, avoidance of unpleasant emotions and memories and other stress-related symptomatology. Clinical manifestations of these neural changes include PTSD, anxiety, and depression (Hart & Rubia, 2012).

The amygdala and prefrontal cortices are also members of other networks, reflecting the theory that multiple models of networks exist within the brain (Cisler, 2017). The mere identification of brain networks is a substantial task, and the precise identification of connectivity, communication, and collaborative functions will continue to challenge science.

Large-Scale Brain Networks

Recently, neuroimaging research has shifted focus toward the conceptualization of large-scale network (LS) models of the brain, a perspective that is attracting significant interest. Studies have shown that the brain is organized into distinct functional networks called 'intrinsic connectivity networks' (ICNs). The perspective of networks that involve multiple structures from various regions to produce specific functions is game-changing to brain scientists. The three most relevant LS networks may be the default mode network (DMN), the central executive network (CEN), and the salience network (SN).

The 'triple network model' of psychopathology was conceptualized by Menon in his investigation of using network analysis to find associations between mental health disorders and aberrant patterns of engagement (and disengagement) between LS networks (Menon, 2011). The three networks are frequently functionally coupled or decoupled during tasks and when at rest (Menon, 2013). Simplified, the CEN is charged with externally focused tasks that tend to involve executive functions and other cognition, and the DMN is tasked with the internal world of less-focused thoughts, such as memories or thinking about the future.

These network collaborations serve multiple functions, and changes in these networks and FC between them has been associated with childhood trauma (Bluhm, et al., 2009) and subsequent psychopathology. Studies show that early trauma can result in a shifting and reconfiguration of neural resources as an adaptation to these environmental experiences. The LS networks become reorganized which is suspected of recalibrating the stress response (Zhang, et al., 2019).

The potential for identifying neural correlates for the healthy and diseased brain offers a glimpse into the future when biomarkers of specific psychopathology will become available. Clinical outcomes of these dysregulated networks include an altered state of self (DMN), cognitive dysfunction (CEN), and problems moderating arousal and engaging in interoception (SN).

The Default Mode Network (DMN)

The most familiar of these networks is the default mode network (DMN). The DMN consists of functionally connected regions including the vmPFC, the dmPFC, and the posterior cingulate cortex (PCC), adjacent precuneus, and lateral parietal cortex. The DMN is a task-irrelevant network that is active during rest periods allowing attention to internal processes. The DMN deactivates during cognitive task engagement (external processes) exhibiting a negative correlation with cognitive networks activation (Rebello, et al. 2018). This pattern of activation is associated with interoception, autobiographical memory retrieval, and self-referential mental processing (Raichle, 2015). The DMN is also involved in multiple complex functions such as attention, social cognition (Iacoboni, et al., 2004), and regulation of emotion (Pan et al., 2018).

This network has drawn increasing attention because of the emerging relationship between alterations within its circuitry and psychological and neurobiological disorders (Tian et al., 2021). Washington and Van Meter (2015) propose that disorders involving social deficits, including neurodevelopment disorders such as autism spectrum disorder (ASD), may reflect disruptions to normal development. The social cognition deficits in ASD have been proposed to be associated with divergent FC within the DMN (between nodes).

Development of the DMN is linked to the disparity between many child/adult behavior patterns. The trajectory of DMN maturity has been implicated in the protracted emergence of conscious awareness of the self and self-referential processes. At age five, as brain function becomes more bilateral, social cognition and mental complexity increase, and the child is more capable of adaptation. Maturation processes continue to around 21 years of age, when the DMN is considered fully integrated (Washington & Van Meter, 2015).

A history of early trauma is believed to disrupt DMN processes that manifest in deficits in regulation, mindfulness, self-referential encoding, and attention shifting (Lanius et al., 2020). When trauma disrupts the DMN, it detaches the individual from their internal world, threatening their sense of coherence and their capacity to connect with others.

The Central Executive Network (CEN)

The frontoparietal CEN is composed of the dorsolateral prefrontal cortex (dlPFC), the posterior parietal cortex (PPC), medial prefrontal cortex (mPFC), and anterior cingulate cortex (ACC). This task-relevant network plays a role in emotion regulation, executive functioning, cognitive control of emotions, goal-directed behavior, attention, verbal learning, and working memory (Seeley et al., 2007), functions that are altered by trauma (Lanius et al., 2015).

The Salience Network (SN)

The SN, consisting of the anterior cingulate cortex (ACC), amygdala, and insula, is involved in detecting and mapping internally and externally salient events (Szeszko & Yehuda, 2019). This network directs attention and behavior to relevant actions (Seeley et al., 2007). The SN is also charged with 'dynamic switching' between the CEN and DMN to meet extrinsic cognitive demands. The SN focuses resources on salient actions by mediating engagement of the CEN and disengagement of the DMN; a regulatory function of shifting between internal and externally focused attention and task-irrelevant and task-relevant processes (Seeley et al., 2007).

The ACC is responsible for multiple functions in the relationship between emotion and cognition including negative emotion processing; integration of relevant information that supports cognitive control, and automatic/interoceptive processing. These functions implicate the ACC in response to threats and the cognitively sourced appraisal strategy used in top-down regulation (Etkin et al., 2011).

Early trauma can result in an attention bias to threat and disrupted salience processing that are served by neurobiological alterations of the SN. These changes may also result in hyperactivity, hypervigilance, and hyperarousal symptoms associated with heightened activation of the amygdala and disruptions within the insula, key components of the SN (Zhang, et al., 2022). Dysregulation of the SN can also alter the perception of fearful and angry faces.

The Importance of Working Together

Another primary process that is critical to function is the capability of networks (between and within) to flexibly shift and switch between activity patterns. Networks need to flexibly transition between activity states to effectively respond to the needs of the individual. Diminished coordination in cooperative, collaborative inter-network function has been found to be characteristic of multiple mental health disorders (Zhao et al., 2021). Empirical evidence from multiple studies also shows that atypical maturation of specific networks, particularly a delayed tract, may increase the vulnerability to psychopathology (Vanes & Dolan, 2021).

The frontolimbic model works well with the LS model, as there are numerous similarities, yet the CEN has been left out of classical models, limiting studies. While some experts view the triple network model as perhaps more valid, an integrated model of classical *and* LS networks should also be considered for its saliency (Ross & Cisler, 2020).

Continued multi-discipline collaborations that conduct multi-modal longitudinal studies following neurobiological and psychological progressions through development are predicted to further the alignment of psychology and the neurosciences. Vanes and Dolan (2021) call for inclusion of refined computational neuroscience and cite the need for preclinical research using animal models for the next step. Questions need to be asked such as 'Why and how do vulnerability factors translate to clinical dysfunction?' And 'Are we able to identify transdiagnostic factors that cross multiple conventional diagnostic categories?' Further investigations, collaboration, and research will hopefully provide clinical insight that can be directed to preventative and much earlier efficacious interventions.

Functional Domains of Impairment

Neurobiological alterations to the structures, function, and FC of the brain produce domain-specific changes in performance. While research is continuing its investigations to identify and link neural correlates to specific psychopathology, the current information serves as a rough guide for clinicians for planning targets and actions of reregulation.

Many functions produced by neural systems involve and enable precise collaboration between geographically disparate regions. If one region becomes dysregulated, or connectivity between regions is dysfunctional, critical communication is disrupted and dysregulation can cascade into other systems and regions. Functional domains are also interdependent and collaborate to produce specific functions. Neural dysregulation can lead to emotional dysregulation, behavioral dysregulation, and beyond.

Emotion Dysregulation

Emotional dysregulation (ED) can result in emotional instability, mood lability, negative and intense emotions, heightened reactivity, and elevated arousal. Children with ED may experience difficulty identifying, recognizing, and differentiating between emotions (in themselves and others). They lack a functional vocabulary for individual emotions and may present as disconnected from their internal world. Children can also be impaired in their ability to accurately interpret facial expressions of emotion, and may display an attention bias for angry faces. Extreme emotional reactivity, lability, irritability, hostility, and fear reflect dysregulation, and mood-related disorders such as depression and anxiety are common.

Maltreated children show increased neural activation during tasks that require sustained attention. They expend more energy than control groups that is reflective of inefficient emotional and physiological control. This level of effort is metabolically taxing (McCrory et al., 2017), and these children are often exhausted and irritable at the end of their school day.

Emotion dysregulation (ED) is the most identified form of impairment that impacts function and mediates risk for psychopathology (PP). Trauma-induced ED is associated with internalizing and externalizing symptoms, and a range of mental health disorders including anxiety, depression, conduct and substance abuse disorders (Aldao, et al., 2010).

Attachment and Relational Function

Children are born with a primal need for safety and security which are key responsibilities of the caregiver. Children with developmental trauma do not feel safe in their homes, in school, and even within their own body. The child with developmental trauma and an insecure attachment is often deprived of attunement, nurturance, and coregulation. They also miss the crucial modeling of appropriate attachment figures that normally demonstrate and teach how to build and maintain relationships. The child is distrustful and suspicious of others and sees the world as a dangerous place. They are uncertain of their own emotions and have difficulty imaging the emotion, thoughts, and intentions of another. When the environment of a dysregulated child is perceived as unsafe and unreliable, the child backs away, and withdrawal leads to avoidance and isolation. For these children, it becomes difficult or even impossible to seek and accept social support.

Behavioral Dysregulation

Dysregulation of the SRS either creates over arousal or dysregulated behavior, as the regions of higher cognition are unable to control or manage higher cognitive functions over subcortical limbic emotion. Impulsivity is one of the primary signs of a child who is reliant upon their limbic system. This manifests as tantrums, aggression, disruptive and high-risk behaviors, and acting out. The inability of the prefrontal cortices (higher cognition) to inhibit amygdala activation (part of the limbic or emotional region) compromises the ability to reduce intense, overwhelming negative emotions. The malfunction of neural systems is what creates neural dysregulation, and that tends to lead to maladaptive strategies and behaviors.

When overwhelmed by emotion, a child may become withdrawn, fearful, and engage in rumination and suppression as regulatory strategies. Other children may act out with impulsivity, aggression, and noncompliance. Older children might engage in self-harm, self-medication, and substance use to deal with unpleasant emotion and memories. Some of these strategies may have worked in a chaotic abusive household, but they become maladaptive in healthy environments. Children with trauma histories engage in reenactment behavior that reflects their earlier experiences. A victim of physical abuse might become a 'bully' and engage in verbal or physical aggression. Sexually abused children may engage in developmentally inappropriate sexual behavior or become avoidant and dissociative.

Young children express their emotions through somatic symptoms and behavior, as they lack language proficiency. When behavioral symptoms serve as primary targets of treatment, the underlying causes remain unresolved and will likely compromise long-term maintenance of positive changes. Oppositional defiant disorder (ODD) has recently become reconceptualized as an expression of emotional dysregulation (Cavanagh, et al., 2014). Behaviorism was the go-to treatment for children for almost half a century, yet conceptualizing behaviors as singular, operationally defined targets can bypass causal history and miss the underlying dysregulation.

When integrated with regulation interventions and social-emotional goals and skills, however, behavioral changes would likely be sustained for longer periods of time.

Cognition

Regions of higher cognition house executive functions (EF), memory, and attention systems, all of which can be compromised by early trauma. Memory can be incompletely or improperly encoded, fragmented, or absent (van der Kolk, 2005). Executive functions, including problem-solving skills, judgment, decision-making, and abstract thinking, might become impaired, and the child may have speech and language problems, learning disabilities, low motivation, and distorted schema. Children with early trauma also suffer a higher risk for a decreased verbal IQ and have higher rates of absenteeism.

Early trauma also results in disrupted connectivity between cortical (PFC) and subcortical limbic structures (amygdala and hippocampus) which disrupt the capability to encode memories contextually. Memory is not just important for academic learning but also for emotional and social learning. Attention is often dysregulated and the child will appear to be inattentive, unmotivated, and/or disinterested. These changes may be partially attributed to the reallocation of all resources to survival. The child becomes consumed with identifying and responding to threats that they now see lurking everywhere.

Somatic

Somatic symptoms are physical manifestations of emotional or psychological distress that can be experienced in most areas of the body. The sensations are real, yet often have no medical explanation. In a well-regulated system, the body communicates information about visceral states to the individual. After trauma, the perception and communication systems of the child can become dysregulated and the body may send false signals or the child may not be able to hear, understand, or manage internal messaging. Children with early trauma experience somatic symptoms at a higher rate and intensity than non-clinical controls. Cardiac symptoms may include dizziness and fainting; neurological symptoms might present as sensory changes or tremors; and stomach aches, constipation, or nausea are common gastrointestinal symptoms.

Somatic symptom disorders have been proposed to be distinct forms of trauma-induced dissociative processes (Luoni, et al., 2018). Dissociation is a protective response to overwhelming trauma as it distances the child from the event. The normal integrated connections between feelings, memories, thoughts, and identity become disconnected. Dissociative behaviors result from disconnection and a disorganization of fear, memory, and social systems of the brain and result in reduced levels of arousal that exist on a continuum from apathetic and withdrawn to depersonalization and derealization.

Physiological Domain

As the stress and fear circuitry can become dysregulated, the child may experience significant alterations of arousal. Hyperactivity, hypervigilance, and an elevated startle response are common symptoms of chronic overactivation of this circuitry. The effects of an over-aroused physiology are disruptive and disturbing to the child, as well as those around them. When over-aroused, the child is unable to access higher cognitive functions, which thus impedes their ability to focus or learn. These children have to expend much more energy than others to maintain attention and behavior in an academic setting and are often exhausted after school. Dysregulation of the stress and fear circuitry can also result in dissociative behaviors, numbing, avoidance, withdrawal, and what looks like inattention.

Social Impairments

Dysregulation can impair social cognition, competence, and behavior. Children have great difficulty making and keeping friends, and experience deficits in reading cues, communicating, and participating in group activities. Impulsive behavior, emotional reactivity, and deficient interpersonal skills diminish their abilities to socialize, make friends, engage in group activities and experience a sense of belonging. Children with DT develop a threat bias and tend to view benign people and situations as dangerous. They misread faces and cannot identify the emotion of others or motivations.

The Self

Early trauma can disrupt the development of a continuous coherent and cohesive sense of self Schore, 2003). Children often suffer from diminished self-esteem, confidence, and lack a sense of self-efficacy. They often feel unvalued, ashamed, isolated, and disconnected. Many children lack interoceptive ability and do not sufficiently sense visceral sensations or make connections between their body and mind. The schema of the child is also disrupted. They lose trust in parents, agencies, teachers, and law enforcement. They view the world as a dangerous place and do not expect to be protected, accepted, or loved.

Conclusion

Childhood maltreatment is capable of altering existing neurobiology and disrupting the trajectory of development, compromising future neural growth, integration, and organization. Functional connectivity, structures (particularly the PFC, amygdala, and hippocampus), function, systems, and networks are all vulnerable to the consequences of maltreatment, particularly during critical periods of neuroplasticity. Neural dysregulation can subsequently disrupt and dysregulate functional domains. The consequences of trauma are mediated by genetics, epigenetics, and other factors of resilience such as interpersonal and social buffering.

While most scientists agree upon the primary anatomy of the human brain, descriptions and even terminology still vary within current literature. Researchers continue to search for a coherent paradigm that explains the neurobiological substrates of regulation (Kelley et al., 2015) as this construct is central to physiological homeostasis and potentially all functions and processes. The current consensus is that regulation involves several specific systems that support regulation, a cumulative result of evolutionarily supported cortical expansion and connectivity across time. Dysregulation is believed to be common in psychopathology and is instrumental in the onset and maintenance of most mental health disorders.

Efficacious clinical treatment for these children requires the support of other living beings and a highly effective source of relational support is the dog. Coevolution provisioned the canine with the capability to provide relational support to humans and offers a bridge to reconnection with others.

The next chapter shares the amazing convergence of humans and wolves, the ancestors of modern dogs. Our interspecies relationship that began during the Ice Age engineered genetic, neurobiological, anatomical, attachment, and social changes that have shaped the canine into a highly efficacious relational agent of healing. While neurobiologically infused canine-assisted therapy is supported by a broad theoretical foundation, our shared evolutionary history made it all possible.

References

Agorastos, A., Pervanidou, P., Chrousos, G.P., & Baker, D.G. (2019). Developmental trajectories of early life stress and trauma: A narrative review on neurobiological aspects beyond stress system regulation. *Frontiers in Psychiatry*; 10: 118. https://doi.org/10.3389/fpsyt.2019.00118

Aldao, A., Nolen-Hoeksema, S., & Schweizer, S. (2010). Emotion-regulation strategies across psychopathology: A meta-analytic review. *Clinical Psychology Review*; 30(2): 217–237. https://doi.org/10.1016/j.cpr.2009.11.004

Bell, P.T. & Shine, J.M. (2015). Estimating large-scale network convergence in the human functional connectome. *Brain Connectivity*; 5(9). Bell https://doi.org/10.1089/brain.2015.0348

Bluhm, R.L., Williamson, P.C., Osuch, E.A., Frewen, P.A., Stevens, T.K., Boksman, K., Neufield, R.W.J., Theberge, J., & Lanius, R.A. (2009). Alterations in default network connectivity in posttraumatic stress disorder related to early life-trauma. *Journal of Psychiatry & Neuroscience*; 34(3): 187–194.

Bremner, J.D. (2006). Traumatic stress: Effects on the brain. *Dialogues in Clinical Neuroscience*; 8(4): 445–461. https://doi.org/10.31887/DCNS.2006.8.4/jbremner

Brieant, A.E., Sisk, L.N., & Gee, D.G. (2021). Associations among negative life events, changes in cortico-limbic connectivity, and psychopathology in the ABCD Study. *Developmental Cognitive Neuroscience*; 52: 101022. https://doi. org/10.1016/j.dcn.2021.101022

Callahan, B.L., & Tottenham, N, (2016). The stress acceleration hypothesis: Effects of early life adversity on emotion circuits and behavior. *Current Opinion in Behavioral Sciences*; 7: 76–81.

Cancel, A., Dallel, S., Zine, A., El-Hage, W., & Fakra, E. (2019).Understanding the link between childhood trauma and schizophrenia: A systematic review of neuroimaging studies. *Neuroscience and Biobehavioral Reviews*; 107: 492–504. https://doi.org/10.1016/j.neubiorev.2019.05.024

Casey, B.J., Oliveri, M.E., & Insel, T. (2014). A neurodevelopmental perspective on the research domain criteria (RDoC) framework. *Biological Psychiatry*; 76(5): 350–353. https://doi.org/10.1016/j.biopsych.2014.01.006

Cavanaugh, M., Quinn, D., Duncan, D., & Graham, T. (2014). Oppositional defiant disorder is better conceptualized as a disorder of emotional regulation. *Journal of Attention Disorders*; 21(5). https://doi.org/10.1177/10870547

Cicchetti, D., & Tucker, D. (1994). Development and self-regulatory structures of the mind. *Development and Psychopathology*; 6: 533–549. https://doi.org/10.1017/s0954579400004673

Cisler, J. (2017). Childhood trauma and functional connectivity between amygdala and medial prefrontal cortex: A dynamic functional connectivity and large-scale network perspective. *Frontiers in Systems Neuroscience*. https://doi.org.10.3389/fnsys.2017.00029

DeBellis, M.D., & Van Dillen, T. (2005). Childhood post-traumatic stress disorder: An overview. *Child and Adolescent Psychiatric Clinics of North America*; 14(4): 745–772. https://doi.org/10.1016/j.chc.2005.05.006

DeBellis, M.D. & Zisk (2014). The biological effects of childhood trauma. *Child and Adolescent Psychiatric Clinics of North America*; 23(2): 185–222, vii. https://doi.org/10.1155/2016/7539065

Doom, J.R., & Gunnar, M.R. (2013). Stress physiology and developmental psychopathology: Past, present and future. *Development and Psychopathology*; 25(4): 1359–1373. https://doi.org/10.1017/S0954579413000667

Etkin, A., Egner, T., & Kalisch, R. (2011). Emotional processing in anterior cingulate and medial prefrontal cortex. *Trends in Cognitive Sciences*; 15(2): 85–93. https://doi.org/10.1016/k/tocs/2010.11.004

Godoy, L.D., Rossignoli, M.T., Delfino-Pereira, P., Garcia-Cairasco, N., & de Lima Umeoka, E.H. (2018). A comprehensive overview on stress neurobiology: Basic concepts and clinical implications. *Frontiers in Behavioral Neuroscience*; 12(127). https://doi.org/10.3389/fnbeh.2018.00127

Gunnar, M.R., & Donzella, B. (2002). Social regulation of the cortisol levels in early human development. *Psychoneuroendocrinology*; 27(1–2): 199–220. https://doi.org/10.1016/s0306-4530(01)00045-2

Hart, H., & Rubia, K. (2012). Neuroimaging of child abuse: A critical review. *Frontiers in Human Neuroscience*; 6:52. https://doi.org/10.3389/fnhum.2012.00052

Herringa, R.J., Birn, R.S., Ruttle, P.A., Burghy, C.A., Stodola, D.E., Davidson, R.J., & Essex, M.J.(2013). Childhood maltreatment is associated with altered fear circuitry and increased internalizing symptoms by late adolescence. *PNAS*; 110(47):19119–19124. https://doi.org/10.1073/pnas.1310766110

Herzberg, M.P., & Gunnar, M.R. (2020). Early life stress and brain function: Activity and connectivity associated with processing emotion and reward. *NeuroImage*; 209: 116493. https://doi.org/10.1016/j.neuroimage.2019.116493

Hibel, L.C., Mercado, E., & Valentino, K. (2019). Child maltreatment and mother-child attunement and transmission of stress physiology. *Child Maltreatment*; 24(4): 340–352. https://doi.org/10.1177/1077559519826295

Iacoboni, M., Lieberman, M.D., Knowlton, B.J., Moinar-Szakacs, I., Moritz, M., Throop, C.J., & Fiske, A.P. (2004). Watching social interactions produces dorsomedial prefrontal and medial parietal BOLD fMRI signal increases compared to a resting baseline. *NeuroImage*; 21: 1167–1173. https://doi.org/10.1016/j.neuroimage.2003.11.013

Ito, Y., Teicher, M.H., Glod, C.A., Harper, D., Magnus, E., & Gelbard, H.A. (1993). Increased prevalence of electrophysiological abnormalities in children with psychological, physical, and sexual abuse. *Journal of Neuropsychiatry and Clinical Neurosciences*; 5: 401–408.

Jeong, H.J., Durham, E.L., Moore, T.M., Dupont, R.M., McDowell, M., Cardenas-Iniguez, C., Micciche, E.T., Berman, M.G., Lahey, B.B., & Kackurkin, A.N. (2021). The association between latent trauma and brain structure in children, *Translational Psychiatry*; 11, 240.

Kebets, V., Favre, P., Houenou, J., Polosan, M., Perroud, N., Aubry, J-M., Van De Ville, D., & Piguet, C. (2021). Fronto-limbic neural variability as a transdiagnostic correlate of emotion dysregulation. *Translational Psychiatry*; 11(545). https://doi.org/10.1038/s41398-021-01666-3

Kelley, W.M., Wagner, D.D., & Heatherton, T.F. (2015). In search of a human self-regulation system. *Annual Review of Neuroscience*; 38: 389–411. https://doi.org/10.2246/annurev-neuro07103-014243

Lanius, R.A., Terpou, B.A., & McKinnon, M.C. (2020). *The sense of self in the aftermath of trauma: Lessons from the DMN in PTSD*. European Journal of Psychotraumatology; 11(1): 1807703. https://doi.org/10.1080/20008198.2020.1807703

Lanius, R.A., Frewen, P.A., Tursich, M., Jetly, R., & McKinnon, M.C. (2015). Restoring large-scale brain networks in PTSD and related disorders: A proposal for neuroscientifically informed interventions. *European Journal of Psychotraumatolog*; 6. https://doi.org/10.3402/ejpt.v6.27313

Luoni, C., Agosti, M., Crugnola, S., Rossi, G., & Termine, C. (2018). Psychopathology, dissociation and somatic symptoms in adolescents who were exposed to traumatic experiences. *Frontiers in Psychology* https://doi.org/10.3389/fpsyg.2018.02390

Lupien, S. J., McEwen, B.S., Gunnar, M.R., & Heim, C. (2009). Effects of stress throughout the lifespan on the brain, behavior, and cognition. *Nature Reviews. Neuroscience*; 10: 434–445. https://doi.org/10.1038/nrn2639

McCrory, E.J., Gerin, M.I., & Viding, E. (2017). Annual research review: Childhood maltreatment, latent vulnerability and the shift to preventative psychiatry-the contribution of functional brain imaging. *Journal of Child Psychology and Psychiatry*; 58(4): 338–357. https://doi.org/10.1111/jcpp.12713

McEwen, B.S. (2012). Brain on stress: How the social environment gets under the skin. *Proceedings of the National Academy of Sciences*; 109: 17180–17185. (PubMed: 20840167).

Menon, V. (2013). Developmental pathways to functional brain networks: Emerging principles. *The Connectome*; 7(12):627–640. https://doi.org/10.1016.j.t ics.2013.09.015

Menon, V. (2011). Large-scale brain networks and psychopathology: A unifying triple network model. *Trends in Cognitive Sciences*; 15(10): 483–586. https://doi.org.10.1016/j.tics.2011.08.003

Moukhtarian, T., Mintah, R., Moran, P., & Asherson, P. (2018). Emotion dysregulation in Attention-deficit/hyperactivity disorder and borderline personality disorder. *Borderline Personality Disorder and Emotion Dysregulation*; 5(9). https://doi.org/10.1186/s40479-018-0086-8

Nemeroff, C.B. (2016). Paradise lost: The neurobiological and clinical consequences of child abuse and neglect. *Neuron*. https://doi.org/10.1016/j.neuron.2016.01.019

Op den Kelder, R., Alithe, L.,Van den Akker, A.L., Geurts, H.M., Lindauer, R., & Overbeek, G. (2018). Executive functions in trauma-exposed youth: A meta-analysis. *European Journal of Psychotraumatology*; 9(1): 1450595. https://doi.org/10.1080/20008198.2018.1450595

Pan, J., Zhan, L., Hu, C.L., Yang, J., Wang, C., Gu, L., Zhong, S., Huang, Y., Wu, Q., Xie, X., Chen, Q., Zhou Huang, M., & Wu, X. (2018). Emotion regulation and complex brain networks: Association between expressive suppression and efficiency in the fronto-parietal network and default-mode network. *Frontiers in Human Neuroscience*; 12. https://doi.org/10.3389/fnhum.2018.00070

Parish-Plass, N. (2022). Personal Communication.

Perry, B.D. (2009). Examining child maltreatment through a neurodevelopmental lens: Clinical applications of the Neurosequential Model of Therapeutics. *Journal of Loss and Trauma*; 14: 240–255.

Phelps, E.A. (2004). Human emotion and memory: Interactions of the amygdala and hippocampal complex. *Current Opinion in Neurobiology*; 14: 198–202. https://doi.org/10.1016/j.conb.2004.03.015

Raichle, M.E. (2015). The brain's default mode network. *Annual Review of Neuroscience*; 38: 433–447. https://doi.org/10.1146/annurev-neuro-071013-014030

Rakesh, D., Allen, N.B., & Whittle, S. (2020). Balancing act: Neural correlates of affect dysregulation in youth depression and substance use-A systematic review of functional neuroimaging studies. *Developmental Cognitive Neuroscience* 42(100775). https://doi.org/10.1016/j.dcn.2020.100775

Rebello, K., Moura, L.M., Pinaya, W.H.L., Rohde, L.A., & Sato, J.R. (2018). Default mode maturation and environmental adversities during childhood. *Chronic Stress* (Thousand Oaks). Jan–Dec;2: 2470547018808295. https://doi.org/10.1177/2470547018808295

Ross, M.C. & Cisler, J.M. (2020). Altered large-scale functional brain organization in posttraumatic stress disorder: A comprehensive review of univariate and network-level neurocircuitry models of PTSD. *NeuroImage: Clinical*; 27(102319). Ross 2020 https://doi.org/10.1016/j.nicl.2020.102319

Sapolsky, R. (2021). Glucocorticoids, the evolution of the stress-response, and the primate predicament. *Neurogenic Stress*; 14: 100320. https://doi.org/10.1016/j.ynstr.2021.100320

Schore, A.N. (2003). *Affect Dysregulation & Disorders of the Self*. New York, NY: WW Norton & Co.

Schuder, M.R. & Lyons-Ruth, K. (2004). 'Hidden trauma in Infancy: Attachment, fearful arousal, and early dysfunction of the stress response system'. In J.D.

Osofsky (Ed.), *Young Children and Trauma: Intervention and Treatment* (pp. 69–104). New York, NY: Guilford Press.

Seeley, W.W., Menon, V., Schatzberg. A.F., Keller, J., Glover, G.H., & Kenna, H, et al. (2007). Dissociable intrinsic connectivity networks for salience processing and executive control. *The Journal of Neuroscience*; 27(9): 2349–2356. https://doi.org/10.1523/neurosci.5587-06-2007

Shine, J.M. (2019). Neuromodulatory influences on integration and segregation in the brain. *Trends in Cognitive Sciences*; 23(7): 572–583. https://doi.org/10.1016/j.tics.2019.04.002

Shonkoff, J. (2016). Capatalizing on advances in science to reduce the health consequences of early childhood adversity. *JAMA Pediatrics*; 170(10): 1003–1007. https://doi.org/10.1001/jamapediatrics.2016.1559

Szeszko, P.R. & Yehuda, R. (2019). Magnetic resonance imaging predictors of psychotherapy treatment response in post-traumatic stress disorder: A role for the salience network. *Psychiatry Research*; 52–57. https://doi.org/10.1016/j.psychres.2019.02.005

Teicher, M.H., Glod, C.A., Surrey, J. Swett, C. (1993). Early childhood abuse and limbic system ratings in adult psychiatric outpatients. *Journal of Neuropsychiatry and Clinical Neurosciences*; 5: 301–306.

Teicher, M.H., Samson, J.A., Anderson, C.M., & Ohashi, K. (2016). The effects of childhood maltreatment on brain structure, function, and connectivity. *Nature Reviews Neuroscience*; 17: 652–666.

Tian, T., Li, J., Zhang, G., Wang, J., Liu, D., Wan, C., Fang, J., Wu, D., Zhou, Y., Qin, Y., & Zhu, W. (2021). Default mode network alterations induced by childhood trauma correlate with emotion function and SLC6A4 expression. *Frontiers in Psychiatry*; 12: 760411. https://doi.org/10.3389/fpsyt.2021.760411

Uddin, L.Q., Yeo, T., & Spreng, R.N. (2019). Towards a universal taxonomy of macro-scale functional human brain networks. *Brain Topography*; 32(6): 926–942.

Van der Kolk, B. (2005). Developmental trauma disorder: Towards a rational diagnosis for children with complex trauma histories. *Psychiatric Annals*; 35(5): 401–408. https://doi.org/10.3928/00485713-20050501-06

Van Essen, D.C., & Barch, D.M. (2015). The human connectome in health and psychopathology. *World Psychiatry*; 14(2): 154–157. https://doi.org/10.1002/wps.20228

Vanes, L.D., & Dolan, R.J. (2021). Transdiagnostic neuroimaging markers of psychiatric risk: A narrative review. *NeuroImage: Clinical*; 30: 102634. https://doi.org/10.1016/j.nicl.2021.102634

Wang, R., Liu, M., Cheng, X., Wu, Y., Hildebrandt, A., & Zhou, C. (2021). Segregation, integration, and balance of large-scale resting brain networks configure different cognitive abilities. *Biological Sciences*; 118(23). E2022288118. https://doi.org/10.1073/pnas.2022288118

Washington, S.D. & Van Meter, J.W. (2015). Anterior-posterior connectivity within the default mode network increases during maturation. *The International Journal of Medical and Biological Frontiers*; 21(2): 207.

Zhao, H., Dong, D., Sun, X.Q., Cheng, C., Wang, X., & Yao, S. (2021). Intrinsic brain network alterations in non-clinical adults with a history of childhood trauma. *European Journal of Psychotraumatology*; 12(1). https://doi.org/10.1080/200008198.2021.1975951

Zhang, W., Hashemi, M.M., Kaldewaij, R., Koch, S.B.J., Beckmann, C., Klump-ers, F., & Roelofs, K. (2019). Acute stress alters the 'default' brain processing. *NeuroImage*; 189: 870–877. https://doi.org/10.1016/j.neuroimage.2019.01.063

Zhang, W., Kaldewaij, R., Hashemi, M.M., Koch, S.B.J., Smit, A., van Ast, V.A., Beckmann, C.F., Klumpers, F.L., & Roelofs, K. (2022). Acute-stress-induced change in SN coupling prospectively predicts post-trauma symptom development. *Translational Psychiatry*; 12 (63). https://doi.org/10.1101/2021.07.03.21259969

Part Two

The Potential of the Dog to Support Healing Dysregulation

Chapter 5 The Coevolution of Humans and Canines

Two thin, tattered men ambled across the ice-patched ground, tugging at their furred capes. They were weary from the chill and gnawing hunger consuming their bodies. The sun was falling in the sky and they had nothing in their hands except sticks.

Glacial movement during the Pleistocene Epoch (Ice Age) was the result of catastrophic climate change, which forced early humans out of their densely forested habitats into the open grasslands of the savanna. The migration led to a higher concentration of numerous and unfamiliar species resulting in increased competition for resources. The new habitat was well suited for carnivorous predators, yet early humans still straddled the division between predator and prey. The profound changes challenged the human brain, and humans would have to adapt in order to survive.

The forest had provided humans with shelter, safety, and an abundance of fruits and nuts. The grasslands were open, with less cover, and their diet shifted to bugs, worms, eggs, and small rodents. Humans discovered that their diet could be supplemented with the meaty leftovers of the abandoned kills of apex predators. This meat was full of fatty acids which nourished brain growth and complexity. The evolving brain is assumed to be the primary adaptation that prevented the human species from joining the large-scale extinction of mammals that occurred during this period. Enabled by a highly evolved visual system, humans began to quietly observe the strength and prowess of the carnivores. While their emotions, thoughts, and actions were consumed with survival, seeds of curiosity, and even admiration began to emerge.

The men felt the earth tremble beneath their feet and recognized the unmistakable sounds of a stampeding herd of caribou. Their bodies were immediately hijacked by an instant acceleration of physiology. They became alert and energized as their musculature was galvanized by increased oxygen and blood flow. Instinctively, they sprinted to hide behind a rock outcropping. The men then saw a pack of wolves that was keeping pace with

DOI: 10.4324/9781003217534-8

the herd and realized what they had predicted as predators were actually prey. They con-
tinued to watch, admiring the wolves' speed, and coordinated movement. The wolves'
behavior held their gaze, and the men noticed that they seemed to be working together. A
fatigued animal was separated from the herd and brought down. A celebratory howl rang
out, and the men hurried back to camp to share their story. They returned with their fami-
lies the next day and salvaged the leftovers.

One can imagine that humans were both frightened *and* mesmerized by the hunting prowess of these commanding predators. The wolves were victorious even though they visibly lacked the size and strength of the large herds. The rhythm and synchrony of the pack represented innovation, cooperation, and intelligence that challenged the inherent human presumption that size and strength always win. These creatures were competent predators yet they were social, cooperative, and doted upon their young.

How and why was human evolution shaped by animals, and in particular, wolves? Meg Olmert (2009) proposes that it all began with *watching*. Surviving such a dangerous environment required the capability to differentiate safety from threat, an ability honed through keen observance and increased knowledge of animal behavior and movement. Watching was initially wrought with fear, then curiosity, and ultimately respect and admiration. It was observation that led to increased knowledge, new skills, and cooperative alliances. The new environment challenged and grew the human brain, increasing sociality which seeded the convergence of humans and wolves. While the increasing complexity of the brain would advantage human evolution, it was possibly this interspecies relationship that may have grown their humanity.

The shared experiences between early humans and wolves fostered a deep connection that fueled the development of the human–animal bond (HAB). Pleistocene history laid the foundation for the powerful interspecies relationship that exists today. An intense mutual connection, the HAB improves the health and well-being of both species and is particularly relevant to canine-assisted psychotherapies. Understanding the history and science of dogs and their unique traits and capabilities will grant clinicians an expanded knowledge that will enhance their work. This chapter will provide a brief review of the coevolution process and dog domestication and identify the relevant empirical evidence that supports an interspecies approach to healing and restoration of humans today.

The Divergence of Canines from Their Ancestors

There has been significant debate on the timing and location of the canine divergence from their gray wolf predecessors, yet some circumstances have been supported by DNA, fossils, bones, and internments. One of the problems with establishing a timeline results from the fact that early dogs probably did not differ morphologically from wolves (Perri, 2021). Existing evidence can be summarized to show that dogs diverged from ancestral wolves in various locations, at various times, and under various circumstances (Pierotti & Fogg, 2017; Schleidt & Shalter, 2018). Archeologists discovered and documented significant genetic and morphological differences between evolved dogs and their ancestors roughly 11,000–16,000 years ago (Axelsson et al., 2013; Perri, 2016), and this time span is fairly ubiquitous throughout the literature. Another source of evidence is the human migration patterns, as it is well accepted that early dogs did accompany humans.

Dogs are believed to be the first animal to be domesticated and are present in almost every community across the world. Domestication of an animal implies human intentional manipulation of a species. Zeuner (1963), however, argued that the dog does not neatly fit into traditional theories of domestication.

The human–canine coevolution (HCE), a phenomenon with considerable consensus among geneticists, archeologists, evolutionary psychologists, and ethnologists, has generated multiple theories that attempt to explain the ontogeny of this interspecies relationship. Two well-known, yet contested hypotheses of the HCE include the *commensal scavenger theory* and the *cross-species adoption theory*. The commensal hypothesis was based on the belief that wolves began to wander into early human encampments to scavenge scraps from garbage dumps. The increasing proximity presumably led to increasing familiarity and decreasing fear. This hypothesis dominated literature for decades as the explanation for how our species came together, yet has been recently challenged. The cross-species adoption theory proposed that humans simply took wolf pups, raised them, and selected those with desirable traits for reproduction (Serpell, 2021). This theory implies that domestication was human-driven. While both of these theories could coexist with other hypotheses, they potentially fall short in acknowledging the role of the wolves and the profound interspecies collaboration

The recent emergence of a more plausible theory is drawing growing consensus among experts. Eminent ethologist Marc Bekoff (2013) described this early relationship as an alliance that was based on mutual respect, seeded in the recognition of sentience in each other and acknowledgment of the mutual benefits of their social and cooperative alliance. While humans were adapting to their new environment and cohabitation, wolves also had to adjust to increased human numbers. Supported by their own neural plasticity, wolves adapted their ecological system to coexist (Cordoni & Palagi, 2019). Emerging evidence implies that each species had a profound effect upon the development of both species (Schleidt & Shalter, 2003). The radical environmental changes placed the two species together, and the relationship that evolved became a catalyst that may have produced a convergent rewiring of both species.

The closest living relatives of humans are chimpanzees (primates). They share 99% of their genome with us, and it would be logical to assume our evolutionary paths might be parallel. However, during the distribution of human groups across Eurasia, the social nature of human groups shifted from the primate model and began to converge with the canid model. This redirected pathway coincided with the increased cohabitation of humans and wolves (Schleidt & Shalter, 2003). Why would humans merge with a species so morphologically different? Chimpanzees are known for their opportunistic, self-focused, aggressive, and competitive behaviors and they do not demonstrate cooperation and loyalty within groups. Wolves presented a contrasting model of group loyalty, cooperation, democracy, and sociality. While the precise cause for this shift may not be known, most would agree humans got the better deal. Konrad Lorenz (1954) thought so and suggested that out of all of the animal species in the world, the dog was the best suited companion for humans. Jane Goodall, the distinguished researcher of primate behavior, also studied wild dogs. She speaks of wolves as affectionate, protective of pups, loyal, and cooperative. Unlike primates who tend to be out for themselves, wolves collaborate and use teamwork to problem solve. Dr Goodall suggests that humans chose traits of sociality over intelligence (Schleidt & Shalter, 2003).

Wolf pack members provide social support for conspecifics, similar to humans helping other humans (Range and Virányi, 2014). The polymorphism linked with high levels of sociality is believed to have been present in wolves prior to domestication (Persson et al., 2017). In fact, it has been proposed that the sociality and cooperative behavior of wolves predated humans by perhaps 'millions of years' (Schleidt & Shalter, 2018). This thinking challenges the concept of domestication, or the intentional behavior of humans to change and direct another species for their benefit. Is it conceivable that wolves domesticated humans? Their influence on human morality, cooperation, and sociality is proposed by Schleidt and Shalter (2018) to meet or surpass human influence on the evolution of the wolf. Yes, humans impacted the evolutionary paths of wolves and canines, but it may have been wolves that gifted us with what we call 'humanity.'

One of the most significant endorsements of the power of animals to effect change in humans emanates from this early coevolution. The very survival of our species was dependent upon the development of attuned, focused attention on animals, especially prior to the ascent of humans to their dominant position in the animal kingdom. What began as survival-based behavior evolved from observation, to curiosity, to increased proximity, and finally a deep relationship that was based on shared sociality, respect, and cooperation and love.

Observation as a Mechanism of Learning

While the primal goal of survival drove early humans to be attentive and vigilant of animals, the increasingly attuned level of observation generated a new, substantial cache of information that was useful beyond survival.

Humans recognized that animals formed alliances and cooperated, and realized that those behaviors were highly beneficial to the success of their groups. Early humans began to refine their ability to decipher actions and sense feelings and motivations within the animals. Underneath, a concurrent neurobiological process was encoding their new abilities on a cellular level.

The modeling of observed behavior has long been recognized as one of the most advantageous methods of learning for humans and animals, yet the mechanisms of this process were not well understood for some time. Then, about 25 years ago at the University of Parma (Italy), Rizzolatti and team revealed a specific neurobiological basis for this amazing process. The discovery of mirror neurons (MN) is believed to be one of the most significant links to brain evolution. One of the most interesting properties of this system is that it does not require conscious thought or intention. The mere observation of another individual's behavior activates the brain cells of the observer, as if they were also performing the action. Early research on MN focused on motor functions, such as hand movements. More recently, MN were found to be involved in the generation of prosocial, empathic behavior (Gallese, 2001). Mirror neurons permit us to understand the emotions, motivations, and behavior of another, by feeling, not thinking (Rizzolatti & Craighero, 2004).

Observations provide visual data that become encoded into an internal representation. Through repetitive experiences, these representations eventually make their way into our DNA. It makes sense that shared learning experiences of early humans and wolves would encode comparable neuronal representations, and this theory has been supported by the multitude of genomic changes in both species that support evolved behavior. There is substantial speculation that the mirror neuron system exists within dogs, although scientists have not yet confirmed this (Ferrari & Coude, 2018).

Observation as a learning mechanism is evolutionarily conserved and is employed within ni-CAP therapeutic interventions today to increase the awareness, knowledge, and connectedness of the child. Evolution remains a central influence upon the neurobiology and behavior of modern humans and provides time-honored lessons. Evolutionary observations supported the continuance of our species and today observation remains a valid, highly effective mechanism for learning, healing, and restoring humans.

Coming Closer

One can only speculate how long humans observed from a distance before the two species wandered closer together. All mammals tend to fear what is unknown, yet many species are highly curious. Research supports the theory that propinquity (increased geographic proximity) can serve as a mechanism for a reduction of fear, increased familiarity, improved tolerance, and the subsequent development of social and emotional affiliation (Zajonc, 2001).

In the 1960s, psychologist Robert Zajonc studied individuals as they were exposed to repeated living or nonliving stimuli. He suggested that these experiences could leave a subliminal neural imprint that stimulates a bond or positive feeling. He labeled this the 'mere exposure effect.'

Zajonc's thinking triggered decades of research, and was replicated and validated by LeDoux (1996). This construct implies that this period of intense coexistence and observation potentially sowed seeds of affection within humans for their animal counterparts (LeDoux, 1996; Zajonc, 2001).

The carnivorous wolf was an apex predator yet also became nature's first pastoralist society living off migrating herds of ungulates including reindeer, horses, and bison. Toward the end of the Pleistocene Epoch, humans adopted the wolves' pastoralist lifestyle and adaptively acquired wolf characteristics of cooperation, shared risks, and the extension of relationships beyond kinship. Sustained and peaceful cohabitation dampened fear circuitry resulting in longer states of felt safety and regulated physiology, and less frequent activation of the stress response system (SRS). The endocrine system plays a key role in both the activation of the SRS and the attenuation of that process. A neuropeptide, oxytocin provides regulatory actions on a multitude of other neural systems. In concert with increased serotonin, a catecholamine, aggression is decreased, resulting in learning and prosocial behavior (McEwen & Morrison, 2013).

Wolf Society

What was it about early wolves that piqued the curiosity in humans? Wolves lived in cohesive family units consisting of a monogamous breeding couple, pups, and older siblings, a structure similar to the human family. They divided their labor fairly including familial tasks such as caring for young, provisioning, play, grooming, and providing protection. Wolves shared risk and worked collaboratively in teams to hunt and distribute the spoils within the pack (Schleidt & Shalter, 2003). They maintained order through a modified democracy and demonstrated a capacity for cooperation that rivals humans today. Wolves relied upon a peaceful and fair system and although conflicts between members did occur, wolves were capable of repair and reconciliation (Cafazzo et al., 2017).

The same behaviors apparent in pup rearing were also strongly reflected in wolves' territorial defense and hunting practices. Wolves were known to cooperatively hunt and were believed to employ strategies. This cooperation required attention, prediction of the other wolves' intentions and behavior, and a plan. Both humans and wolves tracked and hunted herds and observation of the other's methods may have sparked recognition of the potential benefits of combining their skills. (Range & Virányi, 2014). Humans learned hunting strategies through observation (Schleidt & Shalter, 2003), and began to join cooperative hunts. Collaborative hunting perhaps involved human employment of their visual processing and cognitive strengths to learn the patterns of prey. Wolves would give chase, relying upon their speed, endurance, and herding proficiency and would exhaust the herd, separating and disabling their target. At that point, humans might arrive to finish the kill by using their developed weaponry. The partnership would result in nutritional spoils for all (Shipman, 2017).

Wolves have always played, even as adults. Play is rewarding and inspires joy, laughter, and positive connections that lead to strengthened and shared emotional bonds. Humans, wolves, dogs, and other mammalian youth participate in social play which is a crucial developmental mechanism for learning. Neuroscientist Jaak Panksepp (2005) identified play and seeking as two of the primary emotions of mammals He suggested that processes of play and laughter are neurally based, supported by subcortical brain regions and opioids. The context of play provides a fertile milieu for the cultivation of emotional, social, physical, and cognitive skills. Play teaches trust, fairness, sharing, reciprocity, and skills that comprise the building blocks of social relationships and societies. Play lights up the caudate nucleus, the brain region associated with reward and trust. Interspecies play has been suggested as a pathway to peace, as play improves the dynamics of social life and teaches conflict resolution, both requisites of homeostatic coexistence (Palagi et al., 2016).

Wolves then and dogs today, in calm states, provide a sense of safety and security for children. This evolutionarily conserved phenomenon advantages canine-assisted psychotherapy today as distressed children must acquire a sense of safety to progress through therapy. Wolves and dogs have innate protective natures and are highly sensitive to vulnerable individuals, particularly children. As wolves look after their offspring, perhaps they also became shepherds of human children. As affiliation increased, it is plausible that children and pups engaged in pleasurable joint play. Wolves nurtured and protected their young, and extending these behaviors to young children would be natural.

Though humans have superior occipital systems, wolves outshine humans with superior auditory and olfactory systems. Early humans would have recognized the value of wolves as mobile threat detectors due to their sensory prowess. They are also naturally territorial and alert to intrusions of predators and unfamiliar humans. Co-sleeping would allow humans to sleep deeply while vigilant wolves remained on guard (Kortekaas & Kotrschal, 2019).

Successful cohabitation required adaptations in both species that supported the ability to form attachments and social relationships. Both humans and wolves possessed an innate sociality and propensity for cooperation which supported the necessary adaptations to form attachments and enduring social relationships. Each species came to recognize and respect the other as a potential source of survival and social-based learning. This interspecies relationship provided reciprocal social support and a calmer, safer environment, necessary requisites for cognitive and social development.

The Oxytocin Effect on the Interspecies Convergence

The oxytocinergic system (OT) is believed to have played a significant role in the domestication of the dog (Wang et al., 2013). In early evolution OT attenuated fear and anxiety in wolves toward humans. Research suggests that oxytocin plays a primary function in threat perception, in that it attenuates fear circuitry (Herbeck et al., 2022) and reduces aversive avoidance responses. Humans and canines are highly social and seek connections with others, yet their willingness to approach others is mediated by their stress response system. When an encounter does not signal threat, oxytocin will facilitate physiological calming, which supports approach and engagement. Throughout evolution, OT underwent numerous adaptations in response to the changing needs of humans and wolves as they became more social and cooperative. In addition to its function in reproduction, birthing, and attachment, the role of OT expanded to support the development of social bonds, relationships, and cooperation (Herbeck et al., 2022).

It is believed that humans and the evolving canine, supported by internal chemistry, began to form attachment relationships during the coevolution. Attachment security is critical in both species for normal development and serves as a template for interpersonal and social relationships. A neuroimaging study of dogs presented with the scent of a favored human, revealed activation in the canine reward region (caudate nucleus) of the brain, an indicator of implicit rewards from emotional attachment (Berns, 2021).

Cohabitation and socially motivated interaction require communication, and gaze is a powerful tool of emotional interchange. Mutual gaze is a core mechanism in attachment relationships, promoting all aspects of development. The human infant becomes synchronized and attuned with the caregiver and through mutual gaze begins to mimic facial expressions, vocalizations, and movement. Nagasawa and associates (2015) found that oxytocin (OT) promotes face-to-face gazing and motor mimicry which blend to build an emotional bridge that deepens the relationship.

While wolves are not known for frequent eye contact with humans, modern dogs willingly participate in gazing and particularly enjoy the experience. Somehow, during the coevolution, dogs began to take advantage of human caregiver sensitivities to their young by mimicking gestures. Similar to human infants, dogs learned to use eye contact, gazing, and other solicitous gestures to gain human attention and affection (MacLean & Hare, 2015). These behaviors benefited both species with increased oxytocin and caudate nucleus (reward) activation, and positively supported the human–canine relationship.

In a study of human and dog interactions, gazing, and OT, researchers found that oxytocin levels of *both* participants increased during positive interaction and that positive interactions also increased when oxytocin levels rose. These results demonstrate a bidirectional, self-perpetuating process which suggests an exciting potential intervention for treatment of children with dysregulated neurobiology. They identified this pattern as a positive, chemically induced affiliative link, called the 'oxytocin-gaze positive loop' (Nagasawa et al., 2015). When dogs received an intranasal dose of OT, the females increased their gaze. Another study demonstrated that increased oxytocin in dogs during interactions with humans relies upon a *reciprocal* relationship. This result was not evident in a single-direction pathway of either giving or receiving (Romero & Nagawawa, 2014). This implies that the formation of the interspecies relationship was an authentic connection that was nourished by the mutual efforts of both species.

The oxytocin system (OT) can be presumed to have supported stable and affiliative relationships between humans and wolves, as on its key roles is to mediate the social and relational behavior of both species. Similar to humans, wolves engage in strong social and emotional bonds with conspecifics (beyond kinship). Oxytocin also enhances reward via dopamine-dependent mesolimbic reward pathways, and served as a mechanism that supported interspecies cooperation without a need for cognitive interpretation or awareness of potential future benefits. In social contexts that confer safety, OT joins with the dopaminergic system to increase the salience of social cues, support gaze, and proximity seeking, and enhance responses to human gestural communication.

Evolutionary Changes to Canine Sensory Systems (Olfactory, Visual, and Auditory)

The ability of dogs to adapt to the anthropogenic niche of humans has been enhanced by their exquisite sensitivity to human social cues. Dogs have accrued an astonishing array of socio-cognitive skills using their sensory systems, enhanced by an evolved attention bias toward humans (Kis et al., 2017). Modern dogs are capable of detecting of human emotion visually and acoustically (Siniscalchi et al., 2018) through chemical scent (Siniscalchi et al., 2016; D'Aniello et al., 2018a) and observation of human body language (D'Aniello et al., 2018b).

The Olfactory System

The canine olfactory system occupies 2% of brain real estate, compared to a meager 0.03% in humans. Dogs are portable scent detectors capable of discriminating scents in a variety of environments. They can detect bombs, drugs, and follow the trail of a lost child. Dogs have also served human health in disease detection of melanoma, diabetes, and cancer (Kokocinska-Kusiask et al., 2021). The canine olfactory system differs from other sensory systems as their pathways ipsilaterally ascend (the right nostril leads to the right hemisphere). Dogs show clear nostril asymmetries for processing emotional cues. Stressful situations for dogs, such as separation from their human, are processed through the right nostril, while human odors emitted during periods of physical stress and fear are sensed through the left nostril.

While wolves probably depended upon their olfactory prowess for survival, the dogs of today tend to rely on humans for dinner. It is believed that multiple modern breeds may have lost olfactory capability through domestication (Bird et al., 2020). The adage 'use it or lose it' is an accurate depiction of a powerful evolutionary principle (Diamond et al., 1964).

The Visual System

As the gaze between subjects is a key component of social communication and as the coevolution increased sociality in humans and canines, adaptations followed that enabled more complex expression in canines. Visual attention is a construct that is frequently used to evaluate the behavior and cognition of animals. Dogs tend to gaze at features that contain useful information, such as heads and bodies, and novelty sparks their curiosity. Biological anthropologists discovered that dogs are even more capable than our closest primate relatives of recognizing and interpreting human emotional and social cues and behavior (Kaminski & Nitzschner, 2013). While it was well established that primates had a dedicated neural visual system, in the 1990s, scientists discovered similar circuitry in canines, and found that they had a higher level of proficiency over primates (Berns, 2020). The temporal cortex, a component of the ventral visual pathways, was evolutionarily conserved and serves this function (Cuaya et al., 2016).

Dogs are attracted to human faces and look to our facial expressions and vocalizations for assurance, direction, and critical information (Udall, 2015). Facial expressions can explicitly reflect intuitive, internally felt emotional states, and dogs are capable of differentiating positive and negative emotional valence (happy and angry facial expressions) (Muller et al., 2015). Dogs internalize a representation of their human's face (Adachi et al., 2007) and can differentiate between 2D images of faces and familiar from novel faces (Huber et al., 2013). Dogs are recognized for their ability to discern attention states in humans and even follow eye and head direction to find hidden objects (Hare et al., 1998).

Auditory Processing

Andics et al. (2014) found 'functionally analogous' brain regions in humans and dogs for auditory processing. Their study is suggested to be the first study to identify the presence and location of voice areas in dogs and the interspecies coevolution is believed to have been the catalyst for this neural remodeling.

Using fMRI and behavioral data, a study found that the relationship between the human and dog acts as a mediator of neural responses to auditory expressions. Dogs are more sensitive to the praise of a familiar person compared to an unknown human, demonstrated by increased activity in the corticostriatal reward and motivation network (Gabor et al., 2021). Dogs are sensitive to the linguistic content *and* non-linguistic characteristics of speech. Praise compared to neutral content elicits more activation, and positive prosody and tone of the human voice generates robust activation (Gabor et al., 2021). Another interesting find was that dogs are much more attentive when emotion-contextual speech and instructions are directly addressed to them (Jeannin et al., 2017).

Anatomical, Neurobiological, Genetic, Epigenetic, and Emotion, Social, and Cognition Adaptations of Canines

The modern dog has become a preferred subject of study in multiple disciplines, including genetics, evolutionary biology, and neuroscience. The incredible changes they underwent as they diverged from the gray wolf occurred rapidly. Adaptations have been found in the anatomical, neurobiological, genetic and epigenetic, and socio-behavioral domains. The domestication process also increased plasticity, or heightened receptiveness to environmental influences (Udall et al., 2010).

Anatomical Change

The anatomical diversity of canines exceeds all other mammalian species as their size varies 40-fold within their own species (Ostrander & Wayne, 2005). Human selection during domestication has shaped over 350 specific breeds that represent diverse sizes, behavior, and skills. There is incredible heterogeneity between breeds and also between individual dogs.

Anatomical changes occurred in the canine skeleton, musculature, legs, tail, ears, jaw and teeth, and face. Dog sizes, shapes, and color and texture of coats diversified. Facial changes are believed to be associated with the increase in sociality through coevolution, as the facial repertoire of expressions can dramatically expand the communicative and social potential of the dog. The facial changes also had a dramatic effect upon perceived attractiveness. Across the domestication tract, humans likely selected dogs with a more infantilized look, as that feature elicits emotionality. This adaptation in anatomy, however, also changed the traits and maturity levels of dogs. Breeds that are morphologically distant from the wolf tend to be more immature behaviorally and have lost some ability to signal fear states and impending aggression. While upright ears can flexibly signal changes in states, floppy ears tend to telegraph 'happy puppy.'

A study of ten breeds showed that dogs that were morphologically more similar to wolves tended to retain wolf traits and behaviors. The Siberian husky showed 15 (out of 15) wolf behaviors, while the Cavalier King Charles Spaniel showed two. Of note, considering their popularity in therapies, golden retrievers actually retain 12 wolf behaviors (Grandin & Johnson, 2009). Studies are informative, yet produce generalizations. While information *is* useful for the clinician, the determination of an appropriate working therapy dog comes down to the individual dog.

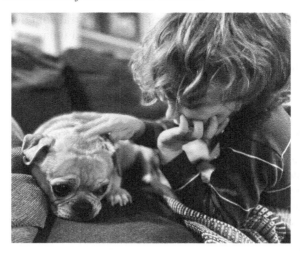

The 'AU101' muscle that produces the inner eyebrow raise was recently identified as an adaptation in the canine eyebrow that gives dogs the appearance of larger, more receptive, and expressive eyes. This muscle is not present in wolves and demonstrates a morphological adaptation in canines that is believed to be linked to the rapid increase in sociality during coevolution. Humans view canines with this feature as more appealing, as it expands their ability to convey emotion during interactions (Kaminski et al., 2019). This now heritable trait is referred to as 'puppy eyes' and elicits an empathic, caregiving reaction from humans. The human response to an infantilized face is believed to be regulated primarily by the autonomic nervous systems which results in heightened activation of brain regions involved in face perception, empathy, attention, reward and emotion processing, and motor control. A recent study revealed that dogs employ the 'eyebrow' lift more frequently when a human is looking at them (Kaminski et al., 2017).

The eyes evolved in humans and dogs to have a white sclera, the area that surrounds the cornea. This shared evolutionary change is in contrast with primates who kept a dark sclera which camouflages the direction of their gaze. Primates require that trait for protection as they continue to primarily exist in the wild. The white sclera is a crucial component of human–dog interactions and likely supported their cooperative hunts in early history. The more visible white sclera increased the ability to convey social information nonverbally with eye movement. It is much easier to determine the direction of another's gaze and dogs today show awareness of human attention and will alter their behavior in response. If a human is not watching, a dog is more likely to 'go against the house rules,' for example, and grab the steak off the table (Kaminski et al., 2017).

Neurobiological: Mental Health and Fear Systems

The evolutionary continuity of the mammalian brain suggests that the limbic brain, the reward system, stress axis, and mirror neuron mechanisms are evolutionary conserved in all mammals (LeDoux, 2012). The social behavior of humans and wolves was, and is, enabled by neural circuitry involved with stress reduction, prosocial contact, and the development of empathic behavior (Beetz et al., 2012).

Of particular interest to the incorporation of canines into treatment for children are the neurobiological similarities shared by both species. Canines share some mental health disorders with humans, and are often treated by veterinarians with psychotropic medications commonly prescribed for humans. This commonality implies shared mechanisms of mood regulation (Berns, 2020). While humans are primarily diagnosed with mental health disorders through identification of symptoms and self-report, dog behaviors require a familiarity with the dog to recognize changes that can be reliably interpreted.

Anxiety, depression, and obsessive-compulsive (OCD) behaviors are three primary disorders seen in canines. Depressed dogs lose interest in eating, reduce activity, lose weight, sleep more, may shed their coat, and are less interested in social interactions and play. They may even refuse treats and rewards. Anxiety is the chronic worry or prediction of fear-inducing stimuli, whereas fear is the more immediate reaction to a threat. Anxious dogs show avoidance, destructive behavior, trembling, reduced play and movement, hiding, and compulsive and/or self-injuring behaviors. They may have separation anxiety when left alone and can also have OCD behaviors.

Dogs with OCD demonstrate repetitive, stereotypic behavior which can be problematic, or simply humorous.

> Derby was a four-year-old terrier mix adopted from a shelter two years earlier. He seemed to adjust relatively well to his new family and he was active and enjoyed playing with the children. His guardian, Amy, mentioned that he did seem 'a little on the nervous side.' One evening, when she walked into the living room, Derby was quietly laying on the floor with a box of Kleenex between his front legs. Next to him was a pile of tissues on the floor, and he was methodically pulling them out of the box, one after another.

Genetic Changes

The expanse of history shared by humans and wolves also resulted in a genomic evolution. Research that studies the role that genetics play in the divergence of canine behavior from wolves through evolution is considered young, though many discoveries have been produced. Similar genes in both species may have undergone changes in response to the shared environmental challenges. Many investigations have found significant variation in the DNA of dogs, with inserted, deleted, mutated, and duplicated genes, complicating the search for genetic-behavioral correlations. Conceivably, this diversity partially accounts for the differences between breeds and even individual dogs in social behavior.

During evolution, behavioral adaptations occur first and then, over time, become encoded into the genome, rendering the behavior heritable. Humans and canines share similarities in genes for metabolism, digestion, neurobiological processes, and cancer. Through rigorous methodology that isolated the top 1% of the genome, Wang and colleagues identified 32 different genes that overlap between humans and dogs today (Wang et al., 2013).

In an extensive study of the divergence of canines from wolves conducted by Axelsson et al., (2013), a whole-genome resequencing of wolves and dogs was conducted using 3.8 million genetic variants to pinpoint 36 genomic regions that could be implicated in dog domestication. Nineteen of these regions contained genes that were critical to brain functions. Eight of those regions belonged to the central nervous system developmental pathways and were proposed to be associated with behavior changes. Ten regions were associated with roles in fat metabolism and starch digestion, implying a substantial change in diet. The diet of dogs changed through evolution from a carnivorous diet to an omnivorous menu that included more starch and fiber, more closely matching the human diet.

While hundreds, or even thousands of specific genes and variations are responsible for personality and behavioral traits, evolutionary biologists are expanding the search for genetic evidence of the canine trait of 'hypersociality.' This distinct trait is a complex phenotype identified by elevated oxytocin levels, sustained face gazing, and proximity seeking (Kujala, 2017).

Recently, a multi-disciplinary research team targeted a chromosomal region that has been implicated in canine sociality, finding several sections of canine DNA that were linked with social behaviors (vonHoldt et al., 2017). Emily Shuldiner, a Princeton alumnus, identified the similarities in genetic architecture between canine sociality and a unique human disorder, the William-Beurens syndrome (WBS). Interestingly, while canine sociality is linked to gene insertions, it is the absence of many of these genes (27 gene deletions) that causes WBS in humans. Humans with WBS experience a cluster of distinct facial characteristics, can have an intelligence disability, and show extreme friendliness, limited social inhibition, and minimal fear of strangers.

Epigenetics

Changes in environmental stress conditions and social behavior can shape brain plasticity, brain structure, and alter gene expression. While specific genetic changes have been identified, recent research has discovered that a significant number of adaptive changes in canines during evolution were mediated through changes in *gene expression*, insinuating epigenetic mechanisms (Sahlen et al., 2021).

An epigenetic process does not change the gene itself; it affects the expression of the gene. The gene is activated (turned on) or deactivated (turned off). The process can be reversed, however, when positively influenced by environmental conditions and behavior. Epigenetic regulation of the HPA axis, a key process of the SRS in wolves, dogs, and humans, reduced the fear axis of both species and enabled approach, proximity, and gradual cohabitation. This allowed the development of social affection (Hare et al., 2012), and is considered a key mechanism that contributed to domestication (Herbeck et al., 2017).

The Gut Microbiome

There is another branch of the nervous system that is not as well known as the sympathetic and parasympathetic systems. The enteric nervous system (ENS) is located in the gastrointestinal system and is home to trillions of bacteria, fungi, virus, and protozoa variations, known as the microbiome. Research conducted by Coelho and team (2013) investigated the gut microbiome of dogs and found a 63% overlap in similar microbes with the human gut. Cohabitation with dogs supports a diverse, resilient microbiome (Se Jin Song et al., 2013) and this exposure can improve immune function and mental and physical health. A downside for dogs that share domestic households, however, is exposure to similar environmental hazards and health conditions as their humans. Dogs have been suggested to function as sentinels of environmental exposure as they may become ill prior to humans from a shared contact with a toxin (such as asbestos/mesothelioma). Dogs that share a 'diabetogenic' lifestyle may also contract diabetes type 2 along with its human (Hernandez et al., 2022).

Emotion, Sociality, and Cognition

Neural adaptations underpin canine capability to express emotion and intent in interpretable form and to recognize and respond accordingly to human emotion (Muller et al., 2015). While historical attitudes have denied or heavily debated the capability of the canine species to experience emotion, research has shown that they do have a range of emotions (Bekoff, 2007; Panksepp, 2004). Dogs can also experience emotional contagion with humans (Yong & Ruffman, 2014). Dogs and other animals have, relatively recently, been granted the status of 'sentience' which acknowledges their ability to experience emotions, consciousness, and intention.

In humans, the substantial increase in sociality is believed to be associated with the enhanced complexity of the brain. In canines, there are mixed views on the precise causal mechanisms that brought dogs to an enhanced level. These changes, however, are genuine, functional, and now genetically and neurobiologically supported, thus heritable. The question arises if two species of such disparate morphology can advance and gain so much from an interspecies affiliation, will our relationship evolve even further?

Several researchers have trained dogs to remain still while unrestrained inside a functional magnetic resonance imaging (fMRI) scanner. This has allowed scientists to view brain activity, opening the door to paradigm-changing studies of the canine. Dogs are believed to be the best model for studying human social behaviors due to the close relationship and abundant similarities. One team of researchers found that dogs do possess neurobiological specialization for social processing. The bilateral temporal cortex, part of the ventral visual pathways, is the neural correlate for canine perception and processing of human faces (Dilks et al., 2015).

Canine cognition has been an increased subject of interest due to their social cognition and amazing capabilities for social behavior and communication with humans. The unique capability of dogs to communicate with humans might imply that dogs possess a high level of cognition. Canines have surpassed primates in multiple measurements of interpersonal skills, yet their skill set is not consistent across domains. Research shows that canine cognition is organized similarly to humans, yet dogs show considerable differences between social and nonsocial capabilities (MacLean et al., 2017). The results of multiple studies lead to the potential conclusion that the exceptionality of canine interspecific social and communicative behaviors is a narrow and specialized cognition. This type of almost 'canine savant' skill set is proposed to be a phenomenon of coevolution and represents more of an exquisite sensitivity and attunement to humans rather than an advanced global cognition (Wynne, 2016). Using the encephalization quotient (EQ), a ratio between the brain and body size, a score of 'EQ=1' indicates an average brain size for body weight. Humans have an EQ of seven and the typical dog score is 1.2.

In spite of differences between humans and dogs, both species share all of the primary brain structures, including the cerebral cortex, cerebellum, and brainstem, amygdala, hippocampus, and basal ganglia (Berns, 2020). The brain of the domestic dog has the primary structures and connectivity that support primary emotion functions. They have a limbic system, nucleus accumbens, a well-connected amygdala, insula, and a cingulate cortex (Kujala, 2017).

Individual breeds and even more so, individual dogs, vary widely in intelligence and traits. Some dogs are highly proficient at learning a word or label for an object. With minimal training, these dogs can quickly associate words and objects, such as 'ball' or 'teddy.' Chaser, a border collie, was able to learn over 1,000 words, methodically taught by John Pilley, a college professor at Wofford College (Pilley & Reid, 2011). Chaser must have also been gifted with patience, attentiveness, and a high level of interest, skills which would be necessary to participate in any long-term training.

Many professionals use cognition test batteries as they have proved highly useful in selecting dogs for working roles. Performance can be associated with specific cognitive measures, and evaluators were able to obtain a 95% accuracy rate in predicting which dogs would pass the proficiency tests for specific jobs *prior* to training (Hare & Ferrans, 2021). Research found six different factors that accounted for variances between dogs, identifying them as 'domains of intelligence.' They included social referencing, inhibition, cooperative communication, working memory, perceptual bias, and discriminatory ability (MacLean et al., 2017). These factors offer a different set of requisites that are unique and separate from compliance, and may be useful in identifying a dog for therapeutic work.

Conclusion

The tract of evolution has produced dramatic changes in the human and canine species that can be identified and generalized in multiple spheres. This process, though, has also produced a considerable heterogeneity within species and individuals, and it is essential to recognize that variants exist in all domains. Humans are highly social beings and require relationships to survive and to thrive. Our health and well-being is directly correlated with positive empathic relationships. The same can be alleged for dogs. Their high sociality, interest and attentiveness in humans, and drive to interact and coexist, evolved from the ancient bond. What began during the Pleistocene Epoch has evolved into a relationship that has a profound potential for healing and restoring regulation and well-being in children impacted by trauma.

References

Adachi, I., Kuwahata, H., & Fujita, K. (2007). Dogs recall their owner's face upon hearing the owner's voice. *Animal Cognition*: 10(1): 17–21. https://doi.org/10.1007/s10071-006-0025-8

Andics, A., Gacsi, M., Farago, T., Kis, A., & Miklósi, A. (2014). Voice-sensitive regions in the dog and human brain are revealed by comparative fMRI. *Current Biology*; 27(8): 1248–1249. https://doi.org/10.1016/jcub.2014.01.058

Axelsson, E., Ratnakumar, A., Arendt, M.L., & Maqbool, K. (2013). The genomic signature of dog domestication reveals adaptation to a starch-rich diet. *Nature*; 495: 360–364. https://doi.org/10.1038/nature.11837

Beetz, A., Uvnas-Moberg, K., Julius, H., & Kotrschal, K. (2012). Psychosocial and psychophysiological effects of human-animal interactions: the possible role of oxytocin. *Frontiers in Psychology*; 3: 234. https://doi.org/10.3389/fpsyg.2012.00234

Bekoff, M. (2007). *The Emotional Lives of Animals*. Novato, CA: New World Library

Bekoff, M. (2013). *Why do Dogs Hump and Bees Get Depressed?* Novato, CA: New World Library.

Berns, G. (2021). Functional MRI in awake unrestrained dogs. *PLoS One*. https://doi.org/10.1371/journal.pone.0038027

Berns, G. (2020). Decoding the canine mind. *Cerebrum*, 2020 Mar–Apr:2020:cer-04–20. Retrieved from PMID: 32395197/PMCID:PMC7192336 Published online 2020 Apr 1.

Bird, D., Buelow, S., Jacquemetton, C., Evans, A., & Van Valkenburgj. B. (2020). Domesticating olfaction: Dog breeds, including scent hounds, have reduced cribriform plate morphology relative to wolves. https://doi.org/10.1002/ar.24518

Cafazzo, S., Marshall-Pescini, S., Lazzaroni, M., Virányi, Z., & Range, F. (2017). The effect of domestication on post-conflict management: Wolves reconcile while dogs avoid each other. *Royal Society Open Science*; 5: 171553. https://doi.org/10.1098/rsos.171553

Cordoni, G. & Palagi, E. (2019). Back to the future: A glance over wolf social behavior to understand dog-human relationship. *Animals (Basel)*; 9: 991. https://doi.org/10.3390/ani0110991

Cuaya, L.V., Hernandez-Perez, R., & Concha, L. (2016). Our faces in the dog's brain: Functional imaging reveals temporal cortex activation during perception of human faces. *PLoS One*; 11(3):e0149431. https://doi.org/10.1371/journal.pone.0140431

D'Aniello, B., Semin, G.R., Alterisio, A., Aria, M., & Scandurra, A. (2018a). Interspecies transmission of emotional information via chemosignals: from humans to dogs (Canis lupus familiaris). *Animal Cognition*; 21: 67–78. https://doi.org/10.1007/s10071-017-1139-x

D'Aniello, M., d'Ingeo, S., Minunno, M. & Quaranta, A. (2018b). Communication in dogs. *Animals (Basel)*; 8(8): 131. https://doi.org/10.3390/ani8080131

Diamond, M., Krech, D., & Rosenzweig, M.R. (1964). The effects of an enriched environment on the histology of the rat cerebral cortex. *The Journal of Comparative Neurology*; 123(1): 111–119. https://doi.org/10.1002/cne.901230110

Dilks, D.D., Cook, P., Weiller, S.K., Berns, H.P., Spivak, M., & Berns, G.S. (2015). Awake fMRI reveals a specialized region in dog temporal cortex for face processing. *Peer J*; 3:e1115. https://doi.org/10.7717/peerj.1115

Ferrari, P.F. & Coude, G. (2018). Mirror neurons, embodied emotion, and empathy. In K.Z. Meyza & A. Knapska (Eds.), *Neuronal Correlates of Empathy: From Rodent to Human* (p. 67–77). Elsevier Academic Press. https://doi.org/10.1016/B978-0-12-805397-3.00006-1

Gabor, A., Andics, A., Miklósi, A., Czeibert, K., Carreiro, C., & Gasci, M. (2021). Social relationship-dependent neural response to speech in dogs. *NeuroImage*; 243: 118480. https://doi.org/10.1016/j.neuroimage.2021.118480

Gallese, V. (2001).The 'shared manifold' hypothesis: From mirror neurons to empathy. In E. Thompson (Ed.), *Between Ourselves: Second-person Issues in the Study of Consciousness* (pp. 33–50). Upton Pyne, Exeter, UK: Imprint Academic.

Grandin, T. & Johnson, C. (2009). *Animals Make Us Human*. New York, NY: Houghton Mifflin Harcourt Publishing Co.

Hare, B., Call, J., & Tomasello, M. (1998). Communication of food location between human and dog (canis familiaris). *Evolution of Communication*; 2(1): 137–159. https://doi.org/10.1075/eoc.2.1.06har

Hare, B., & Ferrans, M. (2021). Is cognition the secret to working dog success? *Animal Cognition*. https://doi.org/10.1007/s10071.021.01491-7

Hare, B., Wobber, V., & Wrangham, R. (2012).The self-domestication hypothesis: evolution of bonobo psychology is due to selection against aggression. *Animal Behavior*: 1–13. https://doi.org/10.1016/j.anbehav.2011.12.007

Herbeck, Y.E., Eliava, E.M., & MacLean, E.L. (2017). Fear, love, and the origins of canid domestication: An oxytocin hypothesis. *Comprehensive Psychoneuroendocrinology*; 9:100100. https://doi.org/10.1016/j.cpnec.2021.100100

Herbeck, Y.E., Eliava, M., Grinevich, V., & MacLean, E.L. (2022). Fear, love, and the origins of canid domestication: An oxytocin hypothesis. *Compr Psychoneuroendocrinol*; 9:100100. https://doi.org/10.1016/j.cpnec.2021.100100

Hernandez, J., Rhimi, S., Kriaa, A., Mariaule, V., Boudaya, H., Drut, A., Jabaoui, A., Mkaouar, H., Saidi, A., Biourge, V., Borgi, M.A., Rhimi, M., & Maguin, E. (2022). Domestic Environment and Gut Microbiota: Lessons from Pet Dogs. *Microorganisms*; 10: 949. https://doi.org/10.3390/microorganisms10050949

Huber, L., Racca, A., Scaf, B., Virányi, Z., & Range, F. (2013). Discrimination of familiar human faces in dogs (Canis familaris). *Learning and Motivation*; 44(4): 258–269. https://doi.org/10.1016/j.lmot.2013.04.005

Jeannin, S., Gilbert, C., Mathieu, A., & Leboucher, G. (2017). Pet-directed speech draws adults dogs' attention more efficiently than adult-directed speech. *Scientific Reports*; 7 (4980).

Kaminski, J., Hynds, J., Morris, P, & Waller, B.M. (2017). Human attention affects facial expressions in domestic dogs. *Scientific Reports*; 7: 12914.

Kaminski, J., & Nitzschner, M. (2013). Do dogs get the point? A review of dog-human communication ability. *Learning and Motivation*; 44: 294–302. https://dx.doi.org/10.1016/j.lmot.2013.05.001

Kaminski, J., Waller, B.B., Digo, R., Harstone-Rose, A., & Burrows, A.M. (2019). Evolution of facial muscle anatomy in dogs. *Proceedings of the National Academy of Sciences*. https://doi.org/10.1073/pnas.1820653116

Kis, A., Hernadi, A., Miklósi, B., Kanizsar, O., & Topál, J. (2017). The way dogs (canis familiaris) look at human emotional faces is modulated by oxytocin. An eye –tracking study. *Frontiers in Behavioral Neuroscience*. https://doi.org.10.3389/frbeh.2017.00210

Kokocinska-Kusiak, A., Woszczylo, M., Zybala, M., Maciocha, J., Barlowska, K., & Dzieciol, M. (2021). Canine olfaction: Physiology, behavior, and possibilities for practical applications. *Animals (Basel)*; 11(8):2463. https://doi.org.10.3390/ani11082463

Kortekaas, K. & Kotrschal, K. (2019). Does socio-ecology drive differences in alertness between wolves and dogs when resting? *Behavioural Processes*; 166, A. 103877. https://doi.org/10.1016/j.beproc.2019.05.024

Kujala, M.V. (2017). Canine emotions as seen through human social cognition. *Animal Sentience*; 14 (1). https://doi.org/10.51291/2377-7478.1114

LeDoux, J. (1996). *The Emotional Brain*. New York: Simon & Schuster.

LeDoux, J. (2012). Evolution of human emotion: a view through fear. *Progress in Brain Research*; 195: 431–432. https://doi.org/10.1016/B978-0-444-53860-4.00021-0

Lorenz, K. (1954). *Man Meets Dog*. London: Methuen.

MacLean & Hare (2015). Evolution. Dogs hijack the human bonding pathway. *Science*; 348(1). https://doi.org/10.1126/science.aab1200

MacLean, E. L., Herrmann, E., Suchindran, S., & Hare, B. (2017). Individual differences in cooperative communicative skills are more similar between dogs and humans than chimpanzees. *Animal Behavior*; 126: 41–51. https://doi.org/10.1016/j.anbehav.2017.01.005

McEwen, B.S. & Morrison, J.H. (2013). The brain on stress: Vulnerability and plasticity of the prefrontal cortex over the life course. *Neuron*; 79(1): 16–29. https://doi.org.10.1016//j.neuron.2013.06.028

Muller, C.A., Schmitt, K., Barber, A.L., Huber, L. (2015). Dogs can discriminate emotional expressions of human faces. *Current Biology* https://doi.org/10.1016/k/cib.2014.12.055

Nagasawa, M., Mitsui, S., En, S., Ohtani, N., & Ohta, M. et al. (2015). Oxytocin-gaze positive loop and the coevolution of human-dog bonds. *Science*; 348: 333–336. https://doi.org/10.1126/science.1261022

Olmert, M.D. (2009). *Made for Each Other*. Cambridge Center, Cambridge: Da Capo Press.

Ostrander, E.A., & Wayne, R.K. (2005). The canine genome. *Genome Research* 15: 1706–1716.

Palagi, E., Cordoni. G., Demuru, E. & Bekoff, M. (2016). Fair play and its connection with social tolerance, reciprocity and the ethology of peace. *Behavior*; 153: (9–11); 1195–1216. Palagi https://dx.doi.org/10.1163/1568539X-00003336

Panksepp, J. (2004). *Affective Neuroscience*. Oxford University Press.

Panksepp, J. (2005). Beyond a joke: From Animal Laughter to Human Joy. *Science*; 308:62–63.

Perri, A. (2016). A wolf in dog's clothing: Initial dog domestication and Pleistocene wolf variation. *Journal of Archaeological Science*; 68:1–4. https://doi.org/10.1016/j.jas.2016.02.003

Perri, A., Feuerborn, T.R., Frantz, L.A.F., Larson, G., Malhi, R.S., Meltzer, D.J., & Witt, K.E. (2021). Dog domestication and the dual dispersal of people and dogs into the Americas. *Anthropology*; 118(6). https://doi.org/10.1073/pnas.2010083118

Persson, M.E., Trottier, A.J., Belteky, J., Roth, L.S.V., Roth, L.S.V., & Jensen, P. (2017). Intranasal oxytocin and a polymorphism in the oxytocin receptor gene are associated with human-directed social behavior in golden retriever dogs. *Hormones and Behavior*; 95: 85–93. https://doi.org/10.1016/j.yhbeh.2017.07-016

Pierotti, R. & Fogg, B.R. (2017). *The First Domestication: How Wolves and Humans Coevolved*. New Haven, CT: Yale University Press. https://doi.org/10.2307/j.ctt1wc7rbm

Pilley, J.W., & Reid, A.K. (2011). Border collie comprehends object names as verbal referents. *Behavioural Processes*; 86(2): 184–195.

Range, F.& Virányi, Z. (2014). Tracking the evolutionary origins of dog-human cooperation. the 'Canine Cooperation Hypothesis' *Frontiers in Psychology*; 5: 1582. https://doi.org/10.3389/fpsyg.2014.01582

Rizzolatti, G. & Craighero, L. (2004). The mirror-neuron system. *Annual Review of Neuroscience*; 27: 169–192. https://doi.org/10.1146/annurev.neuro.27.070203.144230

Romero, T., & Nagawawa, M. (2014). Oxytocin promotes social bonding in dogs. *Psychol & Cognitive Science*; 111(25): 9085–9090. https://doi.org/10.1073/pnas.1322868111

Sahlen, P., Yanhu, L., Su, J., Kubinyi, E., Wange, G-D, Savolainen, P. (2021). Variants that differentiate wolf and dog populations are enriched in regulatory elements. *Genome Biology and Evolution*; 13(4): evab076 Sahlen https://doi.org/10.1093/gbe/evab076

Schleidt, W.M., & Shalter, M.D. (2003). Co-evolution of humans and canids: An alternative view of dog domestication: HOMO HOMINI LUPUS? *Evolution and Cognition*; 9(1): 57–72.

Schleidt, W.M., & Shalter, M.D. (2018). Dogs and mankind: Coevolution on the move-an update. *Human Ethology Bulletin*; 33(1): 15–38. https://doi.org/10.22330/heb/331/015-038

Serpell, J. (2021). Commensalism or cross-species adoption? A critical review of theories of wolf domestication. *Frontiers in Veterinary Science*. https://doi.org/10.3389/fvets.2021.662370

Shipman, P. (2017). *The Invaders, How Humans and Their Dogs Drove Neanderthals to Extinction*. Cambridge, MA: Belknap Press, An Imprint of Harvard University Press.

Siniscalchi, M., d'Ingeo, S., & Quaranta, A. (2016). The dog nose 'KNOWS' fear: Asymmetric nostril use during sniffing at canine and human emotional stimuli. *Behavioural Brain Research*; 304: 34–41.

Siniscalchi, M., d'Ingeo, S., & Quaranta, A. (2018). Orienting asymmetries and physiological reactivity in dogs' response to human emotional faces. *Learning & Behavior*; 46: 574–585.

Song, S-J., Lauber, C., Costello, E.K., Lozupone, C.A., Humphrey, G., Berg-Lyons, D., Caporaso, J.G., Knights, D., Clemente, J.C., Nakielny, S., Gordon, J.I., Fierer, N., & Knight, R. (2013). Cohabiting family members share microbiota with one another and with their dogs. *eLife*, 2, e00458. https://doi.org/10.7554/eLife.00458

Udall, M.A.R. (2015). When dogs look back: Inhibition of independent problem-solving behaviour in domestic dogs (Canis lupus) familiaris compared with wolves (Canis lupus). *The Royal Society*. https://doi.org/10.1098/rsbi.2015.0489

Udall, M.A.R., Dorey, N.R., & Wynne, C.D.L. (2010). What did domestication do to dogs? A new account of dogs' sensitivity to human actions. *Biological Reviews/Cambridge Philosophical Society*; 85: 327–345. https://doi.org/10.1111/j.1469-185X.2009.00104.x

vonHoldt, B.M., Shuldiner, E., Janowitz Koch, I., Kartzinel, R.Y., Hogan, A., Brubaker, L., Wanser, S., Stahler, D., Wynne, C.D.L., Ostrander, E.A., Sinsheimer, J.S., & Udell, M.A.R. (2017). Structural variants in genes associated with human Williams-Beuren syndrome underlie stereotypical hyper-sociability in domestic dogs. *Science Advances*; 3(7). https://doi.org/10.1026/sciadv.1700398

Wang, G., Zhai, W., Yang, H-C., Fan, R-X., Li Zhong, X.C., Wang, L., Liu, F., Wu, H., Cheng, L-G., Poyarkov, A.D., Poyarkov, Jr., N.A., Tang, S.S., Zhao, W.M., Gao, Y., Lv, X-M., Irwin, D.M., Savolainen, P., Wu, C-I., & Zhang, Y-P. (2013). The genomics of selection in dogs and the parallel evolution between dogs and humans. *Nature Communications*; 4 (1860). https://doi.org/10.1038/ncomms2814

Wynne, C.D.L. (2016). What is special about dog cognition? *Current Directions in Psychological Science*; 25(5). https://doi.org/10.1177/0963721416657540

Yong and Ruffman. (2014). Dogs and humans show similar physiological responses to human infant cries. https://doi.org/10.1016/j.beproc.2014.10.006

Zajonc, R.B., (2001). Mere exposure: A gateway to the subliminal. *Current Directions in Psychological Science*; 10(6): 224–228. https://doi.org/10.1111/1467-8721.00154

Zeuner, F.E. (1963). *A History of Domesticated Animals*. New York, NY. Harper & Row.

Chapter 6   The Tao of the Dog

Introduction

The key to understanding the incredible potential of the canine species to heal children is to study the tao of the dog. The word 'tao' is interpreted as the characteristics of dogs that reflect their harmony with nature; their authenticity, elemental perspective, and distinct ability to interpersonally connect. This chapter illuminates the traits, skills, and capabilities of the modern dog through a consolidation of theory, current research, and multidisciplinary literature. Canine mechanisms of change can be understood through multiple lenses and judiciously applied to the healing and restoration of children with dysregulation.

Why the Dog?

Children like Dogs

Scientists at the University of Cambridge conducted a survey of 77 twelve-year-olds to compare the relationship between 'children and their pets' to 'children and their siblings.' The majority responded that they experienced a stronger bond with their pets (Cassels et al., 2017). In a web-based survey of pet owners, responses supported the conclusion that pets provide a consistent source of attachment security and even outrank romantic partners, using multiple measures (Beck & Madresh, 2008). An inference was also drawn that pets of all types surpassed human relationships, in their ability to impart acceptance, calming, and increased self-esteem. Humans with histories of human-inflicted maltreatment will often demonstrate a preference for dogs, as the canine species is widely believed to be safe, trustworthy, and supportive.

Dogs have always fascinated children and the two share a unique kindred relationship. Both share the ability to embrace the moment and love fully and without judgment. Children and dogs can experience life in a realm that is uncomplicated and uncontaminated by adult and worldly concerns. Developmental research has produced substantial evidence of the significance that animals hold for children. According to

DOI: 10.4324/9781003217534-9

research by Melson (2003), animals draw the innate interest of children who instinctively view them as 'like me.' Dogs foster emotional and social development in children through their natural lessons of relationships, life cycles, loyalty, and forgiveness. Children exposed to interspecies relationships have higher self-esteem, empathy, and participation in socially based activities. Dogs have similar socio-behavioral traits as children and cognitively align with particular stages of human development. (Melson, 2003).

Modern children may not grow up within the natural, animal-filled environments of their farming great-grandparents, but their world is inundated with suggestions of animals. Animals are cast as characters in almost all children's books; animals are central to stories and movies; and in schools, colorful posters of animal figures line the walls and are used to enhance lessons. Stuffed animals are typically found in children's arms, upon their beds, or tucked into backpacks. They serve as transition objects and provide security for kids as they expand their worlds beyond their primary caretakers. These supportive *buddies* foster comfort, sooth nerves, and often, the genuine, specific, qualities of the live animal are projected into the toy that portrays protection, confidence, or mystical power to the child.

Dogs can be a Good Friend

Dogs are really good listeners, and they do not talk back. They do not gossip or spread rumors and they will not judge, criticize, or belittle others. Dogs offer a uniquely attuned relationship that permits sharing or coupling of emotional and physical states. It is an affiliation that does not require language, contracts, or contingent behaviors.

Dogs are similar to children as they tend to be uncomplicated and undefended, though the innocence of both can be tarnished by maltreatment and betrayal. Both require interpersonal and social experiences for growth and are highly vulnerable and dependent upon adult humans. Dogs and children have little power and are not typically afforded many choices in their lives.

Many dogs will wait patiently until you are ready to show them attention. They forgive periodic bad moods and behavior, and are loyal in the truest sense of the word. Dogs can make you feel better about yourself and can even make *others* feel better about *you*. They increase confidence, curiosity, and a willingness to engage. Their honest and uncomplicated behavior seeds empathic behavior, kindness, and a desire to care for them. Dogs are often incredibly tolerant, grateful, and forgiving, perhaps even more so than humans. While the majority of child development research has focused upon the child's relationships with other humans, Gail Melson argues for a more *biocentric* approach, incorporating the interspecific relationships that kids have with animals, nature, and all living things (Melson, 2003).

Dogs sense fear, distress, and pain in children and experience a physiological reaction that reflects an emotional response. They can also calm the distressing arousal of others through coregulation, producing feelings of safety and comfort (Parish-Plass & Pfeiffer, 2019). Canine anatomy has evolved (particularly the face) to enhance communication with humans, which facilitates sharing of emotion (Kaminski et al., 2019). The modern dog is also capable of synchronizing emotions, behaviors, and physiological arousal with a child. Synchronization connects and joins the two and creates a unique space for sharing emotions, play, or to access states of calm and safety.

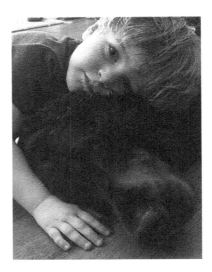

Facilitating positive bonds and interactions between the child and a dog can instill necessary elements for healing. The coevolution and canine domestication resulted in the selection of traits that underlie a profoundly attuned relationship between humans and dogs. The rapid adaptation to our anthropocentric world reflects the dog's incredible receptiveness to human emotional and social communication (Miklósi, 2016).

Most humans would agree that dogs have done some heavy lifting along the journey to our modern relationship. Some would call them 'masters of adaptation,' as they have adapted and morphed to fit into the human world. Dogs have developed a bias toward humans, are socially and emotionally attentive, and seek human attention and approval. Evolution has equipped them with human-like social skills (Hare & Tomasello, 2005). The social behaviors of both species are supported by similar hormonal and neurobiological organizations.

These traits and abilities underlie the capacity of the dog to form healing relationships with children. When a child feels overwhelmed and alone, betrayed by other humans, the dog can offer not just tolerance, but security, coregulation of affect and physiological arousal, friendship, social support, and unconditional acceptance.

Intrinsic Therapeutic Mechanisms of Dogs

Attachment

Through the thousands of years of human–canine coevolution, dogs seem to have drafted social and cognitive systems involved in the attachment process (Hare and Tomasello, 2005), resulting in a shared neurobiological substrate for attachment (Nagasawa et al., 2009). This interspecies relationship mirrors the caregiver–child attachment bond as it reflects attachment-based behaviors evident in human attachments including safe haven, secure-base effects, protest upon separation, and proximity seeking (Kis et al., 2017; Payne et al., 2016; Zilcha-Mano et al., 2011) Attachment relationships coregulate affect and arousal through neurobiological processes that involve oxytocin, the vagal system and finely tuned endocrine cocktails (Porges, 2005). Attachment with a dog creates a powerful source of social support for the child and promotes these physiological and psychological benefits (Jalongo, 2015).

Humans have shaped a dependence in dogs that is similar to children and they rely on us for food, protection, and care. Their behaviors seem to distinctly evoke human attention and response, similar to the infant (Prato-Previde & Valeschi, 2014); and unlike wolves, dogs look to humans for help in seemingly unsolvable tasks (Miklósi, 2016).

The human–canine relationship can be particularly powerful to children who lack a secure attachment with human caregivers (Wanser et al., 2019) and can fulfill the attachment needs of the child (Zilcha-Mano et al., 2012). Of significance to canine-assisted psychotherapy was the discovery that an unhealthy caregiver–child attachment did not translate to the quality of human–pet attachment. Julius and colleagues (2013) also note that the incidence of secure attachment to pets was four times higher than secure human–human attachments. Children who have suffered interpersonal betrayal can become disconnected and distrustful of all humans, and dogs have been shown to be preferable companions to children and can serve as a model for healthy relationships (VanFleet & Faa-Thompson, 2010). Canine participation in an attachment relationship enhances the therapeutic process, instills trust, and invokes a felt safety (Parish-Plass, 2008). This relationship serves as a bridge to treatment and a step toward the objective of reconnecting with humans for social support (VanFleet & Faa-Thompson, 2017). Secure attachments strengthen the resilience of a child by fostering affective and neurobiological regulation and increasing their capacity for supportive relationships (Ulmer-Yaniv et al., 2021).The unavailability of a protective relationship is a substantial factor in trauma outcomes (Shonkoff and Garner, 2012).

The traumatized child must acquire a sense of safety if there is any chance for them to be reset on a healthier trajectory of development. These children need the connection of healthy relationships to help support and coregulate their disrupted neurobiological states. Protection and safety are core provisions of a healthy attachment. Sourcing key components of healthy attachment relationships such as coregulation of affect and arousal, safety, synchronicity, rhythm, and reciprocity, along with sequential mastery of tasks can provide useful targets and guidelines for therapeutic interventions. Observation, interaction, and modeling of animal relational and social behavior can have significant influence upon the child's attitudes, schema, and behavior. These interventions facilitate healthy behavior, neurobiological and domain regulation, and offer the child an alternative template of a healthy relationship. The child is able to view and experience positive relationships which can be internalized as accessible representations that travel with them through life.

Dogs Know What We are Feeling

The seeking of information from other conspecifics and heterospecifics represents a complex and advanced social cognition that was seeded during the coevolution (Nagasawa et al., 2011). The establishment and maintenance of a mutually beneficial social relationship requires communication mechanisms to share emotions, social intentions, and to enable the prediction of behavior. The canine is uniquely capable of reading and interpreting human communication, and these skills support their efficacious therapeutic skills.

Research shows that modern dogs can recognize human emotions through facial expressions, vocalizations, and odor, using visual, auditory, and olfactory systems (Andics et al., 2014; Muller et al., 2015). Dogs were found to be capable of multimodal sourcing, mining and interpreting information from more than one sensory mode inferring a cognitive capability not seen beyond humans (Albuquerque et al., 2016).

Reading our Faces

The dog seeks information from facial expressions and can discern if someone is watching them (paying attention). They understand nodding, and can interpret the meaning of a directed human gaze (Hare et al., 1998). Humans express a great deal of information with their eyes, face, and gestures. Dogs recognize human faces, can discriminate emotions, and can also connect a face with a possible outcome (Nagasawa et al., 2011). A study by researchers at the University of Helsinki investigated eye gaze tracking to evaluate how dogs observe emotional expressions of humans and other dogs. The results indicated that gaze persisted for the longest period of time upon the eyes (Pitteri et al., 2014) though dogs used the entire face to gain social information (Huber et al., 2013). Dogs will attend to human eyes to infer their interest and intention and this skill becomes impaired when the face is masked (Somppi et al., 2016). The facial areas that dogs seek for information can vary depending on the valence. Dogs look at the eyes and mouth of negative expressions (Somppi et al., 2016) and the forehead area during positive emotional expression (Barber et al., 2016).

There is interesting research into hemispheric asymmetry of human and canine emotional expression, processing, and biases with variances between sensory modes. Studies show that dogs have a right hemisphere bias for processing happiness, fear, and anger, and use the left side to process surprise states (Siniscalchi, 2017). Dogs also share a left gaze bias with humans when looking at upright images, a bias not used in observations of other dogs or objects (Guo et al., 2009). The accurate perception of threat is an evolutionarily adaptive skill, thus one that evokes attention bias. Dogs were found to maintain a longer gaze at threatening animal faces, though aggressive human faces do tend to evoke an avoidance response.

Effective training can focus and increase the attention of a dog toward a human, yet as a species, their level of attentiveness goes far beyond simple learned behavior. This trait has become neurobiologically embedded through evolution. Dogs attend and respond to social cues and match their response appropriately with the valence of facial and vocalized expressions of emotions. Dogs have emotionally directed expectations, and are highly sensitive to human emotional states.

Dogs outperform apes in their ability to follow human gestures. They are able to follow a pointed finger or human gaze to determine direction. They match human infants on the interpretation of the intention of gestural signals, showing social cognition (Hare, 2017).The reactions of dogs to various stimuli are typically identified through behavioral observations, yet there are neurobiological correlates to these responses that can now be scientifically measured. Dogs react to emotional and social cues with changes in heart rate, behavior, and variations in cortisol and oxytocin (OT).

Interpreting Vocalizations

Research using fMRI technology found that canines possess neural systems similar to humans that are dedicated to interpretation of vocal sounds, including sensitivity to emotional valence. Like humans, dogs use the left hemisphere to process words, and the right hemisphere to process intonation and emotion. Andics and colleagues also found increased activation in reward regions when intonation was consistent with praise words. Other studies show that dogs can discriminate between familiar and unknown words and will pay increased attention to novel words (Andics et al., 2014). One study investigated dog responses to human crying and found increased cortisol levels and alerting behavior in dogs during exposure. When owners cried, their dog would approach and lick and nuzzle them. The results of this study, consistent with others, revealed that human crying transmits emotional valence to dogs, and they recognize and react with physiological arousal, reflecting a stress response (Yong and Ruffman 2014). Vocalizations that are nonlinguistic emotional expressions are believed to be primeval and evolutionarily conserved (Farago et al., 2014).

Olfactory

Dogs employ their olfactory system for information, communication, identification, interpretation, and decision making. The typical dog possesses around 300 million scent receptors, or about 50 times the number in humans. They can detect a substance concentration diluted to one part per trillion. The proficiency of the canine olfactory system even exceeds modern instrument odorant analytics. In a proof of concept French study, canines demonstrated a sensitivity rating of 97% for identifying COVID-19, beating many 15-minute antigen tests (Devellier et al., 2022).

While most people realize that canines use scent to identify and differentiate between individual dogs, they also apply this skill to humans (D'Aniello et al., 2017). Though dogs also use other sensory systems for identification today, scent remains an evolutionarily conserved primary mechanism to gather information.

Humans transmit emotional states through emitted chemosignals (de Groot et al., 2017), and dogs are now believed to be capable of detecting emotions via these chemical messages (de Groot et al., 2012). Significant research shows that dogs have astute sensitivity to the body odors of humans that are produced during two different emotional states, fear and happiness (Kokocinska-Kusiak et al., 2021).

Dogs are also capable of forecasting behavior through scent. In one study, dogs were found to be predictive of volatility or impending aggressive behavior in hospitalized psychiatric patients. While they identified all of the imminent episodes, however, dogs were not always capable of identifying the specific patient who was culpable. This implied a potential universality of a detectable scent for aggression which could be highly useful in numerous group situations and settings (Bakeman et al., 2019).

Chemosignals occur without intention and below the level of consciousness. Researchers studying emotional contagion between dogs found that the presence of chemosignals in the sender induced a similar emotional state in the receiver (de Groot et al., 2017). The response of dogs to chemosignals is mediated by environmental context and training (Kokocinska-Kusiak et al., 2021). In a therapeutic context with children, a dog with these skills could be highly useful, if trained to signal the clinician of impending shifts in emotional and behavioral states.

How Dogs Communicate with Others

Canines communicate information to others using visual, auditory, olfactory, and tactile signals along with posture and movement. Evolutionarily conserved signals announce the presence of a predator, claim territorial dominance, reveal fear and aggression, and announce the discovery of a food source. Today, dogs employ a similar yet broader repertoire of communication signals with both conspecifics and humans, using their head, face, lips, teeth, and tail for expression. The nuances of postural changes, facial expressions, and proximity are significant cues to the dog's state, yet many humans, particularly the young, do not always learn these signals. Additionally, human actions have diminished the capability of some breeds to signal their emotions and intentions through tail docking, coat selection, and ear stiffening measures (Bradshaw & Rooney, 2016).

Significant numbers of children are bitten each year in the United States by dogs that are reported as 'familiar with no previous history of aggression.' Children with dysregulated behaviors are at higher risk for dog bites for several reasons. There is a higher level of unpredictability in children with disorders of attention, behavior, and impulsivity. When the underlying neurobiology is dysregulated, as it is in children with trauma histories, their heightened arousal and anxiety may be stressful or threatening to dogs with similar histories. Emotional contagion is a mechanism by which a present dog (or another child) picks up the displayed emotion. The child who is highly anxious, agitated, and hyperactive can transmit that state to the dog. This can be troublesome not just for safety, but the dog can be unduly exposed to experiencing and absorbing the stress of the child.

As a core component of canine-assisted programming is to establish a milieu that provides the child with a felt sense of safety, it makes sense that the child's *actual* safety should also be ensured. Beyond the realm of the therapeutic environment, attaining a genuine sense of self-efficacy in personal safety is important to translate into other environments. This is one reason to ensure the child becomes capable in the identification and interpretation of canine communication. This awareness optimizes the ability of the two to bond and form an attachment and if this ability is absent *and* unattainable, can compromise treatment.

Most *components* of language are shared with other species' modes of communication. However, a primary difference between humans and other species is not that we have something to think about, but that we can communicate what we think about (Fitch, 2019). Fitch shares a thought-provoking perspective when he states that the capability to present and manipulate concepts is an antecedent to language and that the understanding of animal communication should be explored through the channels of cognition. The implication is that a lack of capability to communicate what one knows with verbal language does not prove a lack of knowledge (Fitch, 2019). Dogs have come a long way in their ability to communicate with humans, and perhaps it is incumbent upon humans to further *our* ability to interpret what they have to share.

Providing a Bridge: The Canine Mechanism of Connection

Research has provided substantial evidence of the multiple positive effects that dogs have upon humans through human–animal interaction (HAI). Benefits have been linked to multiple domains including psychological, physiological, social, cognitive, behavioral, and intrapersonal (conceptualizing oneself) and interpersonal (relationships and attachment) function. The working psychotherapy dog functions as a coregulator, attachment figure, and citadel of safety, yet these functions are not the end target. They are the scaffold that supports the child in stepping across the chasm between their dysregulated and disconnected state, and a regulated, resilient, and interpersonally connected being. The dog is a living breathing bridge.

Physiological Benefits of Canine Interactions

While most perceptions of the positive impact of a dog are expressed in terms of emotions and perceptions, today, science can provide evidence of physiological benefits, as they are detectable and measurable through biomarkers and advanced neuroimaging. Research shows that the presence of a dog dampens fear and anxiety (Kertes et al., 2017). Dogs also can instill a sense of competency, lower stress levels, and attenuate cardiovascular arousal when facing a stressful challenge (Zilcha-Mano et al., 2012). The child is more likely to relax with canine support and as their system calms, their interest and attention increases, and engagement and participation are enhanced.

A study conducted by Marti and colleagues used functional near-infrared spectroscopy (fNIRS) in a controlled trial to measure prefrontal brain activation in healthy subjects as they interacted with live dogs and plush animals. While activation occurred in both groups, those with the live dog showed stronger attention, higher neural activation, and heightened emotional arousal (Marti et al., 2022).

Parish-Plass and Pfeiffer (2019) write that the incorporation of canines into therapeutic processes with children generates neurobiological stabilization, regulation, and integration. Oxytocin is activated through child–dog interactions which helps restore neural regulation and begins a loop between physiology and socio-emotional, behavioral, and cognitive functional domains. Regulated neurobiology improves domain function and those improvements circle back to help regulate neurobiology. The dog sits at this intersection and serves as a catalyst for this bidirectional process.

Friedmann et al. (1980) conducted a highly referenced study of the physiological effects that the presence of animals and human–canine interaction have upon human physiology. Evidence revealed positive effects of

HAI that included decreases in respiration, heart rate, and muscular tension, indicating a reduction in sympathetic nervous system (SNS) activity. They concluded that these shifts demonstrated a neurobiological mechanism of animals that reduces stress in humans (Friedmann et al., 1980).

Another study of children during medical appointments revealed reduced blood pressure and heart rate with the presence of a dog (Nagengast et al., 1997). Neurotransmitters and hormones, such as serotonin, dopamine, and oxytocin (Beetz et al., 2012) and opioids (Olmert, 2009) also serve as chemical mechanisms that support these physiological benefits. Research that introduced service dogs to children with autism found morning levels of cortisol (a hormonal indicator of stress) were lowered from 58% to 10% with the presence of a dog (Viau et al., 2010). Another study found that short-term interactions between humans and dogs caused a rapid and significant decrease in cortisol levels 15 and 30 minutes after interactions began (Handlin, 2011).

As stress states impair attention, concentration, and learning, regulation of hyper- and hypo-stress arousal levels would logically improve focus, connection, engagement, and participation in therapy interventions. Oxytocin, in collaboration with other neuroendocrine components, regulates numerous mammalian functions. The oxytocin (OT) system has been highlighted in earlier chapters for the role it played through evolution and the continued responsibility it carries for attachment, relationships, and social behavior. Oxytocin is the queen of adaptation and has revised its role innumerable times across 700 million years to support humans and mammals in adjustments to their environment (Olmert, 2009).

Facial expression and mutual gaze, core aspects of the caregiver–infant attachment experience increase oxytocin and are also relevant to the human–canine bond. Research conducted by Odendaal and Meintjes (2003) revealed that oxytocin levels in owners and dogs almost doubled during their positive interactions that involved face-to-face gazing. Increases were also seen in dopamine and beta endorphins in humans. Dopamine has a role in multiple physiological functions including memory, reward, motivation, and movement. Dysregulated dopamine levels have been associated with multiple mental and neurobiological disorders.

Citing supporting research, Meg Olmert (2009) hypothesized that this reciprocal neurobiological process shaped relational and social exchanges and coevolved in humans and wolves, seeding the human–animal bond. Researchers also credit these processes with promoting an emotional *evolution*, subsidized by oxytocin as it attenuated fear and the stress response and supported affiliation and prosocial behaviors (Carter, 2014).

Sufficient levels of OT increase eye contact, mutual gaze, vocal cues, and social touch, essential components of relationships. Oxytocin increases prosocial behaviors and willingness to engage and interact. Trust, social skills, and self-image improve, while negative arousal, depression, and aggression are reduced (Beetz et al., 2012). A groundbreaking study using intranasal administration of OT was found to dampen amygdala reactivity and restore functional connectivity in patients with PTSD, resulting in decreased anxiety (Koch et al., 2016).

In other investigations of the effects of nasal administration of oxytocin, OT was found to increase social sensitivity, attention to human eyes, and prosocial behaviors in canines (Kis et al., 2017). Nagasawa and team (2015) showed that HAI produces OT in both humans and dogs, and that the presence of OT increases human–animal interactions, in what they conceptualized as a bidirectional loop. Beetz and her colleagues (2012) summarized these effects as mechanisms of HAI.

Oxytocin is being studied as a possible pharmacological treatment due its association with positive effects, though there are conflicting results and concerns that might delay its therapeutic use. The release of OT can also be stimulated through behavior, however, which is evidenced through the multiple studies of human dog interactions. The accumulating scientific support for oxytocin that shows its effects on neurobiological processes is exciting and offers a mechanistic theory and option for regulating the damaging effects of trauma. Stimulating OT release through human–canine interactions presents a less complicated approach to mitigating stress effects.

Oxytocin shows significant potential to aid children who suffer from distrust, persistent fear, relational and social deficits, and dysregulation. While additional research is necessary to further develop and enhance efficacious interventions, these early studies of canine-assisted therapy and the potential to confer neurobiological improvements are encouraging. The potential of canine-assisted therapy to reregulate the devastating biological footprint on our most vulnerable population offers a glimpse of what could be the future of trauma treatment.

Accessing the Social Engagement System (SES)

Porges (2017) has predicted that animal-assisted psychotherapy will expand as it is increasingly evident that HAI and the social engagement system (SES) are inextricably linked and are actuated by similar neurobiology. Accessing the SES state does not simply occur if threat signals are absent; it requires the presence of felt safety cues from relational interactions (Porges, 2015). This most recently evolved branch of the stress response system facilitates social connection and prosocial behaviors which promote relationships and social interactions. The dog creates a bridge to the SES as it confers safety, trust, and coregulation, experiences which positively alter neural circuitry. The positive physiological changes conferred by HAI constitute canine mechanisms of change. Interactions with the working psychotherapy dog can recalibrate the child neural circuitry (Carter, 2017) by strengthening functional connectivity between brain regions, improving communication necessary to produce specific functions (Siegel, 2010).

Regulated individuals typically turn to others for social support in times of stress and/or need (Porges, 2005), though children in stress states cannot easily access that form of assistance. When the SES is active, the mobilization and immobilization responses are inhibited allowing the child to feel more regulated and balanced. The reregulation of the stress response system supports the child's willingness and capability to turn toward humans to connect (Porges, 2011). Engaging the SES is a primary goal of ni-CAP as it aligns with the belief that neurobiological regulation is critical for therapeutic participation, progression, and healing. Substantial research has documented many physiological benefits of HAI that provide the substrate for regulation and connection.

Emotional Support

Research studies of HAI have demonstrated improved treatment outcomes (Hunt, 2014) that result from significant reductions in depression, anxiety and negative arousal in children due to canine coregulation (Crossman, 2017). In dysregulated children, the dog serves as emotional support, providing comfort, safety, and increased willingness to share uncomfortable content. The accepting and nonjudgmental nature of the dog assures the child that there will not be consequences for shared thoughts, feelings, or memories. The nurturing tactile support of the proximal dog instills a sense of calm and serves as a safe haven to return to after a difficult experience.

Eliciting Relevant Context

Many traumatized children are unable to verbally present their feelings, memories, or history as the relevant content or memory may be inaccessible. The hippocampus codes explicit memory that can be recalled consciously and has a date or time reference attached to it. Trauma can also be encoded as implicit memory, which exists below consciousness and though it impacts the life of the child, they have no narrative or context that they can connect with explicit feelings. The experience exists in fragments and may produce images or sensations that trigger anxiety, fear, dissociation, or flashbacks. Implicit coding occurs due to the immaturity of the hippocampus (as in preverbal children), elevated cortisol levels during trauma that shut it down, or when dissociation occurs that also hinders hippocampal function. Interaction with dogs can naturally elicit implicit feelings, physiological sensations, thoughts, perspectives, and biases that are not consciously recognized by the child.

Interactions with the dog can facilitate projection which is the process of attributing feelings, traits, and perspectives that are not recognized or believed to be part of oneself, to another. The dog is a living receptacle that is similar to the child, yet not a human, making mentalizing or symbolizing easier. The natural behavior of the dog elicits the internal world of the child. The mirror neuron (MN) system enables the child to subconsciously imagine what another living being is feeling, thinking, or intending. It is a useful therapeutic tool, as the process elicits interpretations and inner content as the child imagines what they would do in a situation.

Cynthia Chandler, in her book, *Animal assisted therapy in counseling (2018)*, describes animal-related symbolism, metaphors, stories, and play as a 'side door' to the inner world of the child. Combining a working psychotherapy dog and play synthesizes the benefits of both, as individually, projection and symbolism will increase. The space between reality and imagination is expanded by the coupling of the two.

The Language of Play is the Same for Children and Canines

Ni-CAP taps the neural circuitry of the brain through employment of the synergistic relationship and interactions of children and dogs. The combination of this synergistically melded duo with play actualizes a formula in which the whole is greater than the sum of the parts; the neurobiological principles of ni-CAP resonate with the neurobiology of play. Bidirectional influences occur that can be viewed as one model potentiating the other. Ni-CAP can be seen as play within the context of relationships or relationships within the context of play.

Dogs are natural partners for children in play; both species have dedicated neural systems devoted specifically to social play. Oxytocin and neurotransmitters (dopamine, opioids, norepinephrine, and serotonin) promote and support social activity and positive experience; mirror neurons support social and motor learning, and engagement of the SES provides regulation and training in self-regulation.

Play experiences are requisite for optimal brain development in human and mammalian youth (Panksepp & Biven, 2012) and provide substantial natural implicit rewards (Vanderschuren et al., 2016). Play develops brain circuitry that supports learning, interpersonal and social relationships, problem solving (Cozolino, 2017), and regulation (Gaskill & Perry, 2014). Social play is one of the most productive mechanisms for the acquisition of regulatory skills and strategies. The absence or the scarcity of these experiences is known to be associated with child psychopathology.

Mammalian play is an evolutionarily derived mechanism that provided early mammals with the capability to shift between the stress response states and calm, resting states. Accurate and rapid differentiation between safety and threat is critical to survival, and mammals need the capability to rapidly shift into a fight or flight state to maintain safety. The decision is instantaneous and occurs before conscious recognition of the threat (neuroception) triggering the behavioral and physiological reaction (Porges, 2004).

Social play with canines facilitates the child's practice of modulating arousal states and increasing tolerance for heightened arousal. 'Mobilization without fear' is defined as a state of arousal that does not trigger the fear response. During a game of tag, heart and respiration rates increase, augmenting blood flow to muscles, and emotions are intensified; the child learns this state does not indicate threat. When a mobilization response occurs during play, both species are able to detect safety (vs. threat) through visual cues. During a game of chase, if a dog is nipped in the tail, they will spin around to look for facial expressions that signal play vs. attack. During 'hide and seek,' the hidden child experiences 'immobilization without fear,' then may instantly shift into arousal when discovered.

The Social Connection of a Canine

Humans are a profoundly social species with a need for affiliation and connection with other humans, animals, and the natural world. Our species relied upon cooperation, affiliated relationships, and social engagement to survive and evolve through time. These traits were shared with Pleistocene wolves, enhanced the interspecies relationship, and are central in the human–canine relationship today. Dogs are believed to be the ideal model for investigation of human social cognition, as they have developed substantial social competence through time and share a profound relationship with humans. Researchers have studied the social cognition of dogs, yet only recently delved into the neurobiological correlates of these behaviors. Several neural systems and circuitry have been identified that support canine interspecific social cognition, particularly the hypothalamic-pituitary-adrenal (HPA) axis which interfaces with oxytocin (Buttner, 2016).

Enabled by advanced neuroimaging technology, study of canine sensory, emotional, social and cognitive competence has expanded, producing illuminating evidence of previously unrecognized competencies. Burgeoning evidence is also being accumulated that demonstrates the profound sensitivity and attention of dogs to humans, along with social, cooperation, and communicative prowess.

This research contributes to the increasing scientific foundation critical to the validation of canine-assisted therapies. A broader, more comprehensive knowledge of canine science, combined with recognition of the influence of the coevolution process will inform and support clinical applications using the ni-CAP framework. The development of this field has been hindered by a lack of science that explains the efficacy of canine mechanisms. In spite of the recent growth of the field and the expanding scientific evidence of recent research, a lingering attitude still persists that the benefits of canine-assisted psychotherapy stem from their mere presence.

It is well known that dogs provide other dogs and humans with a sense of safety, comfort and social support through their affiliations (Cimarelli et al., 2021). Humans feel less isolated and lonely when accompanied by a dog (Antonacopoulos, 2017). The presence of a dog improves well-being and merely thinking about a dog can mitigate the experience of social rejection (Brown et al., 2016).Proximal dogs increase the sense of social competence in humans, and motivation to engage and interact with others. The company of a dog also provides 'social credibility,' increasing the child's attractiveness to others (Gee et al., 2021) and also improves the child's perception of others.

Research of children with autism demonstrated that canine interventions increased language, eye contact, and participation (Prothman et al., 2009). In a group setting, the dog can enhance activities and increase social interaction and attention. Research of children in a classroom setting with an incorporated dog found increased empathy, more social integration, and less aggression in students (Hergovich et al., 2002). These attributes improved learning and reduced disruptive behaviors. A psychotherapy setting that incorporates the dog reaps these same benefits.

Understanding how the brain processes and utilizes social information is an important area of focus for researchers and clinicians, as children with trauma histories *and/or* neurodevelopment disorders seem to suffer deficits in the social arena. As many of these deficits are attributed to a difficulty with interpersonal and social interactions with other humans, the dog can offer an effective alternative for learning, practice, and bridging the child to peers.

Nine-year-old Jimmy, diagnosed with autism spectrum disorder, had struggled with social relationships since he began attending school. In spite of supportive programming, his social competence did not significantly improve. Jimmy desperately wanted a friend and tried to get other children to notice him and play with him. Most of his peers, however, either ignored him or explicitly rejected his attempts.

Jimmy showed an interest in dogs and initiated interactions with Seamus, the school's therapy dog, and asked if he could participate in the junior dog training program. Jimmy was diligent in his efforts and developed competence and confidence in his new skills. He earned the privilege of managing Seamus and would walk him through the school and out to the playground. Jimmy now had an interesting 'topic of conversation' that both attracted other children and provided a shared focus on dogs. The attitude of other students dramatically changed, and they began to approach Jimmy, asking him lots of questions about his 'job' and the dog. Jimmy became an excellent 'trainer' and 'manager,' and he and Seamus became buddies. Jimmy acquired a genuine competency that was respected by his peers and the program expanded with the interest that the pair generated. In middle and high school, Jimmy began to work with horses, showing a profound ability to connect with them. He volunteered at an equine facility for special needs children, and as his confidence grew, he expanded his repertoire of skills and made a few solid human friends. Seamus provided a nonjudgmental and enthusiastic alternative that allowed Jimmy to comfortably learn the necessary skills and mannerisms to socially interact with his peers appropriately and effectively. The experience with the dog provided a bridge to peers by creating a safe space that facilitated social learning, practice, and attainment of genuine competency.

Social learning is a rapid and efficient mechanism for the acquisition of fundamental and necessary relational, emotional, and social skills that support functional success. With social learning, children and dogs learn regulation, problem solving, inhibition, cause and effect, prediction, and social strategies. Social learning requires the behavior to be received through social transmission, observation, perception, and/or interactions with another. These forms of learning serve children *and* dogs, as both are capable of learning from conspecific and heterospecific teachers (Fugazza et al., 2018). Social learning is optimized if enjoyable, positively rewarded, repetitive, and reinforced; necessary requisites for internalization and generalization.

Implicit Rewards

Human interactions with dogs also provide intrinsic rewards to dogs through their attention and provision of choices (Rault et al., 2020). Dogs provide implicit rewards for children and are motivating, engaging, and fun! They provide a mechanism for safe touch and affection and demonstrate healthy relational models. They provide an authentic relational feedback system without judgment or attitude. The dog is a living mood enhancer and naturally promotes a contagion of positivity to children.

A Barometer

The clinician is also better equipped to assess the child initially and throughout treatment. The dog is a natural barometer of emotion and behavior and creates self-awareness in the child through their natural responses and reactions.

Attention and Concentration

Gee and colleagues conducted multiple studies that demonstrated improved performances on different tasks by children in the presence of a dog. Results showed improvements in concentration (Gee, Church, & Altobelli, 2010); a decrease in the number of prompts needed for task completion (Gee et al., 2010), improved compliance with directions (Gee et al., 2009), and increased completion speed (Gee et al., 2007).

Beetz and her team (2012) found an increase in attention, curiosity, motivation, and social interactions in children while in the presence of a dog. The dynamic involvement of the dog improves the child's perception of others and even increases the attractiveness of that child to others.

Children residing in a psychiatric facility reported increased alertness, attention, and adjustment with dog interaction (Prothman, 2015). Several other studies showed improved concentration and task performance in children with a dog present (Hediger & Turner, 2014). Negative arousal states are correlated with reduced PFC function and dopaminergic system disruptions (Biederman, 2005). Dopamine is known to improve attention and concentration and can be substantially increased through human–canine interaction (Odendaal & Meintjes, 2003).

The dog can also serve as an external focus of attention. Dogs seem to seek and genuinely enjoy human attention and are skilled at attracting the attention of the child, and capable of creating a contagion of positive emotion and energy.

Interspecies Synchrony and Mimicry

In literature, imitation is also identified as mimicry and these terms are used interchangeably with synchrony. While they share characteristics, they can be described as individual mechanisms and may occur independently of each other. These systems serve attachment, affiliation and social alignment and reflect an underlying characteristic to be consciously or unconsciously sensitive to another individual (Palagi & Cordini, 2020). Synchronicity can occur in emotional, behavioral, social, and neurobiological domains and the latter can be scientifically measured by hormonal and other physiological biomarkers (Buttner et al., 2016).

Behavioral synchronicity has been evolutionarily conserved due to its advantages to survival, reproduction, and affiliations. During the Pleistocene Epoch, small groups benefited from synchronization as it improved affiliation, communication, and social cohesion. Infant mortality improved as adults worked together to source nutrition and caretaking, and the human–wolf relationship improved survival through synchronous cooperation in defense against predators.

Interspecies synchronization has drawn substantial interest, yet has not been well studied. As synchronization has been conceptualized as 'social glue' in humans, recent findings implicate the behavior as a potential mechanism for human–dog relationships as well (Duranton & Gaunet, 2018). In studies conducted by Duranton and colleagues of nonconscious behavioral synchrony, dogs demonstrated behavioral, temporal, and locomotor synchronization with their guardians. Pairs were observed during a walking activity in an unfamiliar indoor space and the dogs demonstrated behavioral synchrony by moving and stopping with their guardians. They also remained proximal, and shared directional gazing with the guardian. Dogs are capable of behavioral and locomotor synchronization with humans which improves interspecies' social cognition, attachment, and cohesion (Duranton &Gaunet, 2018).

Research by Duranton, Gaunet and team observed similar synchronous behavior in an outdoor family setting and considered the findings to be a 'robust' result. Duranton et al. (2017) suggest that this unique interspecies relationship represents an excellent model, due to the sensitivity of dogs to human emotion and behavior. Synchronization enhances affiliation between individuals, and affiliation increases synchronization, a bidirectional loop (Duranton and Gaunet, 2018).

Studies investigating social referencing found that dogs were tuned into the positive and negative behavioral reactions of humans to an unfamiliar object and matched their approach/avoidance responses. These results also reflect the familiar infant/caregiver behavior process in similar conditions in which the infant references the caregiver's cues (Duranton et al., 2017). The canine capacity to follow human directional signals such as a pointing finger or gaze demonstrates their significant convergence with human communication skills. Social referencing and synchronization are skills that promote social affiliations and serve social learning in humans and are now recognized in dogs.

Mimicry is the conscious or unconscious imitation of another's behavior generated by observation. Social play is an optimal forum for rapid mimicry (Palagi et al., 2015), which increases communication and emotion sharing, and helps interpretation of participant intention. Behavioral mimicry and emotion sharing extend the duration of play sessions. Mimicry is accentuated by existing familiarity (Palagi et al., 2015), yet also promotes affiliations and familiarity.

Mirror neurons (MN) are a mechanism that helps the individual to recognize another's emotions, actions, and motivations. The latter is difficult to discern in humans due to the multiplicity of potential motivations for a single action. While mirror neurons have not yet been proven to exist within the canine species, that paradigm is predicted to be revised soon, as dogs do appear capable of multiple MN functions.

Conclusion

Through evolution and their relationships with humans, the canine species has developed significant potential to support humans in their healing from developmental trauma and dysregulation. The working psychotherapy dog can provide the child with a felt sense of safety, coregulation, and the provisions of a healthy attachment. They can stabilize the child, which is critical prior to deeper therapeutic work and their work positively impacts neural regulation and recalibration. The dog establishes a connection with the child and, through their interaction with the clinician and natural, honest behavior, can enhance the establishment and strength of a therapeutic alliance. Dogs have become highly attuned to humans and are capable of human-like social and cooperative behaviors. Their devotion and dedication to our species makes it imperative that we avoid any exploitation or negative effects of their involvement in a therapeutic endeavor. They are sentient and sensitive creatures and their welfare should be a primary consideration of all who work in this field. The next chapter speaks to their needs and our responsibility to provide for their mental and physical health and fulfillment of their potential.

References

Albuquerque, N., Guo, K., Wilkinson, A., Savalli, C., Otta, E., & Mills, E. (2016). Dogs recognize dog and human emotions. https://doi.org/10.1098/rsbi.2015.0883

Andics, A., Gacsi, M., Farago, T., Kis, A., & Miklósi, A. (2014). Voice-sensitive regions in the dog and human brain are revealed by comparative fMRI. *Current Biology*; 24(5): 574–578. https://doi.org/10.1016/j.cub.2014.01.058

Antonacopoulos, N.M.D. (2017). A longitudinal study of the relation between acquiring a dog and loneliness. *Society and Animals*; 25(4): 1234–1449. https://doi.org/10.1163/15685306-12341449

Bakeman, U., Eilam, H., Schild, C.M., Grinstein, D., Eshed, Y., Laster, M., Fride, E., & Anavi-Goffer, S. (2019). Detection of impending aggressive outbursts in patients with psychiatric disorders: Violence clues from dogs. *Scientific Reports*; 9: 17228. https://doi.org/10.1038/s41598-019-52940-w

Barber, A.L., Randi, D., Muller, C.A., & Huber, L. (2016). The processing of human emotional faces by pet and lab dogs: Evidence for lateralization and experience. *Effects. PLoS ONE*, 11(4), e0152393. https://doi.org/10.1371/journal.pone.0152393

Beck, L., & Madresh, E.A. (2008). Romantic partners and four-legged friends: An extension of attachment theory to relationships with pets. *Anthrozoös*; 21(1): 43–56. https://doi.org/10.2752/089279308X274056

Beetz, A., Uvnas-Moberg, K., Julius, H., & Kotrschal, K. (2012). Psychosocial and psychophysiological effects of human–animal interactions: the possible role of oxytocin. *Frontiers in Psychology* 3: 234. https://doi.org/10.3389/fpsyg.2012.00234

Biederman, J. (2005). Attention-deficit/hyperactivity disorder: A selective overview. *Biological Psychiatry*; 57(11): 1215–1220.

Bradshaw, J., & Rooney, N. (2016). Dog social behavior and communication. *Researchgate*. In: *The Domestic Dog* (pp. 133–159). https://doi.org/10.1017/9781139161800-008

Brown, C.M., Hengy, S.M., & McConnell, A.R. (2016). Thinking about cats or dogs provides relief from social rejection. *Anthrozoös*; 29(1): 47–58. https://doi.org/10.1080/20414005.2015.1067958

Buttner, A.P., Thompson, B., Strasser, R., & Santo, J. (2015). Evidence for a synchronization of hormonal states between humans and dogs during competition. *Physiology & Behavior*; 147: 54–62. https://dx.doi.org/j.physbeh.2015.04.010

Buttner, A.P. (2016). Neurobiological underpinnings of dogs' human-like social competence: How interactions between SRS and OT mediate dogs' social skills. *Neuroscience & Biobehavioral Reviews*; V71: 198–214. https://doi.org/10.1016/j.neubiorev.2016.08.029

Carter. C.S. (2014). Oxytocin Pathways and the Evolution of Human Behavior. *Annual Review of Psychology* 65: 10.1–10.23. https://doi.org/10.1146/annurev-psych-010213-115110

Carter, C.S. (2017). The role of oxytocin and vasopressin in attachment. *Psychodynamic Psychiatry*; 45(4): 499–518.

Cassels, M.T., White, N., Gee, N., & Hughes, C. (2017). One of the family? Measuring early adolescents' relationships with pets and siblings. *Journal of Applied Developmental Psychology*. https://doi.org/10.1016/j.appdev.2017.01.003

Cimarelli, G., Marshall-Pescini, S., Range, F., Berghanel, A., & Virányi, Z. (2021). Relationship quality affects social stress buffering in dogs and wolves. *Animal Behaviour*; 178: 127–140. https://doi.org/10.1016/j.anbehav.2021.06.008

Cozolino, L. (2017). *The neuroscience of human relationships*. New York, NY: WW Norton & Company.

Crossman, M.K. (2017). Effects of interactions with animals on human psychological distress. *Journal of Clinical Psychology* 73: 761–784. https://doi.org/10.1002/jclp.22410

D'Aniello, Semin G.R., Alterisio, A., Aria, M., & Scandurra, A. (2017). Interspecies transmission of emotional information via chemo signals: from humans to dogs (Canis lupus familiaris). *Animal Cognition* https://doi.org/10.1007/s10071-017-1139-x

de Groot, J.H.B., Semin, G.R., Smeets, M.A.M. (2017). On the communicative function of body odors: A theoretical integration and review. *Sage Journal*; 12(2): 306–324. https://doi.org/10.1177/1745691616676599

de Groot, J.H.B., Smeets, M.A.M., Kaldewaij, A., Duijndam, M.J.A., & Semin, G.R. (2012). Chemosignals communicate human emotions. *Psychological Science*; 23: 1417–1424. https://doi.org/10.1177/0956797612445317

Devillier, P., Gallet, C., Salvator, H., Lecoq-Julien, C., Naline, E., Roisse, D., Levert, C., Breton, E., Galtat, A., Decourtray, S., Prevel, L., Grassin-Delyle, S., & Grandjean, D. (2022). Biomedical detection dogs for the identification of SARS-CoV-2 infections from axillary sweat and breath samples. *Journal of Breath Research*; 16: 037101.https://doi.org/10.1086/1752-7163/ac5d8c

Duranton, C., Bedossa, T., & Gaunet, F., (2017). Interspecific behavioral synchronization: Dogs exhibit locomotor synchrony with humans. *Scientific Reports* 7: 12384. https://doi.org/10.1038/s41598-017-12577-z

Duranton, C. & Gaunet, F., (2018). Behavioral synchronization and affiliation: Dogs exhibit human-like skills. *Learning & Behavior*; 46:364–373. https://doi.org/10.3758/s13420-018-0323-4

Farago, T., Andics, A., Devecseri, V., Kis, A., Gacsi, M., & Miklósi, A. (2014). Humans rely on the same rules to assess emotional valence and intensity in conspecific and dog vocalizations. *Biology Letters*, 10: 201309. https://doi.org/10.1098/rsbi.2013.0925

Fitch, W.T. (2019). *Animal Cognition and the Evolution of Human Language: Why We Cannot Focus Solely On Communication*. The Royal Society. https://doi.org/10.1098/rstb.2019.0046

Friedmann, E., Katcher, A.H., Lynch, J.J., & Thomas, S.A. (1980). Animal companions and one-year survival of patients after discharge from a coronary care unit. *Public Health Reports*; 95(4): 307–312.

Fugazza, C., Moesta, A., Pogany, A., & Miklósi, A. (2018). Social learning from conspecifics and humans in dog puppies. *Scientific Reports*; 8 (9257).

Gaskill, R.L., & Perry, B.D. (2014). The neurobiological power of play: Using the neurosequential model of therapeutics to guide play in the healing process. In C.A. Malchiodi & D.A. Crenshaw (Eds.), *Creative arts and play therapy for attachment problems* (pp. 178–194). New York, NY: The Guilford Press.

Gee, N.R., Church, M.T., & Altobelli, C.L. (2010). Preschoolers make fewer errors on an object categorization task in the presence of a dog. *Anthrozoös*; 23: 223–230.

Gee, N.R., Harris, S.L., & Johnson, K.L. (2007). The role of therapy dogs in speed and accuracy to complete motor skills tasks for preschool children. *Anthrozoös*; 20(4). https://doi.org/10.2752/089279307X245509

Gee, N.R., Rodriguez, K.E., Fine, A.H., & Trammell, J.P. (2021). Dogs supporting human health and well-Being: A biopsychosocial approach. *Frontiers in Veterinary Science*; 8: 630465. Gee https://doi.org/10.3389/fvets.2021.630465

Gee, N.R., Sherlock, T.R., Bennett, E.A., & Harris, S.L. (2009). Preschoolers' adherence to instruction as a function of presence of a dog and motor skill task. *Anthrozoös*; 22: 267–276. https://doi.org/10.2751/175303709X457603

Guo, K., Meints, K., Hall, C., Hall, S., & Mills, D. (2009). Left gaze bias in humans, rhesus monkeys and domestic dogs. *Animal Cognition*; 12(3): 409–418. https://doi.org/10/1007/s10071-008-0199-3

Handlin, L., Hydbring-Sandberg, E., Nilsson, A., Ejdeback, M.Jansson, A., & Uvnas-Moberg, K. (2011). Short-term interaction between dogs and their owners: Effects on oxytocin, cortisol, insulin and heart rate-an exploratory study. *Anthrozoös*; 24(3): 301–315. https://doi.org/10.2752/175303711X13045914865385

Hare, B. (2017). Survival of the friendliest: Homo sapiens evolved via SAelection for prosociality. *Annual Review of Psychology*; 68: 155–186. https://doi.org/10.1146/annurev-psych-010416-044201

Hare, B, Call, J., Tomasello, M. (1998). Communication of food location between human and dog (Canis familiaris). *Evolution of Communication*, 2: 137–159. https://doi.org/10.1075/eoc.2.1.06har

Hare, B. & Tomasello, M. (2005). Human-like social skills in dogs? *Trends in Cognitive Sciences* 9(9): 439–444. https://doi.org/10.1016/j.tics.2005.07.003

Hediger, K. & Turner, D.C. (2014). Can dogs increase children's attention and concentration performance? A randomized controlled trial. *Human–animal Interaction Bulletin*; 2(2): 21–39. https://doi.org/10.1079/hai.2014.0010

Hergovich, A., Monshi, B., Semmler, G. & Zieglmayer (2002).The effects of the presence of a dog in the classroom. *Anthrozoös*; 15(1). https://doi.org/10.2752/089279302786992775

Huber, L., Racca, A., Scaf, B., Virányi, Z., & Range, F. (2013). Discrimination of familiar human faces in dogs (Canis familaris). *Learning and Motivation*; 44(4): 258–269. https://doi.org/10.1016/j.lmot.2013.04.005

Hunt, M.G. & Chizkov, R.R. (2014). Are therapy dogs like Xanax? Does animal-assisted therapy impact processes relevant to cognitive behavioral psychotherapy? *Anthrozoös*; 27:457–469. https://doi.org/10.2752/175303714X14023922797959

Jalongo, M.R. (2015). An attachment perspective of the child-dog bond: interdisciplinary and international research findings. *Early Childhood Education Journal*; 43: 395–405. https://doi.org/10.1007/s10643-015-0687-4

Julius, H., Beetz, A., Kotrschal, K., Turner, D., & Uvnas-Moberg, K. (2013). *Attachment to Pets: An Integrative View of Human–animal Relationships with Implications for Therapeutic Practice*. Cambridge, MA: Hogrefe Publishing.

Nagasawa, M., Kikusui, T., Onaka, T., & Ohta, M. (2009). Dog's gaze at its owner increases owner's urinary oxytocin during social interaction. *Hormones and Behavior*

Kaminski, J., Waller, B.M., Diogo, R., Hartstone-Rose, A., & Burrows, A.M., (2019). Evolution of facial muscle anatomy in dogs. *Proceedings of the National Academy of Sciences (PNAS)*; 116929. https://doi.org/10.1073/pnas.1820653116

Kertes, D.A., Liu, J., Hall, N.J., Hadad, N.A., Wynne, C.D.L., & Bhatt, S.S. (2017). Effect of pet dogs on children' perceived stress and cortisol stress response. *Social Development*; 26(2): 382–401. https://doi.org/10.1111/sode.12203

Kis, A., Hernadi, A., Miklósi, B., Kanizsar, O., & Topál, J. (2017). The way dogs (canis familiaris) look at human emotional faces is modulated by oxytocin. An eye-tracking study. *Frontiers in Behavioral Neuroscience* https://doi.org/10.3389/fnbeh.2017.00210

Koch, S.B.J., van Zuiden, M., Nawljn, L., Frijling, J.L., Veltman, D.J., & Olff, M. (2016). Intranasal oxytocin normalizes amygdala functional connectivity in posttraumatic stress disorder. *Neuropsychopharmacology*; 41: 2041–2051. https://doi.org/10.1038/npp.2016.1

Kokocinska-Kusiask, A, Woszcylo, M., Zybala, M., Maciocha, J., Barlowska, K., & Dziecio, M. (2021). Canine olfaction: Physiology, behavior, and possibilities for practical applications. *Animals (Basel)*; 11(8): 2463. https://doi.org/10.3390/ani11082463

Marti, R., Petignat, M., Marcar, V.L., Hattendorf, J., Wolf, M., Hund-Georgiadis, M., & Hediger, K. (2022). Effects of contact with a dog on prefrontal brain activity: A controlled trial. *PLoS One*;17(10): e36197880. https://doi.org/10.1071/j.pone.0274833

Melson, G.F. (2003). Child development and the human-companion animal bond. *The American Behavioral Scientist* 47(1): 31–39. https://doi.org/10.1177/0002764203255210

Miklósi, A. (2016). Current trends in canine problem-solving and cognition. *Current Directions in Psychological Science*; 25(5): 300–306. https://doi.org/10.1177/096372141666606

Muller, C.A., Schmitt, K., Barber, ALA, & Huber, L. (2015). Dogs can discriminate emotional expressions of human faces. *Current Biology*; 25(5): 601–605. https://doi.org/10.1016/cub.2014.12.055

Nagasawa, M., Murai, K., Mogi, K., & Kikusui, T. (2011). Dogs can discriminate human smiling faces from blank expressions. *Animal Cognition*; 14(4): 523–533. https://doi.org/10.1007/s1007-011-0386-5

Nagasawa, M., Mitsui, S., En, S., Ohtani, N., Ohta, M., Sakuma, Y., Onaka, T., Mogi, K., & Kikusui, T. (2015). Social evolution. Oxytocin-gaze positive loop and the coevolution of human-dog bonds. *Science*; 348(6232): 333–336. https://doi.org/10.1126/science.12610

Nagengast, S.L., Baun, M.M., Megel, M., & Leibowitz, M. (1997). The effects of the presence of a companion animal on physiological arousal and behavioral distress in children during a physical examination. *Journal of Pediatric Nursing* 12(6): 323–330. https://doi.org/10.1016/S0882-5963(97)80058-9

Odendaal, J. & Meintjes, R. (2003). Neurophysiological correlates of affiliative behavior between humans and dogs. *Veterinary Journal* 165:296–301

Olmert, M.D. (2009). *Made for Each Other*. Cambridge, MA: Da Capo Press.

Palagi, E., & Cordini, G. (2020). Intraspecific motor and emotional alignment in dogs and wolves: The basic building blocks of dog-human affective connectedness. *Animals*; 10(2): 241. https://doi.org/10.3390/ani10020241

Palagi, E., Nicotra, V., & Cordini, G. (2015). Rapid mimicry and emotional contagion in domestic dogs. *Royal Society Open Science*2(12): 150505. https://doi.org/10.1098/rsos.150505.

Panksepp, J. & Biven, L. (2012). *The Archaeology of Mind: Neural Origins of Human Emotion*. New York, NY: W.W. Norton & Company.

Parish-Plass, N., & Pfeiffer, J. (2019). Implications of animal-assisted psychotherapy for the treatment of developmental trauma through the lens of interpersonal neurobiology. In P. Tedeschi, & M. Jenkins, (Eds.). *Transforming trauma: Resilience and healing through our connections with animals*. (pp. 123–187). Lafayette, IN: Purdue University Press.

Parish-Plass, N. (2008). Animal-asswisted therapy with children suffering from insecure attachment due to abuse and neglect: A method to lower the risk of intergenerational transmission of abuse?. *Clinical Child Psychology and Psychiatry*; 13(1):7–30. https://doi.org/10177/1359914507086338

Payne, E., DeAraugo, J., Bennett, P., & McGreevy, P. (2016). Exploring the existence and potential underpinnings of dog-human and horse-human attachment bonds. *Behavioural Processes*; 125: 114–121. https://doi.org/10.1016/j.beproc.2015.10.004

Pitteri, E., Mongillo, P., Carnier, P., Marinelli, L., & Huber, L. (2014). Part-based and configural processing of owner's face in dogs. *PLoS One*, 9(9), e108176. https://doi.org/10.1371/journal.pone.0108176

Porges, S.W. (2004). Neuroception: A subconscious system for detecting threats and safety. *Zero to Three*; 24(5): 19–24.

Porges, S.W. (2005). The role of social engagement in attachment and bonding. *Attachment and Bonding*; 3: 33–54.

Porges, S.W. (2011). *Norton Series on Interpersonal Neurobiology. The Polyvagal Theory: Neurophysiological Foundations of Emotions, Attachment, Communication, and Self-regulation*. New York, NY: Norton.

Porges, S.W. (2015). *Making the World Safe for our Children: Down-regulating Defence and Up-regulating Social Engagement to 'Optimise' the Human Experience*. Cambridge, UK: Cambridge University Press. https://doi.org/10.1017/cha.2015.12

Porges, S.W. (2017). *The Pocket Guide to the Polyvagal Theory: The Transformative Power of Feeling Safe*. New York, NY: W.W. Norton.

Prato-Previde, E., & Valeschi, P. (2014). The immaterial cord: The dog-human attachment bond. In J. Kaminski & Marshall-Pescini, S. (Eds.), *The Social Dog: Cognition and Behavior* (pp. 165–185). New York, NY: Elsevier. https://doi.org/10.1016/B9787-0-12-407818-5.00006-1

Prothman, A., Bienert, M., & Ettrich, C. (2015). Dogs in child psychotherapy: Effects on state of mind. *Anthrozoös*; 19(3). https://doi.org/10.2752/089279306785415583

Prothman, A., Ettrich, C., & Prothmann, S. (2009). Preference for, and responsiveness to, people, dogs and objects in children with autism. *Anthrozoös*; 22: 161–171. https://doi.org/10.2751/175303709X434185

Rault, J-L., Waiblinger, S., Voivin, X., & Hemsworth, P. (2020). The power of a positive human-animal relationship for animal welfare. *Frontiers in Veterinary Science* 7: 590867. https://doi.org/10.3389/f.vets.2020.590867

Shonkoff, Garner (2012). The lifelong effects of early childhood adversity and toxic stress. *Pediatrics*; 129(1): e232–e246. https://doi.org/10.1542/peds.2011-2663

Siegel, D. (2010). *Mindsight: The Science of Personal Transformation*. New York, NY: Random House.

Siniscalchi, M., d'Ingeo, S., & Quaranta, A. (2017). Lateralized functions in the dog brain. *Symmetry*; 9(5)71. https://doi.org/10.3390/sym9050071

Somppi, S. Tornqvist, H., Kujala, M.V., Hanninen, L., Krause, C.M., & Vainio, O. (2016). Dogs evaluate threatening facial expressions by their biological validity-Evidence from gazing patterns. *PLoS One*, 11(1), e0143047. https://doi.org/10.1371/journal.pone.0143047

Ulmer-Yaniv, A., Waidergoren, S., Shaked, A., Salomon, R., & Feldman, R. (2021). Neural representation of the parent-child attachment from infancy to adulthood. *Social Cognitive and Affective Neuroscience*; 1–16. https://doi.org/10.1093/scan/nsab132

VanFleet, R. & Faa-Thompson, T. (2010). The case for using animal assisted play therapy. *The British Journal of Play Therapy*; 6: 4–18.

VanFleet, R., & Faa-Thompson, T. (2017). *Animal Assisted Play Therapy* (trademarked). Sarasota, FL: Professional Resource Press.

Viau, R., Arsenault-Lapierre, G., Fecteau, Sl, Champagne, N., Walker, C-D., & Lupien, S. (2010). Effect of service dogs on salivary cortisol secretion in autistic children. *Psychoneuroendocrinology*; 35(8): 1187–1193. https://doi.org/10.1016/j.psyneuen.2010.02.004

Vanderschuren, L.J.M.J., Achterberg, E.J.M., & Trezza, V. (2016). The neurobiology of social play and its rewarding value in rats. *Neuroscience Biobehavioral Review*; 70: 86–105. https://doi.org/10.1016/j.neubiorev.2016.07.025

Wanser, S.H., Vitale, K.R., Thielke, L.E., Brubaker, L., & Udell, M.A.R. (2019). Spotlight on the psychological basis of childhood pet attachment and its implications. *Psychology Research and Behavior Management*, 469–470. https://doi.org/10.2147/PRBM.S158998

Yong, M.H. & Ruffman, T. (2014). Emotional contagion: Dogs and humans show a similar physiological response to human infant crying. *Behavioural Processes*; 108C: 155–165. https://doi.org/10.1016/j.beproc.2014.10.006

Zilcha-Mano, S., Miklulincer, M., & Shaver, P.R. (2011). Pet in the therapy room: An attachment perspective on animal-assisted therapy. *Attachment & Human Development*; 13(6): 541–561. https://doi.org/10.1080/14616734.2011.608987

Zilcha-Mano, S., Mikulincer, M., & Shaver, P.R. (2012). Pets as safe havens and secure bases: The moderating role of pet attachment orientations. *Journal of Research in Personality*; 46(5): 571–580.

Chapter 7　Ensuring the Welfare of the Working Psychotherapy Dog

Waiting for a young child to arrive, I looked over at my partner who was sprawled on his back nibbling on a knotted sock. He paused and gazed back, lifting an eyebrow as if expecting me to speak. I asked him if he was up for work today, and he stood up, stretched once, and trotted over. Seamus seemed content and relaxed, yet alert. He was familiar with the pre-session routine that signaled an impending arrival. I stroked his head a few times, and then he climbed up on the chair by the window and looked outside. What he saw triggered a tremor of excitement. Little wiggles began in his tail and worked their way through his whole body. Seamus let out a little squeal as he hopped down and bounded to the door. I concluded that his answer was 'yes.'

For thousands of years, through shifting geography, climate change, and civilizations, dogs have been part of our lives. Through our shared evolution, dogs have converged with humans to the degree that they also require a social environment to thrive. Dogs have become highly attentive and developed amazing capabilities to communicate with us. They can identify and decipher emotions and even make predictions about impending behavior. Boris Levinson, considered the father of animal-assisted therapy, was credited with recognizing how the human–animal bond, shaped by coevolution, positioned the dog as a pivotal agent of human psychological health (Serpell, 2010). That is an incredibly bold statement, particularly with the long-standing resistance among scientists to the early wisdom of Charles Darwin.

Darwin believed that the difference in the minds between humans and other species was 'one of degree and not of kind' (Darwin, 1871). He proposed that humans, other mammals and invertebrates share similar brain regions that are utilized for consciousness and processing emotions (Bekoff, 2013). Up until the late 20th century, the suggestion that animals had emotions was considered an avenue of study that could sink the career of a scientist. Look at how far our human species has come. Is it possible to even consider that our similarities with other animals might outweigh our differences?

DOI: 10.4324/9781003217534-10

Princeton Professor of Bioethics Peter Singer (2009) has long advocated for the ethical and moral treatment of animals and believes that human equality should be extended to animals. Singer interprets the biblical description of God granting human dominion over animals as a human 'obligation' to animals, though apparently much of the population viewed the phrase as permission to do as they pleased. While protective legislation is critical to welfare practices, the higher standard of ethical and moral behavior is to be compassionate for other living beings simply because it is *the right thing to do*.

What is Welfare?

Have humans lived up to that standard? The short answer is 'no'. Compassion has not been enough to ensure positive welfare for animals, so legislation has proved necessary to mandate improvements in animal treatment across the globe. During the 20th century, legislation provided protections to farm and laboratory animals, with an early focus on physical health and comfort (defined as an absence of pain). Donald M. Broom (1986) introduced one of the first modern definitions of welfare, summarizing it as an animal's attempt to cope with their environment. Over 30 years ago, he proposed that an absence of evidence proving poor welfare does not imply the absence of a problem; and it certainly does not imply positive welfare.

The gradual increase in human recognition of animal sentience has become a force behind the current welfare movement. Sentience is the capability of animals to experience consciousness and feel emotions such as joy, fear, and sadness (Platt, 2021). The conceptualization of 'positive welfare' is relatively recent and reflects the movement for human acknowledgment of sentience. The focus on constructs such as canine emotional well-being, cognitive stimulation, and fulfillment of potential are congruous with the burgeoning field of human–animal interactions (HAI) that is illuminating the mutual benefits of interspecies' relationships. There is also increasing consideration that dogs have individual preferences for specific activities, rewards, environmental conditions, and attention. Yeates and Main (2008) identify animal 'needs' and 'wants' as elements of welfare that should be considered. These propensities have substantial relevance for working psychotherapy dogs as there are inherent clinical responsibilities to an animal that is assisting psychotherapy.

The acceptance of these needs or rights has challenged long-held, human-centric thinking, although attitude changes are certainly not universal. The HAI community continues to be challenged in its efforts to establish standards, guidelines, and continuity within the field. The consideration of responsible and positive welfare and what constitutes an optimal experience for participating animals cannot afford to wait for these goals to be met as this issue needs urgent determination (Rault, 2020).

Henry Pollock provided some valuable advice for humans whose nature is to seek and attain *'certainty'* prior to taking action. Certainty is the complete and precise scientific evidence that leaves no room for doubt. The quest for certainty, however, can be used as an excuse for delaying action. Applying this principle to animal sentience and welfare, renowned ethologist Marc Bekoff (2007) believes we should accept the theory that animals are sentient and treat them as such *now*. The current status of animal maltreatment and risk for further harm is obviously of greater consequence if humans delay action, than if we attend to improving welfare immediately.

For now, the clinician might align their perspective to the concept of positive welfare by simply asking themselves, post session, 'Did I encourage agency, fulfillment, choices, and freedom of movement in the dog?' That would elicit a different thought process than the question, 'Did I prevent the dog from being distressed or uncomfortable?' That is the perspective of positive welfare.

What is Stress?

A simple definition of a *stressor* is that which constitutes a genuine or perceived threat to the homeostasis of an organism. The reaction of the organism has been defined as *stress* which involves the triggering of neural, chemical, behavioral, and emotional responses, components of the stress response system (SRS). This reaction is acute, rapid, and automatic, as the body and brain are wired to maintain homeostasis. The canine stress system is comparable to the human circuitry; thus the dog also experiences sympathetic activation that triggers arousal. As in humans, the hypothalamus-pituitary-adrenal (HPA) axis and endocrine system prepare the physiology and behavior to support a mobilization response (fight or flight). When the SRS is repetitively activated, it becomes dysregulated and the dog can become chronically stressed and functionally compromised, just like the child. These physiological changes can be identified through conscientious monitoring and remediated through intentional effort. A fearful, aroused state is not only a risk for safety and effective therapy; it compromises the dog and is highly unethical and unprofessional.

What constitutes a stressor varies between dogs? The determination of what is stressful for an individual dog requires human attunement and awareness of their temperament, tolerances, and history. Research that produces evidence of stressors, stress reactions, and species-specific data is highly beneficial yet represents a 'starting point' in evaluation and monitoring of the individual working psychotherapy dog. While the two primary methods for maintaining optimal welfare in an animal are behavioral observations and physiological biomarkers, it is proposed that it is the attuned relationship that may provide the most accurate assessment.

What Makes Dogs Vulnerable to Stressors?

While our interspecies relationship provides significant bidirectional benefits, dogs remain the most vulnerable as it is an asymmetric affiliation. An inequity of power exists in almost all human–dog relationships. Dogs have become highly social and incredibly attentive and loyal to humans. As mentioned earlier, many actually prefer human company over that of other dogs. Viewing our interspecies relationship through a human-centric lens, one could assume that dogs are quite fortunate to be with us. We provide shelter; feed them; and we keep them safe.

From a dog's perspective, however, they cannot relieve themselves without our permission; they cannot choose their food, when they eat, or how much they may have. Dogs have been bred to create traits that humans desire. Squished noses were bred into bulldogs as it gave the breed a neotinized look, but from the dog's perspective, they now have breathing problems. Human selection of particular breeds and traits has inadvertently caused today's dogs to suffer from diabetes, cancer, cardiac problems, and even depression. Many breeds are subjected to docked tails, braced ears, and a large percentage have their ability to breed 'removed.'

Dogs are deprived of making choices and decisions, some of which would permit a natural avoidance of stressful situations (Serpell et al., 2010).Dogs who participate in therapy settings can become mentally and physically fatigued, be exposed to unpleasant handling, and feel overwhelmed by the noise, activity, and conditions (Haubenhofer & Kirchengast, 2006).

Dogs tend to be patient, forgiving, and rarely complain, though of course, there are exceptions. Non-compliant dogs, like children, do not get chosen for the team and so it can be assumed dogs that pass existing criteria for therapy work are compliant, docile, and devoted. These revered characteristics, however, place them at a higher risk for stress as they may internalize their stress in their effort to please their humans. The weight of stress in a docile, compliant dog is not as visible as it might be in the independent strong-willed dog. Each dog is highly individual and their temperament, tolerances, irritants, and responses vary profoundly. Positive welfare is reflected in the relationship, respect, and familiarity that exist between the members of the clinical team. Attention to the dog's emotional and physical experience of psychotherapy should not simply be the absence of discomfort, boredom, or pain.

The impact of intense emotion can be particularly stressful for any animal, particularly one with the sensitivity of the dog. Known for their focused attentiveness to human states of emotion and arousal, dogs are highly susceptible to emotional contagion (Huber et al., 2017), a primitive form of empathy that does not require a theory of mind or higher cognitive thinking. The phenomenon is believed to have stemmed from interspecies cohabitation in early evolution. Dogs were believed to have alerted humans of approaching predators, a behavior that still exists today (Katayama et al., 2019).Contagion of emotion and behavior goes beyond mere mimicry; it is a *felt* experience that becomes reflected in the physiology of the body. Research revealed that dogs that responded to human crying experienced an elevation in the stress hormone, cortisol, which is indicative of stress system activation (Yong & Ruffman, 2014). The level of contagion in a dog is mediated by the quality and length of relationship with the human.

Dogs are also susceptible to acute and chronic synchronization of stress hormones with humans. If the clinician is anxious or fearful, the dog may *mirror* their state, emotionally and physiologically (Sundman et al., 2019). The polyvagal theory (PVT) is relevant for understanding the states of canines and other animals, as well as humans. Canine nervous systems respond similarly to humans and their physiological status can prevent them from engaging as social beings as well. Today, acute cortisol levels can be measured through blood and saliva samples, though drawing blood is invasive. Recent investigations revealed that concentrations of cortisol can also be found in hair, another promising biomarker that may someday become an assessment tool for animal-supported treatment.

The age and maturity of the dog also require consideration in determining suitability for psychotherapeutic work. Both the young and immature *and* the aging dog are vulnerable. Young dogs under two years old expressed higher rates of behavioral markers of stress than older, more experienced dogs (King et al., 2011). Older dogs potentially become weaker, arthritic, and more easily fatigued, conditions that occur in clinicians, as well.

Stressors that can Impact the Dog

The incorporation of dogs into a treatment environment exposes the animal to a variety of potential stressors that can cause behavioral and/or physiological responses. Mild stress (eustress) can be stimulating. It enhances neural plasticity and learning, and strengthens resilience, positive effects that are central in development and treatment. Welfare considerations focus on the levels of stress that are potentially detrimental. Stress levels that trigger heightened levels of emotion, behavior, and/or physiology can trigger (or reflect) activation of the stress response system (SRS).

The intensity, frequency, and duration of stressors are variables that impact levels of distress and mediate long-term effects. Stressors can be environmental factors, such as a small, hot room or lack of comfortable substrates. Sensory stressors can be auditory, such as high volume of speech, intense tones, and unfamiliar pitch or cadence; olfactory, irritants such as chemicals, perfume, or allergens; tactile stressors can be the experience of tight, restrictive hugging or unexpected, unpleasant touch; and visual triggers might involve lighting or rapid and unpredictable movement. Other stressors that are internal include hunger, thirst, fatigue, an injury, or illness. Individual characteristics of the child may also be perceived as irritating to the dog. These can be difficult to identify, and a highly compliant dog will do its best to be tolerant, so stress cues might be difficult to observe.

Dogs generally seek interactions with humans and experience comfort, safety, and enjoyment through interspecies relationships. However, for some dogs, social interactions can be highly stressful (Ng et al., 2014). Dogs with higher stress levels find it difficult to engage in social contact with unfamiliar individuals (Lind et al., 2017). Research supports the logic that high stress levels in dogs may also impact the *quality* of social interactions between dogs and humans (Glenk, 2017). Again, this infers the relevance of understanding the SRS, polyvagal theory, and physiology and speaks to the importance of an attuned relationship between the clinician and dog.

The lack of autonomy, choice, agency, and the ability to behave naturally are additional categories of stressors. Dogs have evolved to be highly social, yet might prefer a choice of with whom and for how long. Dogs crave social and physical contact, but if there are inadequate breaks or an ability to escape, normally enjoyable interactions can become irritating.

Dogs are comforted and feel secure when they have a predictable routine, thus, a change of routine can be stressful (Rooney et al., 2009). A dog who is typically fed at a specific time will notice if that event has been relegated to a later time. While dogs do not read clocks, they do have awareness of time periods (due to internal signals, light changes, and patterns that precede routines). The opening vignette demonstrates the concept of establishing a routine that informs and prepares the dog for an impending session.

Assessment of Welfare in Working Therapy Dogs

Historically, the assessment of canine welfare has primarily focused on negative emotions, as they tend to be more intense and obvious than positive states. A state of happiness or joy can be achieved through positive experiences, agency, and the freedom to move, behave naturally, and play. Dogs are enriched by abundant opportunities to interact and play with other dogs and humans. An ideal environment is one that is sensory and opportunity rich. Engaging the mind, their curiosity, and providing challenges nourish the dog and support their neurobiological health, as well. The social engagement system (SES) conceptualized by Porges is an ideal neural state for the dog, as is for humans. When the dog feels safe and is coregulated, they are more available and capable of social interaction and that state increases oxytocin and establishes a loop of bilateral benefit (Nagasawa et al., 2015).

The concept and assessment of positive states in working therapy dogs is evolving, yet currently, the two primary methods of evaluation are behavioral observation and physiological markers. While physiological markers sound objective and indisputable, both methods require human interpretation which renders them susceptible to criticism as 'soft' evidence. The physiological markers typically used *are* indicators of stress but are also indicators of positive and pleasurable functions, complicating interpretation (Glenk, 2017). The degree of activation of the sympathetic nervous system (SNS) and parasympathetic nervous system (PNS) branches is subject to regulation which can be envisioned as dials that adjust to increase and decrease arousal and also to establish a balance. An example of this is during play which requires an optimal blending of the SNS and PNS branches to achieve the levels of activation that support a game of tag or hide and go seek, *without* triggering the SRS. It is up to the clinician to monitor and coregulate both the child and dog.

Questionnaires have been suggested as another source of data to be completed by the clinician. Additionally, neuroimaging is being considered as a possible future mode of assessment. A portable system (that is relatively comparable to the fMRI) is being tested, though its use in clinical work has not been determined. Until a single validated method becomes available, measuring the welfare of the dog (including positive indicators) is best served through a multimodal approach (Csoltova & Mehinagic, 2020).

Behavioral Signs of Stress

Signs of emotional stress in dogs, such as fearfulness or anxiety, may be observable as changes in behavior. While observation can be criticized as subjective, it is the familiarity and bond of the relationship that validates this process. Each dog has its own repertoire of behaviors and accurate interpretation of changes does require training in dog science, knowledge of species as well as familiarity, quality of relationship, and intuition. Humans have been noted to be impacted by personal bias of their own dogs.

Canine reactions to stressors can be adaptive or maladaptive, and it is the responsibility of clinicians to recognize their signals and appropriately respond. Literature reports significant variance in clinical attention and response, a potential problem that is relevant to welfare concerns. Workload was positively correlated to stress and higher rates of stress behaviors were found in dogs that interacted with children under 12 years old. Dogs older than age six and/or with two or more years of experience showed fewer stress behaviors. (Marinelli et al., 2009).

Stress behaviors can be categorized as appeasement gestures. Subtle cues of stress are believed to be automatic and hardwired, present throughout evolution, and observable in both intra- and inter-species settings. Appeasement behaviors were defined by Norwegian dog trainer Turid Rugaas as 'calming behaviors' and are believed to be used by dogs and wolves to calm other conspecifics and maintain civility within the group. Over 30 specific behaviors have been identified and can be categorized into appeasement (active submission), deference (passive submission), displacement, and displays of threat and dominance (Rugaas, 2005). While these signals have not been rigorously studied, they are widely accepted as behavioral indicators of stress in canines. The use of behavioral indicators requires attention to context, environment, and other variables that may impact the dog's state. The responsibilities of the ni-CAP clinician may seem daunting, and do require abundant energy and an ability to 'multi-focus.' The attunement, synchrony, training, and experience of the clinical team make it possible.

Active submission is a category of attention-seeking behaviors and includes licking, jumping up, nuzzling or bumping its nose, pawing, crouching, and 'smiling.' These behaviors are often displayed in play situations to signal a non-threatening, friendly intention.

Passive submission contrasts with active and is manifested as tucking the tail, going belly-up, and averting the eyes. When the head is turned to avoid direct eye contact, the dog may look 'sideways' which produces a 'whale eye,' the white of the eye. These behaviors reflect a dog's attempt to disengage. The use of submission behaviors signals, 'I'm not threatening.'

The dog that uses threatening or assertive behaviors feels threatened and is attempting to stop the threat from approaching them. They want to avoid a fight. The dog will stare directly at the threat which (between dogs) often stops the threat. If the threat continues, the dog will curl their lips, and raise the head and ears to a higher position to look larger. If the threat escalates however, the dog will lower its ears and head to protect from bites. Hackling of the hair along the back also increases height but is actually a sign of heightened emotional arousal, not necessarily aggression.

Behaviors that indicate positive emotional states and social engagement include nudging, licking, soft paw lifting (solicitation), belly-up, use of play signals such as play bow, open mouth, and relaxed body language. Does the dog show interest by a willing approach, attentiveness, and increased positive arousal? Does the dog seek proximity with the child? How relaxed is the dog when next to a child or on a lap? Does the dog show enthusiastic anticipation with the child's arrival and greet them enthusiastically? These are a few behaviors that can show positive emotion.

Physiological Signs of Stress in Dogs

Stress can be identified in dogs through physiological markers such as heart rate, respiration, blood pressure, body temperature, and immune indexes. Oxytocin (OT) and cortisol represent two primary hormonal markers of positive and negative physiology in the working psychotherapy dog. They are an example of the complexity of multiple concurrent processes, as OT attenuates the stress response, which may reduce cortisol levels, yet both can reflect positive social arousal. Cortisol is also be associated with positive emotions and activities and is dependent upon the perception of the individual (Haubenhofer & Kirchengast, 2007).

Cortisol, a glucocorticosteroid released in dogs, serves as the primary biomarker and best indicator of stress (Verga & Michelazzi, 2009). Cortisol levels reflect activation of the hypothalamic-pituitary-adrenal axis, reflecting a stress response. Measurable through saliva, urine, plasma, feces, and hair, cortisol markers have complex patterns that vary between individuals in duration, magnitude, and speed of change (Glenk, 2017).

Within individuals, cortisol levels normally rise and fall twice during the day, thus a baseline would be advised for comparative purposes. While short-term variability in cortisol can be considered normal responses to coping mechanisms, chronic elevations of cortisol can dysregulate the immune system (Chrousos, 2000). Elevations of cortisol in dogs were noted on working versus resting days (Haubenhofer & Kirchengast, 2007), yet others reported no changes (Ng et al., 2014). Another study showed no significant differences in salivary cortisol between baseline and AAI sessions among 26 therapy dogs who visited pediatric oncology patients and families (McCullough et al., 2018). While cortisol studies may have discrepant findings, the atypical levels of cortisol deserve consideration, though these differences may be attributable to individual differences and characteristics.

Dogs react to physical touch with physiological responses; the type and location of touch are relevant to these changes. Vagal tone was increased when the dog was touched in the chest area, lower top back, and shoulder area. Dogs experienced physiological calming with these touch locations (Kuhne et al., 2014).

Appeasement behaviors, seen in dogs during stressful conditions, are believed to positively correlate with heart rate and occur *less* under ventral vagal dominance (increased vagal tone), which is mediated by the parasympathetic nervous system (PNS). These types of behaviors can be observed and are linked with neurobiological changes. As positive human–canine interactions (HAI) have been shown to increase oxytocin levels in both species and the primary format in canine-assisted therapy is HAI, oxytocin can be presumed to be a primary hormonal mechanism of this treatment that benefits all involved parties.

Though there are numerous methods to measure stress levels in humans and canines, it is ethical to use noninvasive techniques that do not invoke stress themselves. Heart rate (HR) and heart rate variability (HRV) are examples of mechanisms that can be used to assess physical arousal and stress (Katayama, et al., 2016) and estimate emotions. Heart rate is a good measure of arousal but does not discriminate between positive and negative causation. Exhilaration from downhill skiing and the abject terror from being chased by a large bear will both accelerate the heart. Heart rate variability is the difference between the heart beats during inhalation and exhalation. The larger discrepancy is considered a 'higher HRV' which is indicative of a higher vagal tone. High HRV and high vagal tone are both associated with reduced anxiety, better cardiac function, and good digestive function. Heart rate variability is a measure of the autonomic nervous system balance and systemic health and is also sensitive to the valence and intensity of emotion (Katayama et al., 2016). The index can recognize that something is off, yet it cannot identify the etiology.

Respiration rates are typically easily observed and monitored, providing a viable method to assess stress levels. The rate of respiration is regulated metabolically, yet reacts to emotional valence (Jerath & Beveridge, 2020). Dogs often pant with an open mouth when respiration increases, reflecting anxiety.

Another noninvasive biomarker of stress in a dog is the measurement of temperature. Hemispheric-specific temperatures can be determined through the tympanic membrane, located in the dog's ear. One study found a significant increase in the temperature of the right ear of the dog during a moderate stressor. These results are consistent with the knowledge that stressful experiences are processed in the right hemisphere of the dog (O'Hara & Worsley, 2019).

Any assessment of behavior that involves human interpretation can be challenged as contaminated by subjectivity. Even precise measurements of biomarkers can be questioned, as neurobiology is complex. Single systems have multiple functions and interact with other systems, and it is difficult to analyze interactions between systems. Welfare science needs further study and standardization of endocrine measures as reliable indexes of well-being (Chmelikova et al., 2020) Research of the human and mammalian brain has been propelled forward by technological advancements such as neuroimaging. Use of functional magnetic resonance imaging (fMRI), positron emission tomography (PET), electrocardiogram (ECG), galvanic skin response, and other technology support measuring and monitoring physiology. It is predicted that these mechanisms will someday become more affordable, accessible, and user friendly as they could improve clinical assessments of client response, progress, and outcomes.

Ensuring the Welfare of the Psychotherapy Dog

Responsibilities of the Clinician to the Participating Dog

Canine-assisted psychotherapy can be a highly effective treatment, yet the inclusion of a live animal into the process increases the responsibilities of the clinician. Ethical considerations are now extended beyond the client to the participating animal as well. Animals have emotions, needs, and likes and dislikes that must be identified and addressed. The animal requires adequate attention, consideration, and treatment that meet their needs.

A thorough screening of the child and family is also necessary to identify factors that could be contraindicative to CAP, such as fears, phobias, allergies, illness and immune issues. The previous history of the child and family with dogs and cultural attitudes and practices are also important to vet. Protective measures and standardized protocols should also be in place to protect against pathogens and/or injuries for all participants.

Informed consent must be obtained, backed by transparency and receptiveness to ongoing concerns. 'Goodness of fit' is a central component of good practice and defines the well-orchestrated pairing of the client, their characteristics and needs, and therapeutic objectives with the participating dog (Fine et al., 2019; VanFleet, 2017). Historically, dogs have been chosen based on a certification as a 'therapy dog' *and* availability. However, this practice does not guarantee a suitable synergy for the client, dog, and circumstances. 'Goodness of fit' is directly relevant to treatment outcomes *and* the assurance of ethical welfare practice (VanFleet, 2017). The field of animal-assisted psychotherapy could easily be compromised if these considerations are neglected.

Many clinicians are unable to maintain more than one working psychotherapy dog, as multiple animals require substantial care, attention, and time. Some clinicians supplement their practice with other smaller animals to increase options, such as gerbils, guinea pigs, or birds, yet all animals require a significant commitment plus knowledge of how to best incorporate them. If there is a single dog, it is crucial that the animal is versatile and resilient. The clinician must be objective and forthcoming if the fit between client and dog is not ideal, and be professionally competent in traditional forms of treatment that do not include an animal.

Safeguarding the physical health and safety of the child *and* dog is imperative. Any program that involves dogs and children should have an integrated *dog safety* component. Children brought to the mental health clinician typically have an identifiable disorder and studies show that those with a behavioral disorder are at higher risk for dog bites (Mitchell, et al., 2003). Most of the dogs who bite are known to the child and do not have a history of aggression. A set of established rules provide a structure of expectations and each participant should be aware of these parameters, including the dog.

The Relationship

The relationship between the clinician and the dog is a primary component of good welfare. The clinician and dog should have a healthy bond and relationship that is authentic, mutually fulfilling, and enduring. The relationship should reflect respect, effectual communication, and synchronicity. The pair also serves as a template of a healthy relationship, offering the child an alternative model that may contrast with previous affiliations (VanFleet & Faa-Thompson, 2017). Children should have the opportunity to observe compassion, kindness, and respect between clinician and dog. The inherent inequality in the interspecies relationship requires diligence in the clinician to avoid exploitation in any form. Meeting these conditions conveys an implicit assurance to the child that they will also be respected, valued, and well treated (Tedeschi & Jenkins, 2019).

The clinician also functions as a coregulator of the dog's emotional and arousal states, analogous to the attachment relationship between caregiver and infant. The relationship fulfills the primordial need for safety and functions as a safe haven, offering accessible proximity in times of distress. Felt safety is essential to attachment, the therapeutic alliance, *and* the therapeutic process. Emotionally, the dog that experiences anxiety, fear, or discomfort relies upon the clinician to remediate that state. The clinician must maintain a continuous awareness of the states of both the child and dog and be prepared with strategies that can be rapidly applied. Activation of the SES is a primary objective of the clinician for both the child and the dog.

Training

Puppies do not develop fear until around five to six weeks, making three to six weeks an optimal period for exposure training. The implication of this is that learning within this period becomes encoded as either positive or neutral. Early exposure to a wide variety of experiences will stimulate neural growth and organization, optimizing overall development. Varied early experiences also enhance motor and social development, curiosity and exploration, and confidence. Puppies should not be separated from their mother this early, however, so training must occur with the mother's approval and presence or comfortable proximity.

Positive training practices are founded on the formation of a healthy, mutual relationship, and rely on positive reinforcement, enjoyment, and natural behavior. Canine sensory systems are sensitive. Dogs are able to hear whispered signals and respond to subtle hand signals and nuanced facial expressions. Many dogs can follow a pointing finger as a directional gesture and also are capable of deciphering eye messages that also signal direction. These traits support skills that enhance the human–animal bond (HAB), bidirectional communication, and the ability to function as a team. Training as a team directly impacts the relationship. Punitive practices, such as intimidation, physical force, and anger-based communication have no place in training and can create psychological issues for the dog. This form of training is based on gaining compliance through fear, and this is analogous to aversive parenting. Treating a dog this way and then expecting it to support healing in a child with interpersonal betrayal is not only unethical but contrary to common sense. Direct involvement in dog training contributes to the additional requisites for a clinician who incorporates dogs into treatment. Beyond base educational and licensing requirements for clinical work, the clinician should have additional education, training, and experience in canine sciences, plus sufficient experience in the handling and training of dogs.

Understanding What the Dog is Telling Us

A proficient knowledge of canine communication is a core capability, as the clinician and dog need to be attuned and aware of each other's states. While dogs have evolved to understand human emotion, humans have some catching up to do. Humans have an innate tendency to seek emotional information from faces and if that is to the exclusion of posture, tension, movement, and other nonverbal expressions, the interpretation of emotion might not be accurate. Humans also will anthropomorphize or attribute human characteristics to dogs. This makes sense as we use our human resources to take in, process, and interpret all environmental stimuli. The ability of humans to interpret canine emotion is filtered through our familiarity with the animal, our belief system, and our individual emotional nature (Kujala, 2017). These potential biases and tendencies reinforce the need for additional training and proficiency in canine sciences.

Can You Think Like a Dog?

The clinician needs to be astutely aware of the dog's sphere of emotions, temperament, personality, preferences, triggers, and fears. The interspecies relationship should be on a level of intimacy that supports this awareness along with a proficiency in deciphering the dog's communication signals.

Specific components that maximize the experience for the dog include matching the conditions with their interests and needs, providing abundant opportunity for them to behave as a dog, allowing the freedom to make choices, and ensuring their mental and physical well-being. Dogs require safety, attachment relationships, and abundant social experiences. They deserve novelty, rich sensory experience, and cognitive stimulation. We must be able to consider the world through the *canine lens* to understand their species, and from the perspective of the individual dog, to foster an equitable partnership. The ability to truly understand what the dog needs, what they enjoy, and how they might feel, can probably be summed up in one concept: an attuned relationship. Dogs have evolved to understand us. If we are going to build an authentic relationship with them, then we need to understand them, as well. That is true reciprocity and attunement.

Basic Needs

All dogs deserve a life that provides them safety, attachment relationships, coregulation, lots of social opportunities, exercise, and abundant play. Consistency and predictability are highly stabilizing for dogs, as well as children. Routines should be established that include healthy nutrition, regular veterinary care, exercise, and social experiences with the clinician, other family members, the community, and other dogs and animals. They should be afforded a range of other opportunities (beyond psychotherapy work) that they enjoy. Rituals or the repeated experience of personalized 'events' also enhance the life of the dog. Kerbie rode in the car to get coffee each morning with a family member; Lilley had regular hikes with her human and other familiar dogs; and Cassidy would be taken to McDonald's each year for a birthday hamburger and fries. Apparently, Cassidy convinced his human that anybody's birthday would suffice for that special event. Routines and repeated rituals and activities are valuable to the dog's psyche, well-being, and are reinforcing to the relationship.

The enriching home environment for the dog should be healthy, positive, and be safe and free of verbal abuse, chaos, and physical violence by any residents or visitors. Dogs deserve to be valued as an integral member of a group. Night sleep, naps, eating, digestive, and other basic daily components should be familiar enough that changes in the dog's routines will be easily noticed and remediated. Most dogs are bright, energetic, and hungry when they awaken. These characteristics align with good health and well-being. Behavioral shifts from the norm require attention and remediation.

The Milieu

The milieu of treatment strongly impacts the processes and outcome of treatment, and planning for an optimal environment should accommodate the dog as well as the child. The physical characteristics of the space, whether indoor or outdoor, should be safe, free of distractions, be a comfortable temperature, warmly lit, and spacious. There should be comfortable areas for sitting or lying; space to freely run and play; work areas for activities, and a dedicated space that provides for avoidance or escape. A bed under the desk or in a corner can provide the dog space when not immediately working and it should be out of view of the child. The dog should also *always* have the option to leave the room, relieve itself, and have accessible water. The clinician has the primary responsibility for both the child and dog. The clinician should have energy, enthusiasm, flexibility, and the ability to rapidly shift and multitask.

During the Session

Participation should be enjoyable and enriching for the dog. The animal should receive nourishing praise and positive reinforcement. Their preference to engage will be reflected in their body and energy. Maintaining a positive attitude in the dog will enhance therapy. Along with a safe, welcoming, and healthy setting, rich with options, the milieu will set the stage for productive treatment.

When working with an animal and child, there should be a clear set of rules that ensure safety. The dog should never be placed in harm's way, just as the clinician would never expose the child to harm. Rules that ensure safety can be framed in terms of respect, kindness, and care, and can be intentionally integrated into treatment.

Sensitivity is a valued trait for a therapy dog, yet can create vulnerability to visceral absorption of intense client emotions or negative emotion contagion. Highly compliant dogs may suppress their natural behavior, personality, and energy to please their human. Dogs under stress will show appeasement, displacement, and fatigue, thus the clinician should monitor behaviors and be aware of physiological signs as well. Panting, darting eyes, nervous movement, and proximity seeking or avoidance are indicators of arousal. The dog should be granted agency, choice, and 'be heard' while working. Dogs do communicate their needs and states. It is up to the clinician to 'listen,' be knowledgeable about stress signs, know their normal behavior and notice changes, and be effective in remediating the stress. The dog has the clinician's back, and the clinician should have the dog's back, as well.

Finding Seamus

Seamus was the first dog of the author to participate in psychotherapy, and her interest in this mode of treatment was galvanized by this unique animal. Some animals seem to be born with a purpose and those who can communicate their will and be 'heard' have the opportunity to live a rich and fulfilled life as they fill the hearts of those who come to know them.

Waiting

I told the woman on the phone that I was looking for a very young, brown female pup. A few hours later, she greeted me at her door and led me into a tiny kitchen. It was bright and noisy, and smelled of new puppies. My eyes followed the noisy chaos, and there they were, in a blue plastic swimming tub on the floor. I sat down next to the tub and watched this mass of wiggling little bodies. They crawled up and over each other, melting their individuality into what looked like a bowl of bubbling chocolate.

As I looked closer, trying to study their individual faces, a sudden movement caught my eye, and my attention abruptly shifted to the countertop behind me. Next to a cluttered sink was a much larger pup, vigorously trying to escape the persistent rubbing of a towel across his back. He had obviously just been bathed in the sink, and was completely over that process.

The lady lifted him from the counter, trying desperately to control his flailing limbs and somehow he got to the floor with all four legs underneath him. I was confused, as his coat was marbled in black and white and he was three times the size of the litter in the tub. He charged across the small kitchen, ears flopping up and down and leapt into the tub landing in the middle of the pups, scattering them out of his way. He leapt again and was suddenly face to face with me, little paws on my chest, wiggling and now licking my face.

I smiled, patted him, and set him to my side, eager to see these little brown pups. I picked one up and gazed into her eyes. She wiggled and squeaked, and I set her back into the blob of siblings. I picked up another, and then another, and was disappointed that I wasn't feeling a wave of positive confirmation in my heart. They were young, looked incredibly alike, and none of them seemed to demonstrate any personality.

Meanwhile, the bigger, marbled pup bounded back across my lap and presented himself in my face once again. I felt like he was trying to make his case, though I couldn't immediately decipher his message. I turned to the woman and asked 'why is he so big and different from the others?' I had a brief vision of him stealing all of the puppy food, or maybe he had some kind of mutation. She replied that he was not from that litter. He was two months older and his littermates had all been picked up by their new owners.

He had been passed over, not chosen, and left behind, and I began to see that he knew it. Now he had eight more pups he had to compete with. Did he know that the bigger he grew, the less desirable he would be to people seeking little puppies? He was really working the room, making his case, and trying to win me over. I finally understood.

I let him settle into my lap, and as I stroked him, I became hyper-attuned with of the smooth texture of his coat. I could feel his little heart beating, and studied his head and long floppy ears. I gazed into his bidding eyes and realized he had not only commanded my attention, he had connected to me, and it was undeniable. He didn't have me at 'hello,' but he had woven his way into my heart. I was feeling it now, that wave of confirmation. I did not understand why, but I knew he was mine…or, I was his. As I drove home, my little guy was curled up in a blanket next to me. He seemed content, at peace, like he was in the right place. He had been waiting for me.

Temperament, personality traits, and behavior contribute to the decision of appropriateness for the working therapy dog, yet its capacity for attunement, attachment, and a strong interest in humans are essential. Seamus clearly had the above characteristics and an enthusiasm for his 'job.' He never wavered in his energy for children, yet required and enjoyed his rest and rejuvenation. After a day of being present at the program, even with significant breaks and naps, he would come home and recharge by sleeping up against me. He seemed to 'plug in' and recharge his batteries, and I think he was recharging mine, as well. While other working dogs might recharge through a jog, playtime, or watching television, Seamus chose what I call the 'Ventral Vagal Velcro' technique. We were truly connected and that placed us both in a lovely parasympathetic state

The Benefits of Working as a Psychotherapy Dog

In 2017, when Dr L.M. Glenk conducted a literature search for an article on the effects of therapy work on dogs; she found exactly *nine* peer-reviewed articles (Glenk, 2017). Fortunately, the experience of the dog who participates in psychotherapy is emerging as a critical consideration for AAI, and the response to earlier advocacy for these dogs is growing (Glenk, 2021).

Social Benefits

Socialization helps dogs develop the ability to discriminate between appropriate and inappropriate social behaviors. Dogs who participate in treatment learn social rules, skills, and boundaries; they learn what appropriate behavior is and can also interpret cues to mediate behavior. Dogs are a highly social species and desire, seek, and enjoy social interactions with humans, even showing a preference to our species over interactions with their own (Cobb et al., 2021). The social prowess of dogs has been partially attributed to their ancestors, as wolves were highly social prior to the coevolution; still, dogs have continued to increase their social acumen. Social interaction and play are highly rewarding; so are human attention, affection, and positive touch. Dogs are proficient at solicitation and will actively campaign for implicit and explicit rewards. The treatment session offers abundant opportunities for social engagement and experiences through shared space, games, play, and other interventions.

Behavioral Benefits

The behavior of dogs has been shown to improve with positive HAI, evidenced in improved social behavior (Bergamasco et al., 2010) and increased amenability to training (Valsecchi et al., 2007). Predispositions for traits and skills were selected during domestication, but one has to also consider the propensity of modern dogs to learn. Through observation, mimicry, associative learning, habituation, and training techniques, dogs pick up increasingly complicated skills, most of which benefit treatment. This social skill set improves relationships with conspecifics and other, unknown humans which facilitates increased opportunities for work *and* play opportunities.

Cognitive Enrichment

The animal that has 'a job' feels valued and competent. It can be presumed that most animals, as humans, want to feel loved, appreciated, needed, and useful. A distinct shift in posture, behavior, and focus can be seen in an animal when they step into a role of responsibility. It is crucial that they enjoy their work. Whether it is the water rescue of a swimmer, the detection of a diabetic episode, a planned and goal-directed interaction with a child, or merely a source of comfort and safety for another, all jobs are important. Valued roles are cognitively stimulating, increase a sense of agency, and nourish the overall well-being of the dog.

Dogs need cognitively stimulating activities. Creating challenges for them, problem-solving activities, and puzzles all tap the circuitry that will maintain skills and support further learning. The pairing of the child and dog motivates both and they reinforce each other's curiosity and creativity.

Animals should be valued and encouraged to find their interests and strengths. Dogs are intelligent, curious, and crave social interaction and shared activities. Each has individual potential that when tapped will be reflected in their attitude, energy, and eyes. Canine eyes speak with a unique language. While we can read some of what they signal, it is a communication style that requires attunement and attention. Time spent together and positive training practices increase synchronicity of movement, emotion, and even physiology. The result is a bonded duo that functions as a team and mutually supports the other.

Physiological Benefits

Oxytocin (OT) has been identified as functioning as a substantial regulator in mammalian relational and social behaviors and early studies support its role in human–animal interaction. Oxytocin both encourages social HAI *and* is activated by HAI (Nagasawa et al., 2015). In one study of dogs and humans, positive effects such as bonding and pleasure were evidenced by physiological data showing lowered heart rates and increased oxytocin levels in owners and dogs, but not in controls (Odendaal & Meintjes, 2003). Research by Handlin et al. (2011) investigated the effects of short-term human–dog interaction (HAI) on heart rate, oxytocin, cortisol, and insulin levels in owners *and* dogs. Interspecies interactions provide sensory stimulation including touch, stroking, and pleasurable levels of pressure; along with visual, auditory, and olfactory input (Handlin et al., 2011).

Several studies have investigated the effects of exogenous OT administration upon canine behavior during HAI. The administration of intranasal OT in dogs during affiliative interactions was suggested to facilitate bonding (Romero et al., 2014), social play (Romero et al., 2015), and increased canine sensitivity to human communication (Olivia et al., 2015; Macchitella et al., 2016). Child–dog interactions that involve positive connections, sensory stimulation, and shared proximity enhance oxytocin levels in both subjects which then loop back to reinforce further prosocial and affiliative behaviors.

Oxytocin (OT) studies have garnered substantial interest and enthusiasm for the hormone's positive effects on social behaviors and well-being, yet its processes are complex and often involve multiple components. A recent study by MacLean and associates corroborated earlier studies showing the dramatic response of OT to HAIs, and suggested they may have been the first to examine vasopressin (AVP) in humans, documenting reduced levels during HAIs (MacLean et al., 2017). The effects of OT are dependent upon AVP actions and the two closely linked hormones are frequently involved together in physiological processes, though through different actions. Vasopressin functions to activate the HPA axis, invoking the SRS, while OT attenuates sympathetic action (Buttner, 2016). Oxytocin produces calming and positive social behavior, while AVP is associated with anxiety or aggression (MacLean et al., 2017).

Dogs gain emotional and physical security from the presence of a human (Prato-Previde, 2003). A human that is positively perceived can 'attenuate' stressful experiences in dogs and establish a safe haven effect that encourages exploration (Gacsi et al., 2013; Horn et al., 2013). The clinician's behavior parallels the caregiver in the attachment experience with the infant. Neuroscientist Jaak Panksepp (1998) proposed that mammals have an innate 'seeking' drive that encompasses curiosity and exploration, two behaviors of healthy individuals.

Grooming can be framed as social body care and was investigated for its role in stress buffering (Reinhardt & Reinhardt, 2017). When a dog experiences positive tactile interaction with a human, their cortisol is reduced in both plasma and saliva (Dudley et al., 2015). Stroking a dog also lowers blood pressure and elevates levels of oxytocin, dopamine, and endorphins in both the human and dog (Odendaal & Meintjes, 2003).

Conclusion

Increased awareness and recognition of canine sentience is directing attention beyond basic concerns of health and safety to considerations of quality of experience, emotional health, volition, and the freedom to behave naturally. Science is providing paradigm-changing data that is informing clinicians of canine abilities that were previously unrecognized. The canine species is exceedingly social, relationally focused, and has communication skills that subsidize a proficient capability to interpret human communication. Social animals must communicate to initiate and maintain social relationships, resolve conflicts, and participate in social interactions. Canines are sentient, intelligent, and social. Therefore, if we, as humans, intend to form relationships, interact, and incorporate them into our lives, we owe it to them to learn *their* language and become more mindful of their intelligence and social behavior.

Professor Philip Tedeschi suggested that the Nussbaum capability approach is an excellent statement of what good welfare encompasses. This approach encourages attention, compassion, and justice to children and animals. Developed by theorist Martha Nussbaum and Nobel Prize economist Amartya Sen, this model extends beyond basic freedoms to include opportunities to experience life, health, and bodily integrity; the right to experience emotions, affiliation, and attachments; the freedom to play and experience control; and permission to engage one's senses in thought and imagination (Nussbaum, 2007). Working psychotherapy dogs would surely agree.

References

Bekoff, M. (2007). *The Emotional Lives of Animals*. Novato, CA: New World Library.

Bekoff, M. (2013). After 2,500 Studies, It's Time to Declare Animal Sentience Proven (Op-Ed). Retrieved from http://www.livescience.com/39481-time-to-declare-animal

Bergamasco, L., Osella, M., Savarino, P., Giuseppe, L., et al. (2010). Heart rate variability and saliva cortisol assessment in shelter dog: Human animal interaction effects. *Applied Animal Behaviour Science*; 125(1–2): 56–68.

Broom, D.M. (1986). The scientific assessment of animal welfare. *Applied Animal Behaviour Science*; 20(1–2): 5–19. https://doi.org/10.1016/0168-1591(88)90122-0

Buttner, A.P. (2016). Neurobiological underpinnings of dogs' human-like social competence: How interactions between stress response systems and oxytocin mediate dogs' social skills. *Neurosci Biobehav*; 17: 198–214. https://doi.org/10.1016/j.neubiorev.2016.08.029

Chmelikova, E., Bolechova, P., Chaloupkova, H., Svobodova, I., Jovici, M., & Sedmikova, M. (2020). Salivary cortisol as a marker of acute stress in dogs: a review. *Domestic Animal Endocrinology*; 72: 106428. https://doi.org/10.1016/j.domaniend.2019.106428

Chrouos, G.P. (2000). The stress response and immune function: Clinical implications. *Annals of the New York Academy of Sciences*; 917: 38–67. https://doi.org/10.1111/j.1749-6632.2000.tb05371.x

Cobb, M.L., Otto, C.M., & Fine, A.H. (2021). The animal welfare science of working dogs: Current perspectives on recent advances and future directions. *Frontiers in Veterinary Science*. https://doi.org/10.3389/fvets.2021.666898

Csoltova, E., & Mehinagic, E. (2020). Where do we stand in the domestic dog (canis familiaris) positive-emotion assessment: A state-of-the-art review and future directions. *Frontiers in Psychology*; 11: 2131. https://doi.org/10.3389/fpsyg.2020.02131

Darwin, C. (1871). *The Descent of Man and Selection in Relation to Sex*. New York: Random House.

Dudley, E.S., Schiml, P.A., & Hennessy, M.B. (2015). Effects of repeated petting sessions on leukocyte countries, intestinal parasite prevalence, and plasma cortisol concentration of dogs housed in a county animal shelter. *Journal of the American Veterinary Medical Association* 247(11): 1289–1298. https://doi.org/10.2460/javma.247.11.1289

Fine, A.H., Beck, A.M., & Ng, Z. (2019). The state of animal-assisted interventions: Addressing the contemporary issues that will shape the future. *International Journal of Environmental Research and Public Health*; 16(20): 3997.

Gacsi, M., Maros, K., Serkvist, S., Farago, T., & Miklósi, A. (2013). Human analogue safe haven effect of the owner: Behavioural and heart rate response to stressful social stimuli in dogs. *PLoS One*; 8(3): e58475. https://doi.org/10.1371/Journal.pone.0058475

Glenk, L.M. (2017). Current perspective on therapy dog welfare in animal-assisted interventions. *Animals (Basel)*, 7(2):7.

Glenk, L.M. & Foltin, S. (2021). Therapy dog welfare revisited: A review of the literature. *Veterinary Sciences*; 8(10): 226. https://doi.org/10.3390/vetsci8100226

Handlin, L., Hydbring-Sandberg, E., Nilsson, A., Ejdeback, M., Jansson, A., & Uvnas-Moberg, K. (2011). Short-term interaction between dogs and their owners: Effects on oxytocin, cortisol, insulin and heart rate-an exploratory study. *Anthrozoös*; 245(3). https://doi.org/10.2752/175303711X13045914865385

Haubenhofer, D.K., & Kirchengast, S. (2006). Physiological arousal for companion dogs working with their owners in animal-assisted activities and animal-assisted therapy. *Journal of Applied Animal Welfare Science*; 9(2): 165–172. https://doi.org/10.1207/s15327604jaws0902_5

Haubenhofer, D.K., & Kirchengast, S. (2007). Dog handlers and dogs' emotional and cortisol secretion responses associated with animal-assisted therapy sessions. *Society and Animals*; 15: 127–150. https://doi.org/10.1163/156853007 X187090

Hediger, K., Meisser, A., & Zinsstag, J. (2019). A one health research framework for animal-assisted interventions. *International Journal of Environmental Research and Public Health*; 16: 640.

Horn, L., Huber, L., & Range, F. (2013). The importance of the secure base effect for domestic dogs-evidence from a manipulative problem-solving task. *PLoS One*; 8(5) e65296. https://doi.org/10.1371/j.pne.0065296

Huber, A., Barber, A.L., Farago, T., Muller, C.A., & Huber, L. (2017). Investigating emotional contagion in dogs (Canis familiaris) to emotional sounds of humans and conspecifics. *Animal Cognition*; 20(4): 703–715. https://doi.org/10.1007/s10071-017-1092-8

Jerath, R., & Beveridge, C. (2020). Respiratory rhythm, autonomic modulation, and the spectrum of emotions: The future of emotion recognition and modulation. *Frontiers in Psychology*; 14(11): 1980. https://doi.org/10.3380/fpsyg.2020.01980

Katayama, M., Kubo, T., Mogi, K., Ikeda, K., Nagasawa, M., & Kikusui, T. (2016). Heart rate variability predicts the emotional state in dogs. *Behavioural Processes*; 128: 108–112. https://doi.org/10.1016/j.beproc.2016.04.015

Katayama, M., et al. (2019). Emotion contagion from humans to dogs is facilitated by duration of ownership. *Frontiers in Psychology* https://doi.org/10.3389/fpsyg.2019.01678

King, C., Watters, J., & Mungre, S. (2011). Effects of a time-out session with working animal-assisted therapy dogs. *Journal of Veterinary Behavior*; 6(4): 232–238. https://doi.org.10.1016/j.jveb/2011.01.007

Kuhne, F., Hossler, J.C., & Struwe, R. (2014). Behavioral and cardiac responses by dogs to physical human-dog contact. *Journal of Vet Behav: Clinical Appli and Research*; 9(3): 93–97.

Kujala, M. (2017). Canine emotions as seen through human social cognition. *Animal Sentience*; 2017.013:1–34. https://doi.org/10.51291/237-7478.1114

Lind, A.-K., Hydbring-Sandberg, E., Forkman, B., & Keelings, L.J. (2017). Assessing stress in dogs during a visit to the veterinary clinics: Correlations between dog behavior in standardized tests and assessments by veterinary staff and owners. *Journal of Veterinary Behavior*; 17: 24–31. https://doi.org/10.1016/j.veb.2016.10.003

Macchitella, L., Stegagno, T., Giaconella, R., Polizzi di Sorrentino, E., Schino, G., & Addessi, E. (2016). Oxytocin improves the ability of dogs to follow informative pointing: A neuroemotional hypothesis. *Rendiconti Lincei*; 28(1): 105–115. https://doi.org/10.1007/s12210-016-0579-6

MacLean, E.L., Gesquiere, L.R., Gee, N.R., Levy, K., Martin, W.L., & Carter, C.S. (2017). Effects of affiliative human–animal interaction on dog salivary and plasma oxytocin and vasopressin. *Frontiers in Psychology*; 8:1606. https://doi.org/10.3389/fpsyg.2017.01606.

Marinelli, L., Normando, S., Siliprandi, C., Salvadoretti, M., & Mongillo, P. (2009). Dog assisted interventions in a specialized centre and potential concerns for animal welfare. *Veterinary Research Communications*; 33: 93–95 https://doi. org/10.1007/s,11259-009-9256-x

McCullough, A., Jenkins, M.A., Ruehrdanz, A., Gilmer, M.J. & O'Haire, M.E. (2018). Physiological and behavioral effects of animal-assisted interventions on therapy dogs in pediatric oncology settings. *Applied Animal Behaviour Science*; 200: 86–95. https://doi.org/10.1016/j.applanim.2017.11.014

Mitchell, R.B., Nanez, G., Wagner, J.D., & Kelly, J. (2003). Dog bites of the scalp, face, and neck in children. *The Laryngoscope*; 113(3): 492–495.

Nagasawa, N., et al. (2015). Social evolution. Oxytocin-gaze positive loop and the coevolution of human-dog bonds. *Science*; 348 (6232): 333–336. https://doi. org/10.1126/science.12610

Ng, Z.Y., Pierce, B.J., Otto, C.M., Buechner-Maxwell, V.A., Siracusa, C., & Werre, S.R. (2014). The effect of dog-human interaction on cortisol and behavior in registered animal-assisted activity dogs. *Applied Animal Behaviour Science*; 159: 69–81. https://doi.org/10.1016/j.applanim.2014.07.009

Nussbaum, M. (2007). Human right and human capabilities. *Harvard Human Rights Journal*, 21. Retrieved from chicagounbound.uchicago.edu

O'Hara, S.J., & Worsley, H.K. (2019). A cost-effective, simple measure of emotional response in the brain for use by behavioral biologists. *The Bio-FUT*; 70: 141–148. https://doi.org/10.1556/019.70.2019.18

Odendaal, J.S. & Meintjes, R.A. (2003). Neurophysiological correlates of affiliative behavior between humans and dogs. *The Veterinary Journal*; 165(3): 333–336. https://doi.org/10.1016/S1090-0233(02)00237-X

Olivia, J.L., Rault, J-L., Appleton, B., & Lill, A. (2015). Oxytocin enhances the appropriate use of human social cues by the domestic dog (Canis familiaris) in an object choice task. *Animal Cognition*; 18(3): 767–775. https://doi.org/10.1007/s10071-15-0843-7

Platt, S.R. (2021). Animal sentience: An inconvenient truth? Retrieved from http://todaysveterinarypractice.com/animal-sentience

Prato-Previde, E., Custance, D.M., Spiezio, C., & Sabatini, F. (2003). Is the dog-human relationship an attachment bond? An observational study using Ainsworth's strange situation. *Behaviour*; 140(2): 225–254.

Rault, J-L., Waiblinger, S., Boivin, X., & Hemsworth, P. (2020). The power of a positive human–animal relationship for animal welfare. *Frontiers in Veterinary Science*; 2020: 7. Frontiers Media. https://doi.org/10.3389/fvets.2020.590087

Reinhardt, A., & Reinhardt, V. (2017). *The Magic of Touch*. (2nd ed.).Washington, DC: Animal Welfare Institute.

Romero, T., Nagasawa, M., Mogi, K., Hasegawa, T., & Kikusui, T. (2014). Oxytocin promotes social bonding in dogs. *Psychology Cognitive Science*; 111 (25). https://doi.org/10.1073/pnas.1322868111

Romero, T., Nagasawa, M., Mogi, K., Hasegawa, T., & Kikusui, T. (2015). Intranasal administration of oxytocin promotes social play in domestic dogs. *Communicative & Integrative Biology*; 8(3): e1017157. https://doi.org/10.1080/19420889.2015.1017157

Rooney, N.J., Gaines, S.A., & Hiby, E. (2009). A practitioner's guide to working dog welfare. *Journal of Veterinary Behavior*; 4(3). https://doi.org/10.1016/j.veb.2008.10.37

Rugaas, T. (2005). *On Talking Terms with Dogs: Calming signals* (2nd ed.). Wenatchee, WA: Dogwise Pub.

Serpell, J.A., Coppinger, R., Fine, A.H., & Peralta. (2010).Welfare considerations in therapy and assistance animals. In A.H. Fine (Ed.), *Handbook on Animal-Assisted Therapy: Theoretical Foundations and Guidelines for Practice* (3rd ed., pp. 481–503). New York, NY: Elsevier.

Singer, P. (2009). Speciesism and moral status. special issue: Cognitive disability and its challenge to moral philosophy. *Metaphilosophy*; 40(3–4): 567–581.

Sundman, A-S. et al. (2019). Long-term stress levels are synchronized in dogs and their owners. *Scientific Reports*; 9 (7391). https://doi.org/10.1038/s41598-019-43851-x

Tedeschi, P., & Jenkins, M.A. (2019). *Transforming Trauma: Resilience and Healing Through Our Connections with Animals*. West Lafayette, IN: Purdue U. Press.

Valsecchi, P., Prato-Previde, E., & Accorsi, P.A. (2007). Quality of life assessment in dogs living in rescue shelters. *Animal Welfare; 16*.

VanFleet, R. (2017). Toward greater awareness of welfare in animal assisted interventions: The animal assisted play therapy (trademark) model. *The IAABC Journal*.

Verga, M., & Michelazzi, M. (2009). Companion animal welfare and possible implications on the human-pet relationship. *Italian Journal of Animal Science*; 8(1). https://doi.org/10.4081/ijas.2009.s1.231

Yeates, J.W., & Main, D.C.J. (2008). Assessment of positive welfare: A review. *Veterinary Journal*; 175(3): 293–300. https://doi.org/10.1016/j.tvjl.2007.05.009

Yong, M.H. & Ruffman, T. (2014). Emotional contagion: Dogs and humans show a similar physiological response to human infant crying. *Behavioural Processes*; 108: 155–165. https://doi.org/10.1016/j.beproc.2014.10.006

Part Three

The Structure and Mechanisms of Healing Dysregulation

Chapter 8   The ni-CAP Framework

Introduction: The Conceptual Foundation

The evolutionarily inspired nervous system is shaped by significant relationships and environmental experiences that become encoded into neurobiological hardware. The disruption and dysregulation of neural circuitry manifests symptoms in multiple domains, and these are what bring clients into treatment. When treatment evokes change, the brain itself, an organ of adaptation, changes too (Cozolino, 2017; Siegel, 2015). The ni-CAP framework seeks to facilitate positive changes that become encoded in the neural fabric of the child. A fundamental understanding of the neurobiological mechanisms of development, dysregulation, psychopathology, and treatment informs and equips the clinician with the means to judiciously target objectives and circuitry, and promote enduring change.

Developmental trauma, caused by interpersonal betrayal, causes a deep, primeval injury on the core of the child. Humans have a critical need to connect with others, and if this capacity becomes impaired, the child can become compromised on multiple levels. The paradox of expected care *and* harm coexisting in the caregiver evokes a disconnection of the child from its symbiotic lifeline. Without the scaffolding of social and interpersonal relationships, the child becomes tasked with their own survival, alone and without the resources they would typically acquire through a healthy development. Treatment for these children requires a relational context (Herman, 1997) that is three-pronged. The child must be afforded the safety, coregulation, and nurturance of a healthy attachment experience that fulfills emotional, social, and neurobiological needs. The gaps of disrupted development need to be filled, and the child needs to be equipped with a repertoire of resources to navigate future challenges.

This prescription creates another potential dilemma, as the traumatized child has become disconnected, distrustful, and fearful of other humans. How can trauma be repaired by human relationships when human relationships are associated with betrayal and harm? The answer is the working therapy dog that provides the necessary bridge back to trust, connection, and well-being. The dog that is incorporated into treatment is permitted to behave naturally, which provides an authentic representation of an honest

DOI: 10.4324/9781003217534-12

and reciprocal relationship. The intuition, presence, and skill set of the clinician brings the child into a well-designed milieu that is shaped by neurobiological awareness and intentional, individualized practices. The importance of the authenticity of the dog cannot be over-emphasized, as adverse experiences breed distrust and sensitize the child's radar to continuously scan for deceit, false images, and fakery. The dog is honest, genuine, and attuned, characteristics that are neurally supported by the imprint of evolution.

The brain is a complex system that continuously interacts with the environment to maintain internal homeostasis. Systems require regulation, rhythm, and synchrony to effectively perform a vast array of functions. Dysregulation and impaired rhythm and synchrony create disconnection, dysfunction, and frustration. The roles of synchrony, rhythm, and mimicry in attachment and human relationships have been well researched and found to be associated with healthy development. It is suggested that these are *catalyzing elemental mechanisms* that support and influence neurobiological growth, organization, integration, and connectivity. With that perspective, integrating these mechanisms into treatment with the intent to positively impact neurobiology should improve therapeutic outcomes.

Brain development is sequential and hierarchical and proceeds from simple to complex, neurons to networks. The brainstem and autonomic nervous system (ANS) develop first followed by increasingly complex brain regions. It makes sense to promote reorganization and regulation matching the evolutionarily conserved trajectory of development. Variances in skills and deficits are related to the age of the child, the intensity, frequency, and chronicity of maltreatment, and a host of other factors. Bruce Perry, acclaimed trauma scholar, recognized that these children will typically present with an uneven pattern of development and require a personalized, developmentally attuned treatment plan that meets their unique needs (Perry, 2009).

Children Need Treatment that Meets Their Needs

Interpersonal betrayal consumes trust, safety, and the ability to connect with others. How can a betrayed child acquire the level of safety and trust necessary to even begin therapy? The working psychotherapy dog exudes the necessary components of safety and authenticity at the critical point of entry into treatment.

Neurobiologically infused canine-assisted psychotherapy (ni-CAP) is a developmentally informed framework that integrates psychology with neurobiology, employing implicit (and explicit) mechanisms of change implemented through canine participation. This chapter will provide a conceptualization of ni-CAP identifying the theoretical basis, structure, and mechanisms of change for children with dysregulation. Ni-CAP is designed to be flexible to enable a personalized treatment plan that meets the specific needs of the individual child. As most child-focused clinicians believe, the child should not have to fit into a specific model; the model should fit the child. Intentional integration with components of other models can shape a treatment plan that is comprehensive and individualized.

Over 550 models of child therapy currently exist in the United States (Kazdin, 2000). While many have been shown to be highly effective with children, few are empirically based and when trauma enters the equation, rates of efficacy drop. Several challenges have been identified in traditional models that treat children with developmental trauma and dysregulation. Statistics reflect deficient engagement and participation, high rates of attrition, and poor outcomes (Wamser-Nanney & Steinzor, 2017).

The relative developmental immaturity of children is also a critical consideration of clinicians in the choice of treatment modes. Traditional models are often verbally centered and require self-awareness, a capacity for insight, and the ability to verbally express oneself, all processes of higher cognition. The prefrontal cortices (PFC), tasked with executive functions, language processes, and reflective capacity, have a protracted rate of maturation extending into the third decade (Field, Beeson, & Jones, 2015). Children tend to communicate nonverbally, using behavior and physical movement as means for expression (Goodman, Reed & Athey-Lloyd, 2015).

While developmentally informed treatment is critical for children being treated for any issue, children with trauma history and neurobiological alterations represent a more challenging population. Many clinicians find that children with early trauma history can be especially resistant to treatment. What appears to be resistance in these children, however, can be reframed to be the distinct symptomatology that results from the experience of trauma (Parish-Plass, 2021). Interpersonal trauma causes a rupture of the core relationship that represents the primary influence upon normal development. A betrayed child finds it difficult to trust others; they are anxious and avoidant; and they become disconnected from others *and* themselves.

Dogs Support the Establishment of Therapeutic Alliance

These patterns also hamper the establishment of a therapeutic alliance, which research strongly supports as a salient predictor of treatment outcome (Horvath, 2001).The incorporation of a dog into treatment increases the strength and quality of the therapeutic alliance which was found to form earlier in animal-assisted psychotherapy (Parish-Plass, 2018) than other models. Canine presence facilitates social interaction, and increased treatment 'adherence' in children with trauma history (Signal et al., 2017).

When a child observes the respect, nurturance, and trust between the clinician and dog, a sense of reassurance and safety occurs, opening the window to connection (Chandler, 2017). Incorporating dogs into treatment will activate implicit reward systems, increasing motivation, the rate of attendance, engagement, and participation (Wohlfarth et al., 2013).

The inviting, engaging attention and movement of a dog activates neural mechanisms of interest, attention, and positive arousal. They establish a comfortable safe space that invites the child into an environment enriched by their dynamic presence.

The mechanism behind this is suggested to be the increase in oxytocin from human–canine interactions (Beetz & Bales, 2016; Zoicas, Slattery & Neumann, 2014). Oxytocin improves social perception, increases social interaction, and promotes a sense of safety.

Epidemiological findings have implored mental health disciplines to develop multidimensional models that will efficaciously address the spectrum of debilitating consequences of developmental trauma (DT). Clinicians are responding to these concerns by exploring alternative, creative, and integrated treatments. Animal-assisted therapies (AAT) have garnered increasing interest and approval over the past two decades and more recently, are implemented with children who have suffered from maltreatment and DT (Parish-Plass, 2008; VanFleet & Faa-Thompson, 2014). A survey of 83 US play therapists that incorporated animals into their sessions received a 'universal' positive response that animals could support therapeutic goals (VanFleet, 2007). Studies have shown that adolescents are much more comfortable interacting with a dog compared to adult therapists (Beetz et al., 2012).

A parallel interest in the neurobiological effects of DT has created a synergy between psychology and neuroscience that is rapidly advancing the knowledge base of traumatology (McLaughlin et al., 2015; van der Kolk, 2005). Interest in the potential of animals to positively affect trauma-induced neurobiological insult is also increasing (Parish-Plass & Pfeiffer, 2019). The animal-assisted therapy fields have struggled to obtain a strong empirical base that supports treatment efficacy, and the infusion of neuroscience will likely improve those efforts. It is suggested that multidisciplinary studies of the potential of dogs to restore neurobiological regulation will dramatically increase in the coming years, as neuroscience offers more tangible and measurable constructs that are easier to empirically study.

Ni-CAP does not require cognitive awareness or language proficiency, as it relies upon relationships, mind-body integration, movement, and experiential activities which target the neurobiological basis for prosocial behaviors, regulation, creativity, and emotional expression (Gaskill & Perry, 2014). While these treatment components can be applied explicitly, substantial change with children occurs through implicit mechanisms.

The ni-CAP framework has an exciting potential to reconnect and restore the dysregulated child. This model is not a 'reinvention of the wheel.' It is a reformulation of existing and emerging components that shape treatments. Each of these components has theoretical, empirical, and clinical support, to varying degrees. Some of the science behind these components is, literally, currently emerging.

The primary components of this framework are listed below to give a clear picture of the working parts: principles, theory, neural mechanisms, elemental mechanisms, and components. With further research, an advancing scientific knowledge base and increased clinical input from practice, this framework will presumably be shaped and refined over time, thus should be viewed as somewhat fluid. The flexibility that supports integration of this framework with other model components will likely produce further treatment options that may expand the repertoire of the clinician who treats children. Much of the content below has been introduced in earlier chapters, thus, to avoid repetition, the degree of content will vary.

Primary Principles of ni-CAP

1. Child development, childhood maltreatment, developmental trauma, dysregulation, and psychopathology are best understood using a multidimensional perspective that incorporates neurobiology, attachment, and regulation.
2. Treatment is designed and applied using the same perspective and is shaped to meet the specific individual needs of the child. Treatment is relationally based in an enriched environment, and the dog is a primary agent of change. The unique characteristics of canines function as mechanisms of change and are judiciously incorporated.
3. Ni-CAP is developmentally informed and adheres to a sequential and hierarchical direction of treatment, paralleling early development and the attachment process.
4. Neural dysregulation functions as a link between maltreatment and psychopathology and is a transdiagnostic construct that serves as a primary treatment target.
5. Dysregulation may also occur in multiple developmental domains of the child, including emotion, behavior, physiological/somatic, cognitive, social, and intra- and inter-personal (the self and relationships).
6. Neurobiologically infused CAP can be implemented in a variety of settings with diverse populations and disorders.
7. The interpersonal relationship is a primary mechanism of treatment, and the canine expands the potential number and types of relationships, and supports reconnection and reregulation of the child.

A Proposed Theoretical Basis for ni-CAP Theory

The field of animal-assisted interventions (AAI) has searched for a unifying singular theory that can empirically support the efficacy of human-animal interactions (HAI), yet it remains elusive. Eminent neuroscientist, Eric Kazdin (2017) proposes that no universally accepted single theoretical framework exists. Research that seeks the empirical base continues to be challenged by the heterogeneity of programs, approaches, and applications.

Kazdin proposes that, instead of a singular theory, the evidential support can be found in a set of 'explicit small theories' that together delineate the theoretical foundation.

While ni-CAP aligns well with the primary principles of current canine-assisted therapy and play therapy models, the framework is specifically informed and supported through an integration of the following theories and themes. (These are detailed throughout the book.)

1. The neurobiology of human development, maltreatment and DT, dys-regulation, and psychopathology and the neural mechanisms that support regulation and resilience (listed below).
2. Dysregulation as a transdiagnostic mechanism, link between maltreatment and psychopathology, and target of change.
3. Sculpting the competent social self: acquiring agency, social cognition, and self-efficacy.
4. 'Theory of the Dog'— coevolution, biophilia, canine science, human–animal bond (HAB) and human–animal interaction (HAI).
5. Attachment theory
6. The polyvagal theory (PVT)

The Developmental Direction

Disrupted or incomplete developmental processes can leave children with deficits and gaps in their mastery of developmental stages. Ni-CAP applications are multifactorial and support the regulation, integration, and connectivity of the child following the template of childhood developmental trajectory and attachment. The clinical team is guided by the optimal attunement, responsiveness, and roles of the caregiver who provisions safety, coregulation, care, and nurturance.

Neural systems and regions are targeted in a sequential and hierarchical direction, establishing regulation in the primitive functions of the brainstem as a first step, then addressing limbic system dysregulation, and ultimately recalibrating cerebral cortex processes. Each new stage of growth relies on the successful function of the preceding stage, and bottom-up and top-down interventions are applied that match the child's developmental stage and functional levels. This fundamental approach has been developed and successfully applied by eminent trauma expert, Bruce Perry (2009) in his neurosequential model and is also employed in Linda Chapman's (2014) neurodevelopment art therapy model.

The developmental consequences of DT can become compounded, filtering into multiple domains causing deficits, delays, and symptoms that bring the child to the attention of clinicians. Two possible pathways can be suggested for treatment. One is to address the current symptomatology, seek reduction of symptoms and behavioral change, with the hope that changes will endure. The other process is to address the broad footprint of trauma, revisit and replicate the missing components of development including attachment, and restore regulation of the systems of the child from the bottom up. The latter process should accomplish the goals of the first, as positive neural change will improve symptoms and sustain change. Neural change occurs through efficacious therapy, and a new, more productive trajectory is set that is supported by regulation and resilience.

The Neurobiological Lens

The ni-CAP model reflects the recent increase in collaborations between psychology and neuroscience. While the integration of these disciplines informs and equips the clinician through the increased awareness of the neurobiological imprint upon the child, the most powerful impact may be on treatment design and efficacy.

The primary objective of any psychotherapy is to change the functioning of the brain (Cozolino, 2017; Perry, 2009), as all functions of living beings have neural correlates. Positive relational and social experiences regulate hormones, transmitters, and activate neural processes that recalibrate the nervous system, creating change in regulatory processes, behavior, and social function (Carter, 2017).

While studies have demonstrated the positive effects of therapy (Messina et al., 2016), the identification of specific mechanisms of change has been historically more difficult to delineate. Recent neuroimaging advances that permit observation of brain circuitry activation in real time have supported the development of theories using science to explain function. This study, along with other research attributed positive clinical outcomes from psychotherapy processes as reflecting increased neural regulatory function (Messina, 2016). As with most research, studies answer questions yet generate even more queries reflecting the seemingly indeterminate challenge of deciphering the brain.

Neural change requires activation of neural systems and networks; consider the well-known tenet that 'nerves that fire together wire together' (Hebb, 1949). Treatments seeking to create constructive change in a child may show positive results upon completion, yet a gradual decline often occurs as the effect seems to weaken over time. Enduring change is manifested by integration and internalization of new learning, and generalization to other settings. Change requires patterning, significant repetition, and concurrent activation of neural systems.

Ni-CAP enhances connectivity and integration of neural networks that support relational and social processes. One example of a specific goal of neurobiological change is the enhancement of connectivity and communication between the prefrontal cortexes and the emotional limbic regions. The regulatory competence of the PFC, manifested through inhibition of emotional activity and reactivity in the limbic region (particularly the amygdala), improves emotional and behavioral control. When primitive brain regions are dominant in a child's functioning (as during elevated states of stress), higher levels of cognition are dampened. After initial stabilization and reduction of arousal, therapy can address the emotional systems and then proceed to the cognitive control mechanisms in the prefrontal regions. The PFC is the location of thinking processes that involve self-awareness, social interest, creativity, and regulation of lower regions.

Neural Mechanisms that Support Regulation and Resilience

1. Neural plasticity
2. The PVT, social engagement system (SES) and vagal system
3. The oxytocin system
4. Right-to-right brain coupling and communication
5. Mirror neurons

Brief Overview of Neural Mechanisms of ni-CAP

Neural Plasticity

Critical periods of neural plasticity are essential for the growth, integration, and organization of the young brain. Old paradigms that cited plasticity as time limited have been revised, increasing optimism for the potential of positive changes in neural circuitry throughout most of the lifetime (Kemperman et al., 2002). Studies identified the frontolimbic network, *more than other areas*, retains plasticity similar to early development and that the right hemisphere cycles into growth phases throughout the lifespan (Sapolsky, 2003). These findings imply the potential for brain changes that correlate with functional changes through the use of therapeutic interventions. A key component of therapeutic change is to stimulate neural receptivity to respond to positive, meaningful experiences, as these encode lasting change.

Ni-CAP seeks to incorporate mechanisms that increase the receptiveness of neural circuitry. The concept of an enriched environment as a promoter of neural enhancement and change has been well studied and is an empirically supported mechanism. Physical activity, mindfulness meditation, new learning, creativity, new skills, music, and even adequate sleep are additional mechanisms suggested to open windows of plasticity. Creating an enriched environment and enriching experiences with the canine also stimulate plasticity and expand the potential of other mechanisms.

The PVT, Social Engagement System (SES) and Vagal System

When Stephen Porges initially revealed his polyvagal theory (PVT) to the scientific community in 1994, he did not endorse the theory as apropos to mental health applications (Porges, 1995). The theory was created to explain the collaborative relationship between the brain and body, particularly how the ANS influenced psychological and behavioral processes during times of threat and safety (Porges, 2011). The outstanding reception of the theory by the clinical community propagated interest in 1999 during a conference managed by Bessel van der Kolk that brought the role of neuroscience into clinical understanding of the trauma response. The PVT provides clinicians with the science involved in trauma and dysregulation; science that produces salient targets in trauma treatment.

As explained earlier, the SES provided the highly socialized mammals with a neural substrate that coordinates the heart and bronchi with the striated musculature of the face and head (Porges, 2011). This platform orients the child toward interpersonal connection and prosocial behaviors. When the SES is 'in town,' the mobilization and immobilization defenses are inhibited, establishing a sense of safety. The child cannot access the SES when one of the defense modes is active.

The informed clinician can use their understanding of the psychological, behavioral, and neurobiological aspects of the stress response system to shape and apply interventions. One of the critical initial roles of the clinician and dog is to provide coregulation, supporting the child in stabilizing affect and arousal. The clinical team actuates the effects of social presence, support, and connection to establish a resolute sense of safety and increase receptivity to prosocial behavior. Porges frames HAI as a form of the SES (Porges, 2013).

Regulation is supported by multiple neurobiological components such as parasympathetic activation/vagal tone, right brain coupling/implicit communication, the mirror neuron system, hormones and neurotransmitters, and elemental mechanisms of nature. These components, along with elemental mechanisms of synchrony, rhythm and mimicry, support and accentuate the positive effects of treatment. None of these mechanisms function in isolation. Their benefits are conveyed through complicated collaborations between neural, chemical, and endocrine components. Within the past decade, 'the oxytocin system' has become acclaimed as a powerful hormone that plays a role in a multitude of mammalian functions.

The Oxytocin System (OT)

Meg Olmert noted that children with maltreatment history often have dysregulated OT systems, resulting in lower levels of available, protective quantities. It follows that diminished levels of OT would impair the multitude of functions that it supports, leading to increased vulnerability. Research involving humans and canines has shown that activation of the oxytocin system produces numerous positive effects, including increased trust, calm states, and positive mood; reduced anxiety and subjective sense of stress, and improved social communication and prosocial behavior (Carter & Keverne, 2009). Additionally, OT inhibits and down-regulates the mobilization and immobilization stress responses. The oxytocin system provides a biological resilience that protects the child through its support of social and relational affiliation and competence.

The positive, physiological, and psychological effects of animals also include the activation of the OT system. Touch is a powerful mechanism that activates OT (Carter & Porges, 2016). Mental health clinicians are dissuaded from using touch in human–human therapy, yet dogs provide an ethical and safe modality. Touch is emotional and social support, boosts immunity and growth, and is a key component of healthy attachment. Most dogs respond positively to appropriate, affectionate touch, and OT is activated in them, as well. Human–dog interactions activate a positive loop between the duo, bidirectionally elevating OT levels, which then increase social interaction, creating a circular route of benefits (Nagasawa et al., 2015; Odendaal and Meintjes, 2003).

Right Brain-to-Right Brain Coupling

The primary communication style of the caregiver–infant is becoming recognized as the prototype for the clinician–child duo within treatment. Interpersonal neurobiology research has provided insight into mechanisms of treatment that create change, and Alan Schore has clarified that the right-to-right brain nonverbal, implicit messaging that provides coregulation, implicit learning and nurturance within the attachment relationship, is a mechanism of connection that induces growth and change in treatment (Schore, 2019). The intersubjective nonconscious messaging creates a biological, emotional, and behavioral synchrony and rhythm within the pair. The heart rates of the caregiver and infant synchronize, and within the ni-CAP clinician–dog team, synchronization also occurs on multiple levels.

This form of communication avoids the semantic contamination of motivations, and thoughts; the child is offered a 'felt' experience that transmits acceptance, validation, and coregulation. The experience of 'being felt' provides the critical sense of safety and security (Geller & Porges, 2014; Siegel, 2010). The clinician is able to access the child's emotional journey, and with synchronous, coregulating signaling, can trigger neuroplasticity resulting in neural structural modifications within the child's regulatory systems.

Right-to-right brain communication is a primary component of ni-CAP and other creative, experiential therapies such as play, art, sand play, and other treatments that work with symbolic, nonconscious processes (Schore, 2021).

Mirror Neurons

The MN system helps explain the power of learning through observation and modeling. When we simply observe the actions of another, we unconsciously (and sometimes consciously) learn from them. Firing as if we were performing the same action, behavior, or emotion, mirror neurons give us a visceral insight into the world of another (Rizzolatti & Sinigaglia, 2010). Iacoboni (2008) identified the 'chameleon effect' which is an imitation of another's facial expressions, gestures, and postures. This behavior is an automatic, unconscious attempt to connect or 'match' another. When someone is smiling, we smile as well, as the MN permits us to share and experience an emotion with someone. Contrary to the conceptualizing of MN as mere spectating, the MN system helps facilitate emotional engagement. The MN system is believed to influence social behavior, including the ability to be empathetic. Perceptions of the environment gained through observation generate sensorimotor regions, providing implicit information about the object or action that is observed. Viewing emotional expression in another lights up the MN regions (premotor and parietal), yet also activates the deeper regions of emotion, including the cingulate cortex and anterior insula (Simpson & Ferrari, 2013).

The clinician can tap these processes, increasing the child's realm of positive emotional experience, improving interpersonal connectivity, and entraining their nonverbal body signals to project positivity, confidence, and social messaging. There are suggestions that the MN system is experienced by the clinician during psychotherapy, as well. Observations and interactions with the child elicit neural activation in the clinician. Being keenly aware of their emotional and visceral states will enhance their perceptions of the child.

Catalytic Elemental Mechanisms

1. Synchrony
2. Rhythm
3. Mimicry

Elemental Mechanisms of Nature are Catalysts for Neural Regulation

As treatment of dysregulation involves components of evolution, attachment, and development, it follows that primordial mechanisms of nature would also enhance therapy processes that recalibrate the complex system of a child. 'Elemental mechanisms' are organizing patterns or actions of nature that function as catalysts or guides to all facets of life. They can be framed as mechanisms embedded in the primordial instructions that exist within the world or universe. When humans and animals live by nature's 'primordial instructions' (or guide) that have existed from the beginning of time; processes, functions, and life itself, are enhanced. Synchrony, rhythm, and mimicry are just three examples of elemental mechanisms that can recalibrate the dysregulation of the complex systems of a living being.

Synchrony

Synchrony supports the establishment of the attachment relationship, pro-social behavior, and social cohesion. Synchronous movement promotes trust, empathy (Koehne et al., 2016), and cooperation. Synchrony has a distinct role in the development of emotion regulation, perspective taking, and is influential in rapport building and affiliation. The ability of dogs to synchronize with humans is discussed in Chapter 6.

Movement synchrony couples brains, which is considered 'interbrain synchronization' (IBS), or brain-to-brain coupling (Hasson et al., 2012; Koole & Tschacher, 2016). Brain-to-brain coupling is similar to a Wi-Fi connection. The coupling occurs via sound, light, chemical compound, or pressure (Hasson et al., 2012). Nonverbal expressions that signal information, such as facial expressions and physical gesturing also promote coupling. Coupling occurs implicitly within motor, perceptual, and also cognitive domains (Knoblich et al. 2011).

'Hyperscanning' refers to any brain imaging of more than one person at a time. It is highly useful to the 'two-person' research model. Electroencephalography (EEG), magnetoencephalography, and functional near-infrared spectroscopy (f NIRS) are three modern techniques that allow the study of couples directly engaged in interactions. Interbrain synchronization can be facilitated by the shared activities of a pair that will increase social behaviors, bonds, and affiliations.

In a study of IBS between pairs using hyperscanning, the investigative team found greater synchronization and a higher willingness to help each other in a coordination task, compared to controls (Hu et al., 2017). The results inferred that prosocial behavior was increased by interbrain synchronicity and that result was mediated by a shared intentionality. The scientists also sought to identify the neural substrate that supports interpersonal synchrony and found that the approximate locus of this process correlated with the left medial prefrontal cortex (lmPFC). This region is believed to play a role in the processing of social information (Frith & Frith, 2001) and has shown increased activation during a paired task, when one member simply follows the direction of the other's gaze (Hu et al., 2017).

This study, along with others, demonstrates the potential of interventions that facilitate interpersonal synchronization for children who are dysregulated and disconnected. Synchrony is central in a healthy attachment process, and the facilitation of this process within treatment (between child and clinician) can confer powerful positive effects, particularly if the neural substrate of synchrony is tapped. While research is just beginning to study the potential of humans and animals to neurally sync, the capacity for 'shared intention,' emotional synchrony, and social referencing already exists in canines. Increasing attunement, mindfulness, and focused observation are skills that support the ability to synchronize, join, and connect with others.

Rhythm

Rhythms of the brain and body are central to life itself. Motor movement stimulates cortical spindle oscillations and rhythmic oscillations support movement (Basso, 2021) and the development of cognitive skills, language, and social and emotional learning (Cirelli et al., 2018). 'Interpersonal entrainment' is defined as the moment that rhythmic oscillations are coupled, which occurs in biological, as well as mechanical systems (Schmidt & Richardson, 2008). Synchrony and brain coupling are integral to a healthy attachment relationship and also highly useful mechanisms of treatment.

Rhythmic movement stimulates neural plasticity, facilitates neural network communication, and optimizes brain functionality (Headley & Pare, 2017). Interventions that involve the coordinated movement and activity between the child and the canine can support synchrony and rhythms of nature. Neural integration and organization are optimized through mechanisms of synchrony, rhythm, and mimicry, particularly in the brainstem. Drumming, music, and running are examples of interventions that target the nervous system and serve as stabilizing forces that work from the bottom up.

Automatic Mimicry

Automatic mimicry is an essential component of sociality (Prochazkova & Kret, 2017). It facilitates reciprocity, rapport, emotional recognition, and produces emotional contagion, or the sharing of affect (Niedenthal et al., 2005). Emotional mimicry is the imitation of emotional expressions of others. Emotional expressions can be defined as facial expressions or conceptualized as shared emotion, which is beyond empathy and theory of mind.

Mimicry is proposed to function as a regulator of relationships between individuals (Hess & Fischer, 2014). The act of mimicry requires a degree of attention, openness, interest in another, and perception. Facilitating mimicry opportunities during treatment experiences may have positive neural 'training,' offering new, alternative experiences that may counter previous experience and learning. Mimicry is considered a precursor to the development of empathy and prosocial behavior (Mogan et al., 2017). The capability to engage in mimicry can be strongly impaired in psychological disorders.

Mimicry can be considered as a mechanism of shared emotion and representations (Romero et al., 2013). The mirror neuron substrate supports the ability to recognize and interpret the emotions and intentions of others. Neural activation occurs in the pars opercularis when the child observes and imitates emotional expressions in others. In their investigation of empathy and interpersonal competence in typically developing children, Pfeifer and colleagues correlated MN neural activation with empathy (Pfeifer et al., 2008).

Mimicry occurs more frequently with others that are familiar, possibly because it involves mutual gaze (Seyfarth & Cheney, 2013). Face-to-face gazing is a powerful mechanism in the establishment of attachment and remains so in social relationships throughout life. While mimicry is known to be stronger with affiliates, the behavior also serves the formation of a social relationship, and enhances its quality and depth. The intent to also create joining opportunities can facilitate positively reinforcing experiences from dogs, as well as humans that bolster confidence, self-esteem, and instill feelings of worth.

Mimicry is also more common when the child develops an ability to categorize someone or something else as similar or 'like me,' a capability that is a precursor for the development of social cognition (Meltzoff & Moore, 1989). Children with trauma-induced dysregulation can feel disconnected, isolated, and as if they are different from 'everybody else.' Dogs are seen as 'like me' to most children due to this and the perceived similarities between the two.

Mimicry and synchrony subsidize emotional sharing and activation of empathic pathways, implying a coupling of brains. Information is passed between two individuals without awareness or consciousness and this joining facilitates a shared experience and strengthens the bond (Kret, 2015). Specific emotions can be generated by nuanced and subliminal cues such as postures, movements, and facial expressions, which trigger ANS responses (Prochazkova, & Kret, 2017). Eye contact can be synchronized, and functions as a type of mimicry (Feldman et al., 2011).

Components of ni-CAP Treatment

The Relationship

It truly is 'all about the relationship.' The clinical relationship is the most consistent predictor of change (Norcross & Wampold, 2011). The clinical team of clinician and dog functions as 'intentionally and fully present.' Establishing a state of 'fully present' is necessary to establish the therapeutic relationships and foster effective treatment (Geller, 2017). The coregulation of affect and arousal are embedded in the therapeutic relationship (Geller and Porges, 2014).

The PVT explains how the clinician team's presence creates a 'felt' sense of safety (Porges, 2011). Repeated occasions of safety lead to the experience of safety in other relationships, an example of therapeutic generalization (Geller and Porges, 2014).

An Attachment Partner

The dog–human attachment relationship aligns with the features of the human–human bond: safe haven, secure base, proximity seeking, and separation-induced distress (Zilcha-Mano et al., 2012). Dogs provide functions of attachment, increase engagement, social interaction, and enhance prosocial behavior (Parish-Plass, 2008). Dogs provide social support, camaraderie, affiliation, and increase the sense of value, worth, and self-efficacy in children.

The therapeutic experience, through incorporation of canines, can rework the child's maladaptive internal working model of attachment, establishing a healthier model. The clinician and dog can model a secure attachment by demonstrating attunement, synchronicity, and the provision of needs. The early objectives and processes of treatment parallel the attachment process of early development that establishes the foundation for all future emotional, relational, and social function. Development of the social brain begins at birth and serves as the foundation for future social behavior. Treatment processes target the components of a secure attachment to create, reinstate, and/or strengthen this foundation. Attachment provides the child with internal working representations of their relationships with others and their world (Bowlby, 1969). Internalized models are reflected by the child's patterns and behaviors.

Humans and dogs are capable of bidirectional attachment bonds with each other. Research suggests that the child–animal relationship can be particularly powerful to those children who lack a secure attachment with human caregivers (Wanser et al., 2019). Attachment to a dog is a powerful source of social support for a child and promotes physiological and psychological benefits (Beetz et al., 2012; Jalongo, 2015). Studies also show that a continuing relationship with an animal provides a surrogate that can fulfill similar attachment needs of a human (Zilcha-Mano et al., 2012). The canine participation within an attachment role can enhance the therapeutic process (Parish-Plass, 2008) as they personify a healthy relationship that might contrast with insecure internalized models. Today, the victimized child can experience a strong and healthy relationship with the dog, establishing safety and rebuilding trust. This relationship serves as a bridge to treatment and a step toward the objective of reconnecting with other humans for social support (VanFleet & Faa-Thompson, 2017).

The Dog is the Nucleus of ni-CAP

Neuroimaging studies of the amygdala and hippocampus, limbic structures tasked with emotion and memory, have shown that humans have specific neurons that are selective for specific visual stimuli. The right amygdala was found to have neurons that showed a 'categorical selectivity' for animal images. The neural preference is assumed to be an evolutionarily conserved adaptation and is unrelated to arousal or emotion (Mormann et al., 2011). This rapid processing of animal images implies a biological salience, and can be interpreted as evidence that supports AAIs for children with trauma and dysregulation.

Dogs share an incredible number of traits with the child, including reliance on similar modes of expression and communication. Both species are also dependent upon adult humans, think in relatively simple and concrete terms, and crave attention. One of the most rewarding mutual and bonding characteristics, however, is the strong desire to fulfill the embedded need of our species to play.

The dog embodies authenticity and is virtually incapable of dishonesty, deception, judgment, or exploitation. As a species, humans tend to automatically vet the authenticity of others, even subconsciously. Developmental trauma (DT) can confer in children a pervasive distrust and threat bias to humans that creates suspicion and defensiveness, a response that the dog does not elicit.

The incorporation of a dog fosters empathy, caring and altruistic behavior, and cultivates theory of mind (ToM). Dogs provide a social partner for interactions, play, and strategy practice. Emotional and social skills are enhanced through dog involvement. They also facilitate mind-body and somatic work serving as a social partner to observe, compare, and practice arousal regulation strategies.

The dog provides invaluable influence by providing the child with a sense of safety, lowering anxiety and reducing fear. Dogs are capable of calming distressing arousal implicitly and nonverbally, connecting to a child through visceral mechanisms. The canine-supported therapeutic setting is designed as an enriched environment that incorporates a context of relationships and play.

The capability of canines for reciprocal communication and social interaction has been touted as a powerful promoter of therapeutic success. Canine research has revealed proficiencies in dogs in the use of visual, auditory, and olfactory cues to identify human emotion. They were also found to expressively communicate with humans using specific human

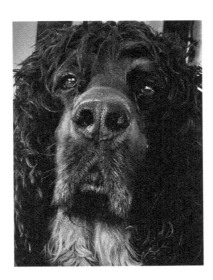

mechanisms, such as eye contact, face-to-face gaze (Maclean et al., 2017), and motor and emotion synchrony.

Enriching Experiences and Enriched Environment

Lou Cozolino describes psychotherapy as an enriched environment as it promotes the development of emotional, cognitive, and social behaviors through activation of the neurobiological substrates of these areas. He states that neural growth, organization, and connectivity correspond to improvements in symptomatology. Enriched environments (EE) have been credited with the reduction of anxiety and stress symptoms (as have canines), and the enhancements of memory processes and cognitive function (Ball et al., 2019).

The ni-CAP milieu is intentionally designed to be an enriched environment (EE) and strives to provide the child with enriching experiences that promote healing, growth, and connection. An EE offers a broad range of sensory-rich stimuli, healthy relationships, movement and creative experiences, and the learning of new skills and strategies, all which support restoration and growth. The assisting canine embodies the elements of EE, and links the child to the restoring power of nature and elemental mechanisms (synchrony, rhythm, and mimicry) that function as catalysts of neural growth and organization.

The restorative effects on neurobiology through EEs have been demonstrated through numerous studies with animals and humans. The results demonstrate that enriched environmental stimuli can increase weight and thickness of brain structures, including the cortex (Diamond et al., 1964) and hippocampus (Kempermann et al., 2002). Enrichment also showed enhanced vascular activity, and increases in neural growth hormones and neurotransmitters (Cozolino, 2017). The effects of EE were found to be most powerful during critical periods when neural plasticity is more receptive to the environment (Nithianantharajah, & Hannan, 2006). Much of the research of EE with children has been in cases of social and sensory deprivation, in which the effects are compensatory.

For children with dysregulation, the enrichment with multisensory stimuli in ni-CAP aims to restore and heal the child, compensating for early harm and deprivation. Ni-CAP seeks to increase curiosity, seeking (Panksepp, 1998), exploration, and engagement with others and the environment. This modality also offers substantial opportunities for controlled experiences of multisensorial stimulation. While all of the senses tend to become engaged by interaction with a live animal, these can be modulated. Children and dogs share the need for movement and play, not just to foster development, but to feel, learn, and more freely express emotions. These forms of positive neural activation introduce new experiences for the child that challenge trauma-induced patterns of thinking, relating, and behaving. When joined with a dog, the child will open their hearts, ears, eyes, and mind to take in the 'canine lessons of life.'

Coregulation and Stress Training

The victimized child often develops a threat bias, seeing danger where it does not exist. Behavior becomes organized around survival and safety. While suspiciousness and avoidance of adults may function as an adaptive mechanism in the context of maltreatment, a threat bias becomes maladaptive within a healthy environment and hinders the establishment of new relationships and experiences. A child who is trapped by stress and fear cannot attend, learn, or engage in healthy social interactions.

Coregulation of Affect and Arousal

The regulation of stress levels and the stress response systems are believed to stimulate neural growth in the prefrontal cortex and amygdala (Panksepp & Biven, 2012). These are key regions that impact homeostasis. Coregulation is one of attachment's primary functions as it establishes a neurobiological foundation of safety through a synchronization of the autonomic nervous systems of the duo. Instilling a sense of safety and through modulation of homeostasis, the coregulator builds trust and connection in the child. Coregulation is a critical building block for the development of the child's functional regulatory competence and provides the necessary resilience to connect with others and optimally function in a social environment. A coregulating attachment relationship of attunement and responsiveness offers protection from early adversity, and within the clinician/dog/child relationship, coregulation offers healing.

The clinical team provides the child with containment of arousal and affect, providing safety and security. Therapeutic coregulation supports the child's capacity to engage, safely revisit sensitive history, and take risks. The clinician is tuned into the arousal levels of the child that are triggered by stress and helps them remain within the 'window of tolerance.'

The Window of Tolerance and Stress Training

Stress that is induced by emotional experiences within treatment can generate neural plasticity by increasing neurotransmitter levels, along with growth hormones that support cortical integration and reorganization. Clinician-regulated moderate stress levels optimize the plasticity for neural 'association' areas of specific regions (such as frontal lobes) that regulate, manage, and integrate numerous neural circuitries (Cozolino, 2017).

A state of calm and receptiveness enhances the child's capacity to tolerate unpleasant emotions (such as anxiety or anger) without retreating into maladaptive behavior patterns. The neural reflection of regulation and adaptive coping strategies is a mild to moderate level of autonomic reactivity when confronted with a stressor. This is a valuable point of reference that can inform clinicians in the assessment of effective interventions. When a child is able to respond to stress with the regulated activation of vagal withdrawal and also engage the vagal brake, in response to changing environmental conditions, their actions are reflecting flexibility and increased regulatory capacity (Porges, 2007).

Clinicians tend to agree that, as with early development, an optimal level of stress supports growth and maturation. Within treatment, optimal levels of stress are coregulated by the clinician and dog to help the child remain within a 'window of tolerance' (Siegel, 2015). Mild stress blended with nurturance creates an environment that is growth-inducing; one that supports and challenges the child. The temporal modulation of stress for a child in therapy enables them to work on sensitive content while maintaining safety (Steele & Malchiodi, 2012).

This safe space represents a physiological level in the child that supports a sense of safety yet permits the addressing of relevant content (Ogden, Minton, & Paine, 2006). This window permits the safe processing of uncomfortable material (Ogden et al., 2006), sculpting the optimal milieu for enhancing neural plasticity and integration (Cozolino, 2017). An increased tolerance of stress levels promotes the activation of higher brain regions, facilitating the capacity to handle emotional and cognitive topics, such as narratives, identity, shame, and guilt (Heller & LaPierre, 2012).

The Importance of Play for Children and Dogs

Interspecies play represents a mode of communication with the self and others. As dysregulation can cause disconnection between children and other humans due to distrust and discomfort, dogs offer a healthy substitute and step toward this goal. The immaturity of language skills in children make reciprocal verbal therapies difficult to employ, thus interspecies play, with its symbolic nature and developmental fit, is highly suitable for children. Symbolic play allows the child to safely distance from difficult emotions, experiences, and memories. Using symbolic reenactment can reduce disruptive behaviors, support a mastery over fears or experiences, and improve regulatory competence (Crenshaw & Hardy, 2007). Play creates opportunities for children to learn, practice, and refine skills and the tolerant and enthusiastic nature of the dog endorses their suitability as playmates and partners. Children express their emotions and worries through behavior, and trauma is typically reenacted in play. When the dog is present and/or participates in play, the child experiences 'felt' safety and is able to work through their trauma.

The grandparents of two young sisters drowned when their boat capsized in Lake Huron. Upon beginning canine-assisted psychotherapy the five and seven-year-old girls spent their first two sessions cuddled up to Bucky, a large St. Bernard. Bucky had enough real estate to fully support both little bodies, and he seemed happy to shelter them. In the third session they both approached the toy shelf and the older child picked up a large blue plastic sailboat. They placed some figures on the boat and sailed it around the room a few times until they 'ran into bad weather.' The figures tried very hard to save the boat and each other, but it was looking bleak. They repeated this scene over two sessions, stopping play without an ending. In the next session, Bucky was invited into the story and performed an amazing rescue. He 'swam' to the boat and the figures jumped up on his back and were taken to an island. The girls said that the island was far away and they could only visit their grandparents one time 'because they had to stay there.' They asked Bentley if he would stay with them and protect them, and smiled when 'he said yes!'

The experience of social play occupies a central, critical role in the development of a child's emotional, cognitive, and physical health and serves as a mechanism for communication with others and the self (Winnicott, 1971). Play is crucial for canine development, as well. Social play for both species offers an enriching context for sharing emotions, learning social rules, and developing interpersonal and relational skills. Play and affiliative behaviors will decrease blood pressure in both species and increase their oxytocin, dopamine, and beta-endorphins (Odendaal & Meintjes, 2003).

Marc Bekoff (2007) writes that canines offer an incredible model for moral and social development, as their repertoire of communication, skills, and 'rules' present a highly appropriate model for humans. Humans and dogs are believed to share a neural anatomy for morality in that dogs are fair, cooperative, and show components of empathy in their play; dogs will self-handicap (which is behavioral inhibition) to even the field and use a variety of social cues to communicate their intent. Play offers the opportunity to utilize symbolism through 'pretend' scenarios. Play offers the opportunity to test new behaviors, symbolically rewrite painful past experiences, and connect with other living beings. Dogs and children will not play if they are anxious, burdened, or do not feel safe. Severe early trauma can impair the child's ability to play, which can rob them of joy, freedom, social learning, and friendships. As play and social relationships improve regulation of neurobiology and behavior (Odendaal & Meintjes, 2003), an absence of play can deprive the individual of supportive neurocircuitry. Per the polyvagal theory, children cannot freely engage in play if they are trapped in a survival state which shifts all of their resources to threat and defense. When experiencing mobilization or immobilization responses that activate the sympathetic nervous system (SNS) or the parasympathetic primitive branch (PNS), the child cannot access the SES without a calming of those systems. Canines are able to support the child in play by helping shift their threat state into a social state (Porges, 2011). Once activated, the threat responses are inhibited, and the child is free to engage, play, and participate in treatment.

Canine-assisted psychotherapy (CAP) and play therapy (PT) models are similar and easily blend on multiple levels. Both children and dogs communicate most comfortably with their bodies and both instinctively love to move and play. Both depend on others for survival; and they are both biologically predisposed to pay attention to each other. Canine-assisted psychotherapies and play therapies are both supported and guided by a set of similar principles, mechanisms, and theory (VanFleet & Faa-Thompson, 2017).

Core Objectives of ni-CAP

These core objectives are a primary set of goals that are fundamental to most treatments, yet are particularly critical for victims of developmental trauma.

1. Create a resolute sense of safety
2. Provide coregulation of affect and arousal to stabilize
3. Establish the therapeutic alliance
4. Establish or enhance attachment security
5. Sensory integration
6. Regulate neurobiology
7. Improve interoception

Conclusion: Ensuring Enduring Change

The traditional treatment schedule of one session per week has been demonstrated to positively impact functioning, yet adhering to principles of neural change may require reconsideration of that format. Residential or day treatment models would theoretically be more efficacious in achieving lasting neural changes, assuming programming fits the requisites. Repetition and reinforcement over days, weeks, and months have a clear advantage over one hour per week. Positive changes increase when treatment involves a comprehensive and inclusive approach that involves the family, schools, and other professional services.

As children progress through developmental stages, challenges and family circumstances may change, and periodic 'refresher' sessions could be advantageous. As efficacious treatment is centered on relationships, perhaps more clinicians will expand to an intermittent schedule that follows the child through life stages.

Efforts should address the tendency of the mental health field to frame trauma consequences as pathological, particularly as we note that they can lead to *psychopathology*. When the processes of the body are dysregulated, it becomes more difficult for a child to 'feel normal,' and this can create a sense of helplessness. Framing the child as central in their own healing by establishing resources they can draw upon, instilling agency and choices, and bringing them back 'into the fold' of human support are all mechanisms of restoration. The canine serves as the bridge back by helping rebuild the necessary components of attachment, safety, coregulation, and resilience. The child gains a coherent sense of self and builds genuine competencies and self-efficacy. The dog supports this healing through the bond, relationship, play, and being themselves a live, breathing animal. What could be more normal than that?

The next chapter provides a template that will bring the components of ni-CAP together to craft interventions that effectively incorporate the dog and specifically address the unique needs of the child. Dysregulation is a transdiagnostic component of most disorders, and the recognition of the neural correlates of function, behavior, and all other domains is proposed to become an integral part of clinical work going forward. The template serves as a guideline to be mindful of the goal to integrate psychology and neuroscience.

References

Ball, N.J., Mercado III, E., & Orduna, I. (2019). Enriched Environments as a potential treatment for developmental disorders: A critical assessment. *Frontiers in Psychology* https://doi.org/10.3389/fpsyg.2019.00466

Basso, J.C. (2021). Dance on the brain: Enhancing intra- and inter-brain synchrony. *Human Neuroscience* https://doi.org/10.3389/fnhum.2020.584312

Beetz, A., & Bales, K. (2016). Affiliation in human-animal interaction. In L.S. Freud, S. McCune, L. Esposito, N.R. Gee, & P. McCardle (Eds.), *The Social Neuroscience of Human-Animal Interaction* (pp. 107–125). American Psychological Association.

Beetz, A., Julius, H., Turner, D., & Kotrschal, K. (2012). Effects of social support by a dog on stress modulation in male children with insecure attachment. *Frontiers in Psychology*; 3(352): 352. https://doi.org/10.3389/fpsyg.2012.00352

Bekoff, M. (2007). *The Emotional Lives of Animals*. Novato, CA. New World Library.

Bowlby, J. (1969). *Attachment: Attachment and Loss*. Vol.1. Loss. New York: Basic Books

Carter, C.S. (2017. The oxytocin-vasopressin pathway in the context of love and fear. *Frontiers in Endocrinology* https://doi.org/10.3389/fendo.2017.00356

Carter, C.S., & Keverne, E.B. (2009). The neurobiology of social affiliation and pair bonding. In D.W. Pfaff, A.P. Arnold, A.M. Etgen, S.E. Fahrbach, & R.T. Rubin (Eds.), *Hormones, Brain and Behavior* (pp 137–165). Elsevier Academic Press. https://doi.org/10.1016/B978-008088783-8.00004-8

Carter, C.S. & Porges, S.W. (2016). Neural mechanisms underlying human-animal interaction: An evolutionary perspective. In L.S. Freund, S. McCune, L. Esposito, N.R. Gee, & P. McCardle (Eds.), *The Social Neuroscience of Human-Animal Interaction* (pp.89–105). American Psychological Association. https://doi.org/10.1037/14856-006

Chandler, C. (2017). *Animal-Assisted Therapy in Counseling*. New York, NY: Routledge.

Chapman, L. (2014). *Neurobiologically Informed Trauma Therapy with Children and Adolescence*. New York, NY: W.W. Norton & Co.

Cirelli, L.K., Trehub, S.E., & Trainor, L.J. (2018). Rhythm and melody as social signals for infants. *Annals of the New York Academy of Sciences* https://doi.org/10.1111/nyas/13580

Cozolino, L. (2017). *The Neuroscience of Psychotherapy: Healing the Social Brain* (3rd ed.). New York, NY: W.W. Norton.

Crenshaw, D.A., & Hardy, K.V. (2007). The crucial role of empathy in breaking the silence of traumatized children in play therapy. *International Journal of Play Therapy*; 16(2): 160–175. https://doi.org/10.1037/1555-6824.16.2.160

Diamond, M., Krech, D., & Rosenzweig, M.R. (1964). The effects of an enriched environment on the histology of the rat cerebral cortex. *The Journal of Comparative Neurology*; 123(1): 111–119. https://doi.org/10.1002/cne.901230110

Feldman, R., Magori-Cohen, R., Galili, G., Singer, M, & Louzoun, Y. (2011). Mother and infant coordinate heart rhythms through episodes of interaction synchrony. *Infant Behavior and Development*; 34(4): 569–577. https://doi.org/10.1016/j.infbeh.2011.06.008

Field, T.A., Beeson, E.T., & Jones, L.K. (2015). Neuroscience-informed cognitive-behavior therapy in clinical practice: A preliminary study. *Journal of Mental Health Counseling*; 38(2): 139–154. https://doi.org/10.17744/mehc.38.2.05

Frith, U. & Frith, C. (2001). The biological basic of social interaction. *Current Directions in Psychological Science*; 10(5): 151–155. https://dx.doi.org/10.1111/1467-8721.00137

Gaskill, R.L., & Perry, B.D. (2014). The neurobiological power of play: Using the neurosequential model of therapeutics to guide play in the healing process. In C.A. Malchiodi & D.A. Crenshaw (Eds.), *Creative arts and Play Therapy for Attachment Problems* pp. 178–194. New York, NY: The Guilford Press.

Geller, S.M. (2017). *A Guide to Cultivating Therapeutic Presence*. Washington, DC: American Psychological Association.

Geller, S.M., & Porges, S.W. (2014). Therapeutic presence: Neurophysiological mechanisms mediating feeling safe in therapeutic relationship. *Journal of Psychotherapy Integration*; 24(3): 178–192.

Goodman, G., Reed, P. & Athey-Lloyd, L. (2015). Mentalization and play processes between two therapists and a child with Asperger's disorder. *International Journal of Play Therapy*; 24(1): 13–29. https://doi.org/10.1037/a0038660

Hasson, U., Ghazanfar, A.A., Galantucci, B., Garrod, S., & Keysers, C. (2012). Brain-to-Brain coupling: A mechanism for creating and sharing a social world. *Trends in Cognitive Sciences*; 16(2): 114–121. https://doi.org/10.1016/j.tics.2011.12.007

Headley, D.B., & Pare, D. (2017). Common oscillatory mechanisms across multiple memory systems. *NPJ Science of Learning* 2(1). https://doi.org/10.1038/s41539-016-0001-2

Hebb, D.O. (1949). *The Organization of Behavior. A Neuropsychological Theory*. New York: John Wiley & Sons, Inc.

Heller, L., & LaPierre, A. (2012). *Healing Developmental Trauma*. Berkeley, CA: N Atlantic Books.

Herman, J. (1997). *Trauma and Recovery*. New York: Basic Books.

Hess, U., & Fischer, A. (2014). Emotional mimicry: Why and when we mimic emotions. *Social and Personality Psychology Compass*; 8(2): 45–57. https://doi. org/10.1111/spc3.12083

Horvath, A.O. (2001). The alliance. psychotherapy: Theory, research, practice, *Training*; 38(4): 365–372.

Hu, Y., Hu, Y., Li, X., Pan, Y., & Cheng, X. (2017). Brain-to-brain synchronization across two persons predicts mutual prosociality. *Social Cognitive and Affective Neuroscience*; 12(12): 1835–1844. https://doi.org/10.1093/scan/nsx118

Iacoboni, M. (2008). *Mirroring People: The New Science of How We Connect with Others*. New York, NY: Farrar, Straus & amp; Giroux.

Jalongo, M.R. (2015). An attachment perspective on the child-dog bond: Interdisciplinary and international research findings. *Early Childhood Education Journal*; 43: 395–405.

Kazdin, A.E. (2000). Understanding change: From description to explanation in Child and Adolescent Psychotherapy research. *Journal of School Psychology*; 38(4):337–347. https://doi.org/10.1016/S0022-4405(00)00040-6

Kazdin, A.E. (2017). Strategies to improve the evidence base of animal-assisted interventions. *Applied Developmental Science*; 21(2): 150–164. https://doi.org/10. 1080/10888691.2016.1191952

Kemperman, G., Gast, D., & Gage, F.H. (2002). Neuroplasticity in old age: Sustained fivefold induction of hippocampal neurogenesis by long-term environmental enrichment. *Annals of Neurology*; 52(2): 135–143. https://doi.org/10.1002/ana.10262

Knoblich, G. Butterfill, & Sebanz, N. (2011). *Psychological Research on Joint Action: Theory and Data On the Psychology of Learning and Motivation*. B. Ross (Ed.). (pp. 59–101). Academic Press.

Koehne, S., Behrends, A., Fairhurst, M.T., & Dziobek, I. (2016). Fostering social cognition through an imitation-and synchronization-based dance/movement intervention in adults with autism spectrum disorder: A controlled proof-of-concept study. *Psychotherapy and Psychosomatics*; 85(1): 27–35. https://doi. org/10.1159/000441111

Koole, S.L., & Tschacher, W. (2016). Synchrony in psychotherapy: A review and an integrative framework for the therapeutic alliance. *Frontiers in Psychology* https://doi.org/10.3389/fpsyg.2016.00862

Kret, M.E. (2015). Emotional expressions beyond facial muscle actions. A call for studying autonomic signals and their impact on social perception. *Frontiers in Psychology*; 15 https://doi.org/10.3389/fpsyg.2015.00711

MacLean, E.L., Herrmann, E., Suchindran, S., & Hare, B. (2017). Individual differences in cooperative communication skills are more similar between dogs and humans than chimpanzees. *Animal Behavior*; 126: 41–51. https://doi. org/10.1016/j.anbehav.2017.01.005

McLaughlin, K.A., Peverill, M., Gold, A.L., Alves, S., & Sheridan, M.A. (2015). Child maltreatment and neural systems underlying emotion regulation. *Journal of the American Academy of Child and Adolescent Psychiatry*; 54(9): 753–762.

Meltzoff, A.N. & Moore, M.K. (1989). Imitation in newborn infants: Exploring the range of gestures imitated and the underlying mechanisms. *Developmental Psychology*; 25(6): 954–962.

Messina, I., Sambin, M., Beschoner, P., & Viviani, R. (2016). Changing views of emotion regulation and neurobiological models of the mechanism of action of psychotherapy. *Cognitive, Affective, & Behavioral Neuroscience*; 16: 571–587. https://doi.org/10.3758/s13415-016-0440-5

Mogan, R., Fischer, R., & Bulbulia, J.A. (2017). To be in synchrony or not? A meta-analysis of synchrony's effects on behavior, perception, cognition and affect. *Journal of Experimental Social Psychology*; 72: 13–20. https://doi.org/10.1016/j.jes.2017.03.009

Mormann, F., Dubois, J., Kornblith, S., Milosavljevic, M., Cerf, M., Ison, M., Tschiya, N., Kraskov, A., Quiroga, R.Q., Adolphs, R., Fried, I., & Koch, C. (2011).A category-specific response to animals in the right human amygdala. *Nature Neuroscience*; 14(10): 1247–1249.

Nagasawa, N., Mitsui, S., En, S., Ohtani, N., Ohta, M., Sakuma, Y., Onaka, T., Mogi, K., & Kikusui, T. (2015). Social evolution. Oxytocin-gaze positive loop and the coevolution of human-dog bonds. *Science*; 348 (6232): 333–336. https://doi.org/10.1126/science.12610

Niedenthal, P.M., Barsalou, L.W., Winkielman, P., Krauth-Gruber, S.A., & Ric, F. (2005). Embodiment in attitudes, social perception, and emotion *Personality and Social Psychology Review*; 9(3): 184–211. https://doi.org/10.1207/s15327957pspr0903_1

Nithianantharajah, J., & Hannan, A.J. (2006). Enriched environments, experience-dependent plasticity and disorders of the nervous system. *Nature Reviews. Neuroscience*; 7: 697–709.

Norcross, J.C., & Wampold, B.E. (2011). Evidence-based therapy relationships: Conclusions and clinical practices. *Psychotherapy*; 48: 98–102.

Odendaal, J.S., & Meintjes, R.A. (2003). Neurophysiological correlates of affiliative behavior between humans and dogs. *Veterinary Journal* 65: 296–301.

Ogden, P., Minton, K., & Pain, C. (2006). *Trauma and the Body: A Sensorimotor Approach to Psychotherapy*. New York: W.W. Norton & Co.

Panksepp, J. (1998). *Affective Neuroscience: Foundations of Human and Animal Emotions*. New York :Oxford University Press.

Panksepp, J., & Biven, L. (2012). *The Archaeology of Mind: Neuroevolutionary Origins of Human Emotions*. New York: WW Norton & Co.

Parish-Plass, N. (2008). Animal-assisted therapy with children suffering from insecure attachment due to abuse and neglect: A method to lower the risk of intergenerational transmission of abuse? *Clinical Child Psychology and Psychiatry*; 13(1): 7–30.

Parish-Plass, N. (2018). The influence of animal-assisted psychotherapy on the establishment of the therapeutic alliance with maltreated children in residential care (Unpublished master's thesis). U. Haifa, Haifa, Israel. https://www.researchgate.net/publication/323944061

Parish-Plass, N. (2021). Animal-assisted psychotherapy for developmental trauma through the lens of interpersonal neurobiology of trauma: Creating connection with self and others. *Journal of Psychotherapy Integration*, 31(3): 302–325. https://doi.org/10.1037/int0000253

Parish-Plass, N., & Pfeiffer, J. (2019). Implications of animal-assisted psychotherapy for the treatment of developmental trauma. In M. Tedeschi & M.A. Jenkins. (Ed.), *Transforming Trauma*. W. Lafayette, IN: Purdue University Press.

Perry, B.D. (2009). Examining child maltreatment through a neurodevelopmental lens: Clinical applications of the neurosequential model of therapeutics. *Journal of Loss and Trauma*: 14: 240–255.

Pfeifer, J.H., Iacoboni, M., Mazziotta, J.C., & Dapretto, M. (2008). Mirroring others' emotions relates to empathy and interpersonal competence in children. *NeuroImage*; 39(4). https://doi.org/10.1016/j.neuroimage.2007.10,1032

Porges, S.W. (1995). Orienting in a defensive world: Mammalian modifications of our evolutionary heritage. A Polyvagal Theory. *Psychophysiology*; 32(4): 301–318.

Porges, S.W. (2007). The polyvagal perspective. *Biological Psychology* 74(2): 111–143.

Porges, S.W. (2011). *Norton Series on Interpersonal Neurobiology. The Polyvagal Theory: Neurophysiological Foundations of Emotions, Attachment, Communication, and Self-regulation*. New York, NY: Norton.

Porges, S.W. (2013). Human-animal interactions. A neural exercise supporting health. Plenary speech at the annual conference of IAHAIO International Association of Human-Animal Interaction Organization.

Prochazkova, E. & Kret, M. (2017). Connecting minds and sharing emotions through mimicry: A neurocognitive model of emotional contagion. *Neuroscience & Biobehavioral Reviews*, 80: 99–114. https://doi.org/10.1016/neubiorev.2017.05.013

Rizzolatti, G., & Sinigaglia, C. (2010). The functional role of the parieto-frontal mirror circuit: Interpretations and misinterpretations. *Nature Reviews Neuroscience*; 11(4): 265–274. https://doi.org/10.1038/nrn2805

Romero, T., Konno, A., & Hasegawa, T. (2013). Familiarity bias and physiological responses to contagious yawning by dogs support link to empathy. *PLoS One*; 8, e71365. https://doi.org/10.1371/journal.pone.0071365

Sapolsky, R.M. (2003). Stress and plasticity in the limbic system. *Neurochemical Research* 28(11): 1735–1742. https://doi.org/10.1023/a:1026021307833

Schmidt, R.C., & Richardson, M.J. (2008). Dynamics of interpersonal coordination. In A. Fuchs & V. Jirsa (Eds.), *Coordination: Neural, Behavioral and Social Dynamics*. New York: Springer.

Schore, A.N. (2019). *Right Brain Psychotherapy*. New York: Norton.

Schore, A.N. (2021). Right brain-to-right brain psychotherapy: Recent clinical and scientific advances. *Journal of Symbols & Sandplay Therapy*; 12(2): 1–22. https://doi.org/10.12964/jsst.21007

Seyfarth, RM & Cheney, DL (2013). Affiliation, empathy, and the origins of theory of mind. *Proceedings of the National Academy of Sciences of the United States of America*; 110: 10349–10356. https://doi.org/10.1073/pnas.1301223110

Siegel, D. (2010). *Mindsight: The Science of Personal Transformation*. New York, NY: Random House.

Siegel, D. (2015). *The Developing Mind: How Relationships and the Brain Interact to Shape who we are*. New York: Guilford Publications.

Signal, T., Taylor, N., Prentice, K., McDade, M., & Burke, K. (2017). Going to the dogs: A quasi-experimental assessment of animal assisted therapy for children who have experienced abuse. *Applied Developmental Science*; 21: 81–93.

Simpson, E.A. & Ferrari, P.F. (2013). Mirror neurons are central for a second-person neuroscience: Insights from developmental studies. *The Behavioral and Brain Sciences*; 36(4): 438. Simpson https://doi.org/10.1017/S0140525X12002051

Steele, W., & Malchiodi, C.A. (2012). *Trauma-Informed Practices with Children and Adolescents*. Routledge/Taylor & Francis Group.

Van der Kolk, B.A. (2005). Developmental trauma disorder. *Psychiatric Annals*; 35(5): 401–409. https://doi.org/10.1038/472298a

VanFleet, R. (2007). *Preliminary Results from the Ongoing Pet Therapy Study*. Boiling Springs, PA: Play Therapy Press.

VanFleet, R., & Faa-Thompson, T. (2014). Animal assisted play therapy to empower vulnerablechildren. In E. Green & A. Myrick, (Eds.), *Play therapy with vulnerable populations. No child forgotten* (pp. 85–103). Lanham, MD: Rowman & Littlefield.

VanFleet, R., & Faa-Thompson, T. (2017). *Animal Assisted Play Therapy* (trademarked). Sarasota, FL: Professional Resource Press.

Wamser-Nanney, R. & Steinzor, C.E. (2017). Factors related to attrition from trauma-focused cognitive behavioral therapy. *Child Abuse & Neglect*; 66: 73–83. https://doi.org/10.1016/j.chiabu.2016.11.031

Wanser, S.H., Vitale, K.R., Thielke, L.E., Brubaker, L., & Udell, M.A.R. (2019). Spotlight on the psychological basis of childhood pet attachment and its implications. *Psychology Research and Behavior Management*; 12: 469–479. https://doi.org/10.2147/PRBM.S158998

Winnicott, D. (1971). *Playing and Reality* (pp. 1–156). London: Tavistock Publications.

Wohlfarth, R., Mutscher, B., Beetz, A., Kreuser, F., & Korsten-Rek, U. (2013). Dogs motivate obese children for physical activities: Key elements of a motivational theory of animal-assisted interventions. *Frontiers in Psychology*; 4: 796. https://doi.org/10.3389/fpsyg.2013.00796

Zilcha-Mano, S., Mikulincer, M., & Shaver, P.R. (2012). Pets as safe havens and secure bases: The moderating role of pet attachment orientations. *Journal of Research in Personality*; 2012. https://dx.doi.org/10.1016/j.jrp.2012.06.005

Zoicas, I., Slattery, D.Z., & Neumann, I.D. (2014). Brain oxytocin in social fear conditioning and its extinction: Involvement of the lateral septum. *Neuropsychopharmacy*; 39: 3027–3035.

Chapter 9   Melding Mechanisms

Introduction

This chapter adds further detail to the relevance of neural, elemental, sensory, attachment, and canine mechanisms for ni-CAP, and illuminates how they support treatment. Understanding and applying neurobiological principles to treatment design helps identify the specific mechanisms of change that will subsidize more efficacious applications. Therapeutic interventions support increased regulation of neurobiology and functional domains, and they require planning and intention. A template is shared that supports the clinician in integrating specific elements and mechanisms to design specific interventions.

There are many modes of psychotherapy that can improve the lives of individuals who have suffered from early adversity, dysregulation, and psychopathology. Over 550 treatments exist for children and adolescents alone (Kazdin, 2000). While all of these treatments seek to reduce symptoms and improve function and many succeed, do we know *why* they are effective? Can we identify the specific mechanisms of change? Our traditional focus on symptom reduction can fall short of what is 'true healing.' Imagine an adolescent soccer player has a sore knee. They are advised to ice it and take an anti-inflammatory medication for a week. They follow the advice and the pain goes away. Over the next few months, or even years, however, the knee remains an issue that becomes increasingly debilitating. This is a simple example of treating symptoms rather than the cause. The knee pain may have been caused by an earlier injury. If it is not resolved, serious arthritis can set in, and the pain becomes debilitating and enduring.

A large majority of children who are victims of early maltreatment do not come to the attention of school personnel, clinicians, or law enforcement until years later. They appear defiant, are over reactive, hyperactive, and are underperforming at school. It makes sense that they might be diagnosed with ADHD, ODD, anxiety, and other disorders based on symptoms. Identifying early maltreatment may be nearly impossible at that point, but if that history caused neural and multidomain dysfunction and dysregulation, we now have a viable current source of causation that is more amenable to change.

DOI: 10.4324/9781003217534-13

All psychotherapy is purported to alter neurobiology, but much of the literature frames that as almost a 'side effect,' rather than implementation of an intentional plan to address the entirety of the child. The future of psychotherapy has been suggested by numerous scientists and clinicians to become more efficacious through the integration of neurobiology and psychology. While further research is clearly necessary to establish a more comprehensive base for this conceptualization of neurobiologically infused treatment, we can begin taking steps toward these objectives.

Top-Down and Bottom-Up

Current trauma treatment models tend to use two distinct categories of approach that begin with either cognitive or somatic processing. These approaches are known as 'top-down' and 'bottom- up'. Top-down processing is seen in traditional forms of talk or verbal therapy. This format targets the dorsolateral prefrontal cortex (dlPFC), an area of higher cognition and executive functions. The regions of the prefrontal cortex can be framed as the logical 'thinking' hub that uses cognitive control to regulate the subcortical limbic regions, the 'feeling' hub. Unfortunately, this region tends to go offline during trauma, and top-down approaches may not developmentally match children.

Bottom-up interventions address the physiological dysregulation, somatic distress, and visceral responses of trauma. Targeting the subcortical limbic or 'emotion system' seeks to regulate the sensory and emotional fallout from trauma that becomes imprinted in the body. These interventions use mechanisms such as synchrony, rhythm, and movement/exercise. Bessel van der Kolk (2014) suggests that mind-body or somatic interventions improve communication and valance between the thinking and feeling regions of the brain through the medial prefrontal cortex (mPFC), also known as the orbitofrontal OFC. Children who have dysregulated autonomic nervous systems are unable to engage, participate, and gain from interpersonal and social interactions. They are unable to attend and learn. Bottom-up interventions can stabilize the child, preparing them for further work. When a child is capable of top-down work, further integration of systems can be achieved, but the direction and graduated timing of these processes need to match developmental and functional levels.

Mechanisms

The biological need for relationships *is* powerful, and begins with the infant whose neural development is dependent upon the caregiver. A healthy attachment relationship is associated with regulation and resilience, and provisions the child with a foundation for all future relationships. The relationship in treatment is also powerful and associated with healing the child with trauma history and dysregulation and the canine increases the number of potential relationships.

The Initial Connection

Research validates the therapeutic alliance as an unequivocal covariate of change in psychotherapy (Norcross & Wampold, 2011). The child requires trust and a sense of safety to establish this alliance, however, which can be disabled by developmental trauma. 'One hundred milliseconds' is how long it takes a human to determine safety upon viewing another's face (Willis and Todorov, 2006).The inclusion of a working psychotherapy (WP) dog into treatment should increase oxytocin (OT) levels which dampens the stress response system and increases social interaction. The clinician and working therapy dog establish a setting that exudes a palpable sense of safety in the child by modeling a healthy, reciprocal relationship that is attuned, synchronous, and genuine. The energy, movement, and presence of the dog are captivating and impossible to ignore. The child is able to observe the authentic kindness and respect directed at the dog by the clinician, which increases the potential of the child to trust. This is welcoming to the child who may subconsciously imagine joining or being the recipient of that care.

The deficient social cognition seen in children with dysregulation typically manifests as a lack of friends. This is often the number one complaint of children of all ages who are experiencing profound loneliness and a disconnection from others. The almost immediate effect on a child, who has made a reciprocal connection with the dog, is one of hope. The lonely child now has someone in their corner that is interested in them, values their attention and will not judge. The establishment of an alliance with the dog may precede the therapeutic alliance with the clinician, as the neural mechanisms of canines are implicit, rapid, and unconscious. Being therapeutically and authentically present is a key component of establishing the therapeutic alliance, and the dog may have the jump on that role. This connection slips the child into a relationship that will rarely fail.

Mick was a typical 14-year-old teen who was highly resistant to the idea of therapy. His mom parked and as he slowly exited the car, he pulled his hood as far forward as he could, stared down at the ground and literally dragged his feet. The clinician opened the door and Kerbie went to work. This little dog had one 'special power' and she performed it magnificently. Kerbie was a 'greeter.' She ran out to meet Mick and ran rapid circles around him that forced him to notice her. Her speed and energy were captivating, and Mick had to pay attention to her, if for no other reason, to keep from tripping. She literally herded him through the door and into the room. As he sat down she jumped onto his lap and began licking his face. Her wiggling drew his hands to her, and as he began to vigorously pet her, his hood slipped off and he smiled. The little dog had shifted Mick from a state of anxious resistance to one of curiosity and engagement.

Presence

According to the polyvagal theory (Porges, 2011), the clinician and canine who are present and receptive convey safety that is experienced at a neurobiological level (Geller, 2017; Geller & Porges, 2014). The clinician and canine function as a clinical team and are grounded, attuned, and able to sync with each other, and that transfers to the child as a genuine invitation to join. The child vicariously imagines what it would be like to be part of that relationship. Porges states that the sensation of safety is not established by the mere absence of threat. There must be manifestations of safety, as reflected in the dog's calm and attentive presence, the clinician's gentle tone and prosody, open and receptive posture and gestures, and kind facial expressions (Porges, 2011). Being present is an intentional effort to be 'all in,' focusing energy into the creation of a welcoming and nurturing space.

When the clinician shifts away from a left-brain, intellectual, verbal style of interactive approach into a more right-brain intersubjective, nonverbal style, they are able to open up a channel of communication similar to attachment. The clinician becomes more attuned and receptive to the emotional state of the child and through this implicit, unconscious interaction can enable interbrain synchronization. This 'therapeutic presence' gives the child the experience of being joined in their space and understood. Face-to-face interaction is one of the most powerful mechanisms that link humans and communicating with full attention creates a connection and 'interpersonal context' (Schore, 2022). This implicit nonverbal style of communicating also reflects the attuned relationship between a human and dog. While dogs are capable of learning the meaning or inferences of words, the 'felt' communication that is unspoken is more likely to be understood.

Attachment

Humans and canines are capable of establishing an attachment bond with each other, a mutual relationship that benefits both parties. Many healthy attachment behaviors can be experienced during treatment such as face-to-face gazing, touch, proximity, and coregulation. The child–dog relationship is enhanced through the neurobiological substrate of attachment, which includes increased levels of oxytocin and reductions in cortisol, activation of the social engagement system (SES), and decreased indices of arousal. The therapeutic relationship may initially serve as transitional, yet can grow in depth, endure, and support the subsequent formation of human-to-human attachments. This is another example of the dog functioning as a bridge.

While the caregiver–child attachment relationship places the child in the position of 'care recipient,' the child–dog attachment promotes a bidirectional flow of care. The child is able to both receive care *and* provide

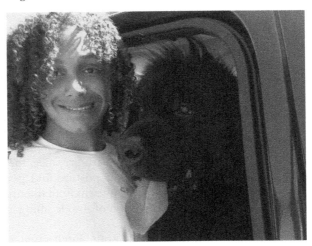

for another, an experience of reciprocity. Caring for another is often a new role for children who have experienced a lifetime of being the 'care receiver.' Children with complex needs can be captive in that role as they may receive multiple forms of treatment and service. Being charged with the responsibility of another living being offers a new level of confidence that increases self-worth and can lead to an upwelling of compassion for others. Louis Cozolino (2017) suggests that 'guided altruism' can confer a broad range of benefits through activation of neurobiological circuitry. The orbital prefrontal cortex (OPFC) becomes more proficient regulating/calming the amygdala (emotion structure) which increases the child's capacity to accept relational regulation of fear and anxiety. Altruistic experiences also increase neuroplasticity, agency, perspective-taking, empathy, and confidence. The new experiences of empathy and compassion may also lead to the child extending that kindness to their self (Cozolino, 2017).

Right Brain-to-Right Brain Communication and Coupling

The implicit communication between the infant and caregiver involves an unconscious right brain-to-right brain coupling that is a key mechanism in the attachment relationship. A primary principle of interpersonal neurobiology is that the neural development of the child's brain requires a coupling of their brain to a mature brain. The right brain-to-right brain (RB-RB) coupling promotes the ability to coregulate and share emotional states. The coupling can be of emotion, behavior, and physiology and is enhanced by elemental mechanisms of synchrony, rhythm, and mimicry.

The treatment protocol that parallels the attachment experience can also be enhanced by coupling, yet research is just emerging that explains this phenomenon. It might be presumptuous, yet attuned clinicians may have been coupling with young clients for decades, attributing their success to intuition. Although proposed in 1994, scientific evidence of the actual process of interbrain synchronization during a therapy session was recently obtained through hyperscanning research (Zhang, 2020). Hyperscanning is advanced technology that can scan two or more subjects at one time, during an interaction. This technology supports the 'two-brain' model that neuroscience has adopted.

This implicit pairing enables the clinician to join the child in their space and resonate back to the child that they are 'felt' (Schore, 2022). Schore explains that through implicit attunement, the clinician recognizes their own emotional and physiological reaction to the child and interprets that input to more accurately 'read' the state of the child.

The concept of implicit, nonverbal communication that is actuated by right brain-to-right brain coupling can be hypothesized as a similar pathway that enables humans and animals to communicate with each other. Through decades of work with children diagnosed with autism spectrum disorder, the author noticed that many of those children have an incredible ability to connect and communicate with dogs and horses. Taking into account the portrayal by Temple Grandin of her thought patterns as 'thinking in pictures' and speaking with others who have established a credible ability to 'read' animals, it is logical to consider that these capabilities might enable a more effective way to connect, couple, and communicate with animals (Grandin & Johnson, 2005). The relevance of this for canine-assisted psychotherapy is substantial and may explain the success of canine support in accessing, understanding, and healing the child. Continued research will hopefully continue to investigate the interspecies bonds and relationships and gain further insight into the avenues of communication.

Coregulation of Arousal and Affect

The human brain is evolutionarily programmed to seek homeostasis. When systems become dysregulated, the brain seeks to 'right' itself. The dysregulated child often feels helpless, powerless, and disconnected from their body. Increasing awareness of internally generated cues is a key goal in reconnecting the child with their inner world. Called interoception, children can regain equilibrium through increased attunement and attentiveness to visceral sensations.

Ni-CAP aligns with mind-body models, as it also strives to maximize the individual's interoception and ability to regulate their physiological symptoms and bodily functions. Ni-CAP is informed by polyvagal conceptualizations of the autonomic nervous system, stress responses, and regulation of these systems to decrease arousal and correlated symptoms. The body, brain, and mind constitute a highly complex system, and healing requires attention to all components, targeting regulation and integration.

Right brain-to-right brain (RB-RB) coupling between the clinician and child and can be propagated by synchronization of the pair's motor activity. As behavioral synchrony is established, physiological harmony can manifest in breathing patterns, and even heart rates. Coupling and synchronization create a neural platform that augments coregulation.

Regions of complex cognition (such as the prefrontal cortices) serve as regulators of subcortical areas. The frontolimbic network is a traditional focus for models of trauma-induced dysregulation and is central in many treatments that are shaped to promote reregulation. The frontolimbic system plays a significant role in the stress response system (SRS), whose dysregulation is also believed to be a common consequence of developmental trauma. The inability to successfully regulate levels of arousal can be debilitating. A state of trauma-induced hyperarousal directs the child's resources away from learning and social interaction to survival.

The dog has been recognized as capable of effective coregulation by itself, and paired with specifically designed interventions, is even more proficient at calming and stabilizing the child. The establishment of safety, relationships, and therapeutic team alliance coregulates the child and activates the ventral vagal pathway and social engagement system (SES).

> Jasmine had attended her new school for a few days when she suddenly experienced a heightened anxiety episode when it came time for her to leave her mother. She began to tremble, hyperventilate, and sweat, and she clung to her mother unable to separate. The school therapist was summoned with a special request for Seamus, an English Cocker. The dog was familiar with this type of reaction, and upon exiting the school he walked over to the child and sat at her feet. She immediately acknowledged him, yet her visible anxiety continued. The therapist asked her if she would join them in an empty classroom 'to relax' with Seamus. Jasmine agreed and tearfully left her mother. The therapist had the child sit down in a large, overstuffed chair and asked if she wanted the dog to sit with her. She agreed and Seamus hopped up onto her lap, but it immediately became obvious she was not calming down. Jasmine was breathing erratically and her legs were moving back and forth. The small dog tried to sit down but had to step back and forth to keep from falling.
>
> The therapist suggested that perhaps Seamus was a little nervous too, and asked Jasmine if she could help him relax. She blurted out 'How do I do that? I don't know how!' The therapist asked if she would like to learn and Jasmine agreed. She was asked to 'breathe with the therapist.' After her breathing slowed and became regulated, the therapist spoke softly and relaxed her posture, settling back into her chair, and Jasmine matched her. Once her body relaxed, Seamus quickly sank into her and laid his head upon her shoulder. As she stroked the now profoundly quiet dog, she reveled in her new skill.
>
> After processing her experience, Jasmine recognized that she was capable of calming down and identified herself and Seamus as a 'team.' Work continued over the next few weeks and Jasmine's confidence and emotional control improved significantly. She went on to become a peer counselor and worked with supervision to teach other students how to

This intervention has served the needs of many children in multiple settings, over years. The dog will often mirror the child's arousal state due to the contagion effect. They provide a natural and honest response to the experience that redirects the child's focus and offers an opportunity to shift roles. The dog-supported intervention with Jasmine occurred in a day-treatment setting and provided a short-term solution-based response.

When a child with a history of trauma is treated, disabling physiological arousal must be initially addressed to prepare the child for further treatment. The polyvagal theory clarifies the neurobiological processes at work beneath trauma and dysregulation that can be targeted when seeking stabilization of arousal and affect. A calm regulated state supports further treatment and healing processes.

Following a natural progression, later sessions might include interventions that enhance the child's mind-body connection and interoception, emotional 'intelligence' and learning and practicing strategies of regulation. Each child, setting, and needs are unique and require personalizing. The dog functions as an anchor for the child, providing a source of safety, implicit strength, and predictability. Called 'grounding' the dog provides the child with a viscerally felt state of calm. The working psychotherapy dog is a live entity and, thus, is capable of neural coupling and implicit messaging that is coregulating and soothing.

The Social Engagement System (SES)

To briefly summarize the SES: as mammals evolved and began to display social behavior, a second vagal path developed with the capacity to inhibit the existing primitive defenses, the mobilization and immobilization responses. This ventral vagal pathway that emerged was coined 'the social engagement system' (SES) (Porges, 2011). During this major adaptation, deep in the brainstem, the structures that regulate this section of the vagus became linked with structures that regulate the striated musculature of the face and head (Porges, 2018). This coupling is known as the 'face-heart' connection and was identified when the heart became linked with head and facial musculature. The myelinated ventral vagus regulates social gestures like facial expression, head turns, gesturing, listening, and vocalization. These gestures serve the maintenance of eye contact, use of rhythm, prosody and tone to convey emotions vocally, and the ability to interpret facial expression, vocal qualities and other nonverbal gestures (Porges 2011).

The original function of the SES was to support the timing and coordination of suckling, swallowing, breathing, and vocalizing of the infant. These functions were necessary for survival as mammals began to nourish their offspring through lactation. The competence of these functions was necessary for attachment, growth, future social function, and emotion regulation. The face-heart connection provides mammals with the ability to differentiate between a calm, safe state in another (who is safe to approach) versus an agitated aroused individual who represents a threat.

Relationships impact physiology and coregulation during attachment or within psychotherapy and establish a physiological base of safety that allows the child to access the social engagement system (SES). A dominant SES inhibits the 'fight, flight, and freeze' levels of the SNS and PNS, reflecting its power to establish a neural sensation of safety. Accessing the SES enables the child to achieve a state of calm, engage in treatment, socially interact, and learn. When the child feels safe, they can participate in social interaction and play. The clinician that incorporates the gestures served by the ventral vagus will support the child in entering the SES and will activate these benefits.

Using Polyvagal Theory to Regulate

Research investigations suggest that emotional and behavioral disorders can stem from problems with regulation of the SRS neural systems (Heim et al., 2008). This inability to maintain ventral vagal regulation reflects dysregulation. It is incumbent upon the clinician to provide coregulation while helping the child to gradually acquire the skills to establish their own regulatory competence (RC). Regulatory skills can be learned and facilitate self-esteem and social and academic success. They also support the child's control of their attention, feelings, thoughts, and behavior (Blair & Raver, 2014).

Elements of the SES can be employed in therapeutic interventions using an integration of canine mechanisms, mind-body techniques, and mindfulness. The natural intuitiveness of many clinicians enables them to utilize passive pathways of social support through gentle eye contact, comforting postures and movements, and softened prosody and intonation. These are calming mechanisms and accentuate social receptivity and engagement. The judicious application of these mechanisms impact the child's neurobiology as the ventral vagus is accessed.

Neural Regulation During Social Play

Participation in play promotes emotional and social growth, communication, and regulation, and resilience. Social play is a sensorimotor experience; it nourishes the entire sensory system and promotes movement and social connection. Ni-CAP allows the child to express their feelings and thoughts through social play with the dog that is typically a willing and enthusiastic participant.

Social play and the stress response system (SRS) share the same substrate, the autonomic nervous system. During play, the child can experience sympathetic activation and metabolic increases to enjoy active play activities. The vagal brake releases to allow this arousal, yet maintains the innervations below the level of a stress response. This is called 'mobilization without fear.' These state experiences teach the child how to tolerate increased arousal levels and how to shift between states (Kestly, 2014). The graduated response/dial permits experience of negative emotion or experience without instigating withdrawal or aggression. Low arousal states during play, such as in hiding or pretending to sleep or die, are mediated by the dorsal vagal branch of the parasympathetic branch, a state called 'immobilization without fear.' The child experiences pleasure and fun while remaining out of reach of a full stress response.

Rapid shifts between engagement and disengagement with the environment are necessary for switching between defense states and social, safe states. Accessing the SES during canine–child play interactions provides coregulation of the stress responses, allowing the child to safely participate without dysfunctional states of arousal. The clinician can guide the session, encouraging state shifts from calm to defensive and back again (safety to threat to safety). This practice of flexible rapid shifting is also stress training, flexibility, and creates practice for self-regulation of arousal states. The face-to-face interactions with the dog provide safety, calming, and regulation. The ultimate goal is to provide the child with the ability to rapidly shift states on their own accord. Dog play with another dog also involves the SES, as they also rely on the capability to rapidly shift between states. Face-to-face interaction for dogs also signals safety, as they use cues to convey that message, preventing escalation into a confrontation.

Pendulating Stress to Expand the Window of Tolerance

Clinician-managed pendulation of stress is a useful intervention technique that requires attunement and coregulation to manage. The intentional modulation of mild to moderate stress periods that are interspersed with nurturing and regulating moments expand the window of tolerance (Dana, 2018). Management of these states requires significant attunement and close monitoring of the child. Moderate levels of stress can trigger the release of neurohormones that positively impact neural reorganization (Myers, et al., 2000). The canine can be incorporated into interventions that support play experiences that stimulate neural growth and integration, leading to increased regulation (Porges, 2013). Natural ruptures in the child–dog relationship occur which will trigger stress, yet the repair of the rupture is a healing experience. Episodes of rupture and repair are also common in the child–clinician relationship. In those cases, the dog can help ease the repair process for the child.

Increasing Vagal Tone

The longest nerve of the body is the vagus which connects the brain to the heart, lungs, and gut, face and head. A core component of the PNS, the ventral vagus, regulates heart rate, breathing, and digestion. High vagal tone is a marker of health and well-being and is also correlated with heart rate variability (HRV). The vagal nerve connects with eyes, ears, facial musculature, and the vocal cords. Humming, singing, chanting, and even gargling increase vagal tone. Conscious relaxation of the muscles around the eyes as part of progressive relaxation also increases PNS tone.

One of the most effective techniques for activating the vagal system is the conscious control of breathing. Inhalation activates and exhalation inhibits, extending and slowing the in and out rates directly affecting vagus activation. When the clinician incorporates even simple breathing exercises, the results are typically rapid. One of the most commonly used methods is '6-4-6' which is slow inspiration for six seconds, holding the breath for four, and a slow, full exhalation for six seconds.

Singing and rhythmic patterns of speech influence breathing and recruit additional regulatory components of the SES. The child becomes capable of activating their facial musculature, eye movement, and vocal elements. Vocalizations can be considered active pathways that regulate the autonomic nervous system (ANS). Repeated practice shapes and reinforces neural patterns, thus interventions which stimulate neural activations are reinforcing neural strength (Cozolino, 2017).

Regulating stress levels and response systems is believed to stimulate neural growth in the prefrontal cortex and amygdala, particularly functional connectivity that improves messaging between structures. These regions support empathic behavior, the perception of emotionality in others, and regulation (Panksepp & Biven, 2012). It follows that successful coregulation will recalibrate the child's frontolimbic system enabling the prefrontal cortex to become more proficient at regulating the amygdala and limbic system. As discussed earlier, the prefrontal regions are the last to mature, which is why even typical young children need the support of coregulating relationships to maintain a homeostatic state.

Stimulating Oxytocin

Oxytocin (OT) is released in both species during human–dog interactions, and also promotes social interaction, prosocial behavior, and attachment. A safe pleasant touch, face-to-face interactions, mutual gaze, play, affection, and proximity all increase OT, which then increases vagal tone and

HRV, biomarkers of autonomic nervous system regulation. Oxytocin down regulates the stress response system and increases trust, empathy, and prosocial behavior. Interactions with the working therapy dog increase OT levels in both species which facilitates and strengthens their bond, relationship, and willingness to engage. The child–dog interactions produce increased levels of OT and decrease cortisol, neurobiological conditions which support accessing the SES and increasing social interaction. While OT has garnered significant excitement as a primary mechanism in many processes, neurochemistry is far more complicated. Human animal interaction also increases dopamine, prolactin, and beta-endorphins (Odendaal & Meintjes, 2003) yet the precise secretion levels and compounds require further scientific insight.

Observation

The biophilia theory describes how the fascination with animals that developed in humans was actually seeded in their core drive for survival. Humans developed into a species that required astute observation to survive the predator-rich Ice Age. Their ability to watch the behavior of animals during this period supported continuing life as they became familiar with animal patterns of behavior. The amygdala, known for its role in emotional responses and processes developed a 'preferential response' to animals, possibly as a result of this history. A neuroimaging study by Mormann et al. (2011) supports the biophilia theory and the amygdala has been proposed as a direct inroad or 'portal' into the internal world of the child (Parish-Plass & Pfeiffer, 2019). Interestingly, the most productive method of learning today is through observation, which is supported by the mirror neuron system. Intervention activities that involve observation of animal behavior can produce a multitude of content and emotion from the child's inner world. This exercise can be shaped into an activity with specific goals, or simply be casual observation.

Observation requires being present and mindful. Attention is focused upon another living being and their observed behavior activates the mirror neuron (MN) system of the child. The MN system allows an observer to experience similar emotion, actions, and also increases understanding. Simply by viewing a behavior, the observer's MN system triggers the same neural circuitry of the other who performed the action (Rizzolatti & Craighero, 2004). This system may underlie projection, or the insertion of one's own emotions and intentions into the other, a powerful therapeutic process (Keysers & Gazzola, 2014). The emotion felt by the animal can become 'felt' by the child (Gendlin, 1978). An excited, energized dog that is enjoying a game will implicitly share that feeling, and if the child mimics the movement patterns of the dog, then that shared feeling is intensified (Shafir et al., 2016).

Fifteen-year-old Paul and I were standing at the fence, watching Rusty in his corral. I had to re-home my Arabian gelding as I could not ride anymore, and he loved the trails. I felt some pangs of sadness and shared that I was torn over giving him away, and hoped it was the right thing for him. Paul was quiet for a moment and I suddenly realized the door I had inadvertently opened. The 14-year-old teen had been adopted at birth due to his biological mother's drug addiction. Keeping his eyes on Rusty, Paul said, 'He knows and he'll be ok. You're doing the right thing for him.' Paul had avoided discussing his adoption for months, but he decided that day to walk through the door that Rusty opened.

Observation offers a state experience of quiescence that is unusual for children today. The continuous bombardment of distractions in modern society prevents periods of mindfulness interoception. There are few opportunities for uninterrupted thought and it is increasingly rare to see preteens and teens without a phone or headphones. Observation shares similar characteristics with mindfulness. The child learns to become aware and attuned with the moment, their environment, and their body. Thoughts and emotions often spontaneously emerge during periods of calm.

A child will recognize that they have an impact on animals (and other humans), and can begin to identify and process the effects that the animals have upon them. They become aware of emotions such as excitement, joy, and fear, notice energy shifts and come to understand reciprocity, caring for another, and how to shape their behavior to draw the interest of another. The child becomes more aware of the physical sensations of their body. Does their heart beat faster? Are they excited, nervous, or overwhelmed; and how does their body change with different feelings? The clinician is also able to learn a great deal about the child by their observation and shared experience. The clinician also picks up information from the responses of the animal to the child.

Dogs at play elicit a significant amount of social content, opening up many opportunities to experience and process, through play or talk. The child will also learn about relationships, the dog's individual personality and come to see animals as unique sentient beings. Through focused observation, children also have the opportunity to learn about various aspects of 'real life,' such as anatomy.

Eight-year-old Jay had a serious and concerned look on his face as he stared down at Seamus who lay on his back, his furry underbelly exposed. After a few minutes of intent visual study, he turned to me with a question. Pointing to the dog's belly, he asked 'Is that his penis?' I cleared my throat and quietly stated that yes, it was. He quietly continued to focus on the belly and then empathetically said, 'Don't worry, Seamus, mine is small too.'

Trying on Hats

Trauma dysregulates the functional domains of the child and the 'intrapersonal' domain involves establishing and maintaining a coherent and stable sense of self. Children with dysregulation need new experiences that enrich and stimulate all aspects of their lives. New learning and new experiences trigger neuroplasticity and neural growth. 'Trying on hats' is an intervention format that allows children to take on a role as scientist, doctor, vet, animal trainer, caregiver, or teacher, allowing them to be creative, tap imagination, and engage in symbolism that offers opportunities to re-enact implicit memories. Depending on their age and maturity, they can dress up, use a stethoscope, binoculars, a clipboard, and work with the animal in a role play/story that they create. This form of intervention is flexible and serves a wide variety of goals and experiences. 'Trying on hats' places the child into a position or role of competence, control, and even authority creating a 'pseudo-paradox.' The word 'paradox' is derived from the Greek word that means 'contrary to expectation.'

> While working in an elementary school, I was asked to address a playground problem. A small group of fourth-grade boys were frequently breaking rules, teasing others, and being defiant. I met with them and informed them that I was creating a new set of playground rules for safety, and I needed them to be my assistants in teaching the new rules to the younger children. As their eyes widened in disbelief, I added that I knew they had experience with rules and consequences and I needed guys with their level of expertise. Through a well-planned process, the boys became stellar models and helped teach and monitor younger students to follow the playground rules.

Interoception is a Body to Mind Status Report

Emotion regulation (ER) requires interoception (Craig, 2015), a functional awareness of internal sensations that provides essential feedback about the state of the body. The body is supposed to relay visceral information to the brain. Recognizing afferent signals, processing their meaning, and establishing accurate mental representations of these body signals provides critical information necessary for decision-making (Damasio, 1994). The ability to self-regulate to decrease physiological arousal, for example, requires the ability to feel the emotion and observe oneself (Siegel, 2012). These physical sensations arise from internal receptors, whereas external stimuli activate cutaneous receptors, a process called exteroception. The two can intermingle (Strigo & Craig, 2016).

Emotion is believed by many theorists to arise from physiological states, and awareness of these states can support the individual in changing their emotions. Deficient interoception has been linked with several forms of psychopathology, including body-related disorders such as eating, panic, and somatic trauma. The latter describes trauma that manifests in specific somatic symptoms. Developmental trauma can cause disruptions to the signaling patterns between the brain and body. Many of the systems and processes that are perceived to become dysregulated by trauma confer unpleasant psychophysiological sensations that become confusing and even disabling. The dysregulation of the HPA axis (of the stress response system) can create a persistent state of anxiety, hyperarousal, and an attention bias to threat. These conditions are potentially distracting and consuming to the child and likely dull sensitivity and awareness to interoceptive signals. Children with dissociation and emotional detachments that may arise from unresponsive parenting may also suffer from impaired interoception (Oldroyd et al., 2019). While dissociation numbs the child to painful emotions, it can diminish the sense of joy and the vibrancy of being alive.

Therapeutic work that helps the child become more attuned to visceral signals is a step toward learning how to manage states *and* emotions. This type of work fosters integration of their brain, mind, and body. The child who lacks interoceptive awareness can become more familiar with the functions and sensations of the body beginning with a focus on the dog. An intervention that encourages children to listen to the hearts of animals while they are calm and after exercise and arousal, introduces the basic concept, and this leads into mind-body work and increasing attunement to one's internal world. Goals that support increasing interoceptive awareness also increase the child's tolerance of uncomfortable emotional and arousal states. The minds of fearful children will often develop complex and terrifying pseudo-memories that, if not shared and reframed, can lead to increased disconnection with the body.

Human animal interaction (HAI) is a form of Mindfulness

Mindfulness is being aware and intentionally focused on the present moment. It is contrary to rumination, fear, and thoughts of the past and future. Mindfulness is also an acceptance (without judgment) of the self and experience. Mindfulness applications have been shown to improve emotion regulation. The practice reduces anxiety, mood lability, depression and distress (Hoffman & Gomez, 2017). The techniques of mindfulness strengthen PNS tone, mediate amygdala responsiveness, and increase cortical thickness (Lazar et al., 2005) and gray matter density (Hotzel et al., 2011).

Human animal interaction is a form of mindfulness as animals draw the attention of the child and require focus on the present. Interacting with dogs draws in and contains focus almost automatically. Teaching and supporting children to be mindful and focused in conjunction with awareness and attunement to animal needs, supports the development of 'theory of mind,' leading to empathy, and a probable positive impact on future behaviors toward other humans. As children observe, interact, and play with animals, they make assumptions and predictions about animal behavior. The process stimulates their thought processes as they attempt to interpret the animal's behavior. Piaget (1962) conducted perspective-taking studies, investigating the child's capacity to comprehend others' thoughts, feelings, and intentions, recognizing they may be different than their own. Focusing on another living being, allowing oneself to be drawn into their world, and the natural comparison of similarities and differences can strengthen individuation and differentiation.

Mind-body techniques enhance the resilience of the child by strengthening the higher level neural circuitry, reducing reliance on autonomic, more primitive systems. Unconscious, automatic response patterns are reduced, supporting increased confidence and a sense of control. Combined with the positive effects of human–canine interaction, the potential for growth and integration is enhanced when combining these elements.

The Body is an Unedited Story

Clinical perspectives are gravitating toward a more inclusive and holistic mind-body approach in psychology. Theories and models have begun to address the mind and body as a unified and integrated system. Still, these new models have been perceived as alternative, nontraditional, and lacking empirical evidence. Psychotherapy for dysregulation should address the entirety of the child, attending to the mind, brain, and body as an integrated system. The neurobiological dysregulation of trauma is easier to comprehend when the child is perceived as a complex system. Dysregulation and trauma do not discriminate; all systems of the child are vulnerable to their effects.

Along with the brain and mind, the body is also a repository for trauma and psychological distress (van der Kolk, 2014). It is not a new concept that traumatic experiences, implicit memories, sadness, grief, and other emotions are held within the fibers of the body. Gestalt Therapy frames the body as a container of that which requires expression to release psychological distress (Peris, Hefferline & Goodman, 1951). Implicit, preverbal memories are encoded and referenced in the nervous system, neurobiology, and neurochemistry. They are expressed in postures, gestures, mannerisms and compulsions (Erskine, 2014). The significant interest in the consequences of developmental trauma is already focusing research on the neurobiological impact on children. Hopefully, research will expand investigations of animal-assisted, mind-body, somatic, creative arts, and movement therapies, moving them from 'alternative' to mainstream.

According to Koch, therapies that are based on movement reduce distress and suffering, activate resources, and improve health. Body movements provide proprioceptive feedback to regions of higher cognition, detailing the relationship between body position and movement to the central nervous system. The meaning of movements is stored with learning memory. Rhythmic qualities of movement impact emotion and attitudes, and also regulate approach/avoidance (motor) patterns (Koch, 2014).

Exercise positively impacts respiratory, cardiovascular, immune, emotional and social systems and increases the growth hormone in the brain, supporting mitochondria and cognition. Severe and frequent early trauma can cause dysregulation of the stress response system (SRS) causing a pervasive stress arousal that can be highly activated or hypoactive. The child who is 'stuck' in a stress response feels disconnected from their emotions and body, and is governed by the more primitive brain regions. Exercise recalibrates the dysregulation of arousal, and promotes an integrated resilient state. Exercise can burn off the energy of high arousal and also reverses the immobilization of hypoarousal (Schiraldi, 2021).

Regular exercise down-regulates the SNS and HPA axis, reducing stress response activation and arousal (Meeusen, 2005. This type of movement also impacts neurotransmitter levels and increases growth factors (Shafir et al., 2016). Aerobic exercise improves neural structure and function, enhances brain connectivity (Li et al., 2017), increases brain volume, and promotes neurogenesis (Voss et al., 2019).

Physical activity is tightly coupled with learning and cognition (Kempermann et al., 2010). A study at Kobe University, using fMRI technology, revealed that children who are physically active (through age 12) showed higher cognitive functioning in later years. The link was evidenced in the modular segregation of brain networks, increased cortical thickness, stronger connectivity between hemispheres, and lesser levels of arborization in dendrites (Ishihara et al., 2020). Exercise increases brain volume which improves cognitive functioning (learning and memory); increases antioxidants which are neuroprotective; and increases the health and connectivity between neurons which also improves learning and attention (Schiraldi, 2021). Exercise has been found to be comparable to psychotropics and other treatments for depression (Kvam et al., 2016). Incorporating movement into a multidimensional treatment plan can positively impact the brain regulation, and using it as an adjunct to those interventions would be a powerful supplement and provide additional social opportunities.

Multiple forms of exercise can be done with canine participation. The dog adds a unique, genuine, and responsive addition to learning and offers a multisensory experience that is more likely to be integrated into memory. Active play with dogs elicits ANS activation and provides cardiovascular and neural benefits. Active movement with a dog or other humans also supports social and intrapersonal domains. While exercise is not currently considered a typical component of treatment for DT, it should be given serious consideration, as there is significant science that supports its effects on the mind and body.

Yoga

Yoga is an ancient practice that can improve the well-being and health of individuals with dysregulation. The practice encourages interoceptive awareness of internal states, promoting increased tolerance for physical and sensory experiences of fear and vulnerability. The use of mindful controlled breathing and relaxation poses decreases SNS activation and cortisol levels and promotes regulation and self-acceptance (West et al., 2016).

Sullivan and team collaborated with Dr Porges and proposed a yoga therapy model that links with the polyvagal theory. This framework demonstrates the fit between the two distinct platforms which emphasize resilience and regulation. (For more information, see Sullivan et al., 2018.) There are increasing examples of dogs synchronizing with their humans by mimicking their specific yoga moves. This is a previously unknown canine behavior.

Template for ni-CAP Interventions

The following is a template that creates a structure for individualizing treatment for a child. The categories support the clinician in creating specific interventions that address the child's needs. Thinking in terms of equations can be useful in choosing and integrating elements for specific goals. For example, if a clinician wants to employ supportive neural mechanisms to achieve a calm and receptive state in the child, enabling them to participate in a role play, the equation might look like this:

> *Dog and child interaction=increased oxytocin=safety/coregulation=accessing the SES=increased receptivity and social engagement=productive role play and positive interactions with dog =perceived social competence and confidence.*

An example of a template-designed intervention is in *italics*.

The ni-CAP Template

Child Name: *Jordan*   **Setting**: *Office and outdoor area*   **Date**: *1/1/2023*

Treatment Goal: *Improve interoceptive ability to become more aware of internal world. Make connection between emotions and body sensations and learn language, definitions, and characteristics of emotion. Learn to self-soothe.*
Session Goal: *Learn the relationship between the heart and movement. Become aware of the sensation of the heartbeat in the dog and self.*
Role of the Dog: *The dog is the patient in a role play.*

Function of Dog: *The dog serves as recipient of care, play partner, supports the child in gaining awareness and competence, increases awareness of canine species and similarities to self, and adds movement, play, and fun.*

Neural Mechanisms: *Oxytocin, the social engagement system (SES).*

Elemental Mechanisms: *Rhythm and synchrony*

Incorporated Modalities: *Mind-body, play, movement and exercise, mindfulness, and therapeutic education*

Neuroplasticity: *Activated by movement, mindfulness, and learning new skills*

Sensory Components: *Tactile, auditory, visual, proprioception*

Setting and Specific Equipment: *Set up 'veterinarian office'; stethoscope and/or heart monitor; clipboard for keeping track of data, lab coat. Prep outdoor area for play and running.*

Special Considerations and Concerns: Safety, Health, and Other: *Prior to session, assure that the dog is familiar and comfortable with heart rate monitoring.*

Describe Intervention: *Child takes role of veterinarian and the dog comes in for a checkup. The dog's owner (clinician) is concerned that its heart rate goes too high during exercise and wants to rule out a problem. The child vet gives the dog a 'checkup' by listening to the dog's heart and/or taking pulse, while sitting, after active play, and following a calming session. The vet is responsible for calming the dog for the final session (using calming or soothing techniques) and reassures the owner that humans and dogs are similar, and that the dog is healthy. If relatively successful, Jordan also checks her own pulse and heart rate for comparison.*

Outcome and Thoughts: *Jordan has learned calming and soothing techniques to calm dogs in earlier sessions and has established a positive and reciprocal relationship with the dog. This type of intervention can be repeated using a bunny and a horse for further comparison and increased self-awareness. Jordan will check her heart rate during future sessions to increase her interoception and progress to connecting visceral sensations with emotions and activity/experiences.*

Therapeutic Education

When a child understands some of the systems and processes of their body, they feel a sense of mastery and their fear of the unknown is decreased. Children from around five years' old and up can learn about their nervous system and stress responses. This knowledge can reassure the most fearful child that their body is not occupied by an unmanageable force.

A valuable intervention for all children is to teach them (in a developmentally appropriate way) about their bodies and mind. Awareness of the stress response system along with acquiring strategies to regulate their responses is empowering and increases a sense of control and self-efficacy. Recognition of heart rate, breathing, muscular tension, and somatic sensations can be a hands-on experience with animals. Listening to the beating heart with an ear pressed against the side of a dog or horse, or using a stethoscope offers an experience that connects the child to a primordial life function. The child learns the steps for a calm, safe approach that relaxes the animal even though their own heart rate is heightened by excitement or anxiety. The child is also taught self-soothing strategies to calm and regulate their breathing and body, finding ways to also soothe the animal.

Children also experience a visceral response that is enhanced by multiple senses. Up close the child smells the animal, feels their breath on their face and shoulder, and feels the texture of their fur. Best of all, their whole system is triggered by the sounds that enter through auditory channels; there is a rhythm and synchrony between themselves and the animal. The child will also become aware of their beating heart and may notice a reduction of rate that coincides with a sense of calming.

Social cognition and a fundamental set of social skills are crucial for all children, and are particularly vital for those with dysregulation, trauma history, and most traditional mental health disorders. The author has conducted canine-assisted therapeutic social skills for many years in multiple settings, with observable and measurable results. A research grant was obtained by the University of California Irvine for Project Positive Assertive Cooperative Kids (P.A.C.K.), a study using canine-assisted social skill interventions. Based on our successful canine-assisted therapeutic social skills program children who received the canine-supported programming showed improvements in social skills, prosocial behavior, and experienced reductions in problematic behaviors (Gee et al., 2017).

Conclusion

Any clinical work with children requires collaboration with the relevant others in their lives, particularly parents. While many factors weigh into this, including confidentiality and family stability, the adults in a child's life have phenomenal impact and should ideally be part of an integrated program. If, for example, the goal is to change a specific behavior, reinforcement needs to occur in all settings. When multiple therapies, such as speech and language, occupational, medical, and others are involved, it is critical to operate as a 'team' along with the teacher, parents, and when possible, the child. When the child feels supported by a collaboration of advocates, the effect can be substantial.

References

Blair, C., & Raver, C.C. (2014). School readiness and self-regulation: A developmental psychobiological approach. *Annual Review of Psychology*; 66: 711–731. https://doi.org/10.1146/annurev-psych-010814-015221

Cozolino, L. (2017). *The Neuroscience of Psychotherapy: Building and Rebuilding the Human Brain*. New York: W.W. Norton.

Craig, A.D. (2015). *How Do You Feel? An Interoceptive Moment with Your Neurobiological Self*. Princeton, NJ: Princeton U. Press.

Damasio, A. (1994). *Descartes' Error: Emotion, Reason and the Human Brain*. New York: Grosset/Putnam.

Dana, D. (2018). *The Polyvagal Theory in Therapy: Engaging the Rhythm of Regulation*. New York: W.W. Norton & Co.

Erskine, R. (2014). Nonverbal stories: The body in psychotherapy. *International Journal of Integrative Psychotherapy*; 5(1).

Gee, N.R., Griffin, J.A., McCardle, P. (2017). Human-animal interaction research in school settings: Current knowledge and future directions. *AERA Open*; 3(3): 233285841772434. https://doi.org/10.1177/233285841772434

Geller & Porges, (2014). Therapeutic presence: Neurophysiological mechanisms mediating feeling safe in therapeutic relationships. *Journal of Psychotherapy Integration*; 24(3): 178–192. https://doi.org.10.1037/a0037511

Geller, S.M. (2017). Therapeutic presence and polyvagal theory: Principles and practices for cultivating effective therapeutic relationships. In S.W. Porges, & Deb Dana (Eds.), *Clinical Applications of The Polyvagal Theory: The Emergence of Polyvagal-Informed Therapies*.

Gendlin, E.T. (1978). *Focusing*. New York, NY: Bantham Books.

Grandin, T., & Johnson, C. (2005). *Animals in Translation: Using the Mysteries of Autism to Decode Animal Behavior*. New York, NY: Simon & Schuster.

Heim, C., Newport, D.J., Mletzko, T., Miller, A.H., & Nemeroff, C.B. (2008).The link between childhood trauma and depression: Insights from HPA axis studies in humans. *Psychoneuroendocrinology*; 33(6): 693–710. https://doi.org/10.1016/j.psyneuen.2008.03.008

Hoffman, S.G., & Gomez, A.F. (2017). Mindfulness-based Interventions for Anxiety and Depression. *Psychiatric Clinics of North America*; 40(4): 739–749. https://doi.org/10.1016/j.psc.2017.08.008

Hotzel, B., Carmody, J., Vangel, M., Congleton, C., Yerramsetti, S.M., Gard, T., & Lazar, S.W. (2011). *Psychiatry Research*; 191(1): 36–43. https://doi.org/10.1016/j.psychresns.2010.08.006

Ishihara, T., Miyazaki, A., Tanaka, H., & Matsuda, T. (2020). Identification of the brain networks that contribute to the interaction between physical function and working memory: An fMRI investigation with over 1,000 healthy adults. *NeuroImage*; 221: 117152. https://doi.org/10.1016/j.neuroimage.2020.117152

Kazdin, A.E. (2000). Psychotherapy for children and adolescents. *Annual Review of Psychology* 54: 253–276. https://doi.org/10.1146/annurev.psych.54.101601.145105

Kempermann, G., Fabel, K., Ehninger, D., Babu, H., Leal-Galicia, P., Garthe, A., & Wolf, S.A. (2010). Why and how physical activity promotes experience-induced brain plasticity. *Front. Neurosci.* https://doi.org/10.3389/fnins.2010.00189

Kestly, T.A. (2014). *The Interpersonal Neurobiology of Play: Brain-building Interventions for Emotional Well-being*. New York, NY: W.W. Norton & Co.

Keysers, C., & Gazzola, V. (2014). Hebbian learning and predictive mirror neurons for actions, sensations and emotions. *Philos Trans Royal Soc. B: Biological Sciences*; 369: 20130175. Keysers https://doi.org/10.1098.rstb.2013.0175

Koch, S.C. (2014). Rhythm is it: Effects of dynamic body feedback on affect, Attitudes and Cognition. *Frontiers in Psychology* 5:537. https://doi.org/10.3389/fpsyg.2014.00537

Kvam, S., Kleppe, C.L., Nordhus, I.H., & Hovland, A. (2016). Exercise as a treatment for depression: A meta-analysis. *Journal of Affective Disorders*; 202: 67–86. https://doi.org/10.1016/j.jad.2016.03.063

Lazar, S.W., Kerr, C.E., Wasserman, R.H., Gray, J.R., Greve, D.N., Treadway, M.T., McGarvey, M, Quinn, B.T., Dusek, J.A., Benson, H., Rauch, S.L., Moore, C.I., & Fischl, B. (2005). Meditation experience is associated with increased cortical thickness. *Neuroreport*; 16(17): 1893–1897. https://doi.org/10.1097/01.wnr.0000186598.66243.19

Li, M.Y., Huang, M.M., Li, S.Z., Tao, J., Zheng, G.H., & Chen, L.D. (2017). The effects of aerobic exercise on the structure and function of DMN-related brain regions. A systematic review. *The International Journal of Neuroscience*; 127(7): 634–649. https://doi.org/10.1080/00207454.2016.1212855

Meeusen, R. (2005). Exercise and the brain: Insight into new therapeutic. *Annals of Transplantation*; 10: 49–51.

Mormann, F., Dubois, J., Kornblith, S., Milosavljevic, M., Cerf, M. Ison, Tsuchiya, N., Kraskov, A., Quiroga, R.Q., Adolphs, R., Fried, I., & Koch, C. (2011). A category-specific response to animals in the right human amygdala. *Nature Neuroscience*; 14(10): 1247–1249. https://doi.org/10.1038/nn.2999

Myers, W.A., Churchill, J.D., Muja, N., & Garraghty, P.E. (2000). Role of NMDA receptors in adult primate cortical somatosensory plasticity. *The Journal of Comparative Neurology*; 418: 373–382.

Norcross, J.C., & Wampold, B.E. (2011). Evidence-based therapy relationships: Conclusions and clinical practices. *Psychotherapy*; 48: 98–102.

Odendaal, J.S. & Meintjes, R.A. (2003). Neurophysiological correlates of affiliative behavior between humans and dogs. *The Veterinary Journal*; 165(3): 333–336. https://doi.org/10.1016/S1090-0233(02)00237-X

Oldroyd, K., Pasupathi, M., & Wainryb, C. (2019). Social antecedents to the development of interoception: Attachment related processes are associated with interoception. *Frontiers in Psychology*. https://doi.org/10.3389/fpsyg.2019.00712

Panksepp, J. & Biven, L. (2012). *The Archaeology of Mind: Neuroevolutionary Origins of Human Emotions*. New York, NY: W.W. Norton & Co.

Parish-Plass, N., & Pfeiffer, J. (2019). Implications of animal-assisted psychotherapy for the treatment of developmental trauma. In M. Tedeschi & M.A. Jenkins (Eds.), *Transforming Trauma*. W. Lafayette, IN: Purdue University Press.

Peris, F.S., Hefferline, R.F., & Goodman, P. (1951). *Gestalt Therapy: Excitement and Growth in the Human Personality*. New York, NY: Julian Press.

Piaget, J. (1962). *The Moral Judgment of the Child*. Glencoe, IL: The Free Press.

Porges, S.W. (2011). *Norton Series on Interpersonal Neurobiology. The Polyvagal Theory: Neurophysiological Foundations of Emotions, Attachment, Communication, and Self-regulation*. New York, NY: Norton

Porges, S.W. (2013). Human-animal interactions. A neural exercise supporting health. Plenary speech at the annual conference of IAHAIO International Association of Human-Animal Interaction Organization.

Porges, S.W. & Dana, D. (Eds.). (2018). *Clinical applications of the polyvagal theory: The emergence of polyvagal-informed therapies.* W.W. Norton & Company.

Rizzolatti, G., & Craighero, L. (2004). The mirror-neuron system. *Annual Review of Neuroscience*; 27: 169–192. https://doi.org/10.1146/annurev.neuro.27.070203.144230

Schiraldi, G.R. (2021). *The Adverse Childhood Experiences Recovery Workbook*, Oakland, CA: New Harbinger.

Schore, A.N. (2022). Right brain-to-right brain psychotherapy: Recent scientific and clinical advances. *Annals of General Psychiatry*; 21(46). https://doi.org/10.1186/s12991-022-00420-3

Shafir, T., Tsachor, R.P., & Welch, K. (2016). Emotion regulation through movement: Unique sets of movement characteristics are associated with and enhance basic emotions. *Frontiers in Psychology* 6: 2030. Shaf 16 https://doi.org/10.3389/20165.02030

Siegel, D.J. (2012). *The developing mind: How relationships and the brain interact to shape who we are* (2nd ed.). New York, NY: Guilford Press.

Strigo, I.A., & Craig, A.D. (2016). Interoception, homeostatic emotions and sympathovagal balance. *Philosophical Transactions of the Royal Society of London. Series B, Biological Sciences*; 371: 20160010. https://doi.org/10.1098/rstb.20160010.

Sullivan, M.B., Erb, M., Schmalzl, L., Moonaz, S., Noggle Taylor, J., & Porges, S.W. (2018). Yoga therapy and polyvagal theory: The convergence of traditional wisdom and contemporary neuroscience for self-regulation and resilience. *Frontiers in Human Neuroscience.*

van der Kolk, B. (2014). *The Body Keeps Score: Brain, Mind, and Body in the Healing of Trauma.* New York, NY: Penguin Group.

Voss, M.W., Soto, C., Yoo, S., Sodoma, M., Vivar, C., & van Praag, H. (2019). Exercise and hippocampal memory systems. *Trends in Cognitive Science*; 23(4): 318–333. https://doi.org/10.1016/j.tics.2019.03.015

West, J., Liang, B., & Spinazzola, J. (2016). Trauma sensitive yoga as a complementary treatment for posttraumatic stress disorder: A qualitative descriptive analysis. *International Journal of Stress Management*; 24(2). https://doi.org/10.1037/str0000040

Willis, J., & Todorov, A. (2006). First impressions: Making up your mind after a 100-ms exposure to a face. *Psychological Science*; 17: 592–598.

Wolpe, J. (1954). Reciprocal inhibition as the main basis of psychotherapeutic effects. *A.M.A. Archives of Neurology and Psychiatry*; 72(2): 205–226. https://doi.org/10.1001/archneurpsyc.1954.02330020073007

Zhang, M., Jia, H., & Zheng, M. (2020). Interbrain synchrony in the expectation of cooperation behavior: A hyperscanning study using functional near-infrared spectroscopy. *Frontiers in Psychology* https://doi.org/10.3389/fpsyg.2020.542093

Conclusion

The brain is an incredible and dynamic complex system that has been touted as the 'last frontier' of science. Within the past few decades, neuroimaging technology has profoundly increased our knowledge of the human brain. The ability to peer 'under the hood' of human emotion, social and cognitive behavior to witness the generation of typical and atypical function is fascinating and has answered many questions, yet many remain.

The development of the brain is now understood to be the result of a complex interface of evolutionary influence and environmental experiences (nature *and* nurture). Evolutionary forces organized the nervous system with a preset timetable for development and coded specific neural regions to be experience-expectant and experience-dependent upon the environment.

Fields of psychology and neuroscience have historically studied brain development independently, yet a convergence is occurring that will hopefully lead to a more comprehensive and complete understanding of human brain development, dysfunction, and dysregulation that lead to psychopathology. A foundation for this convergence is provided by the 2000 Nobel Prize winner Eric Kandel through his research that shows all mental processes have a neural basis seated in the brain, and that learning and environmental experiences impact neural connectivity. Kandel (1998) also states that psychotherapy has the potential to change behavior by altering gene expression through mechanisms of neural activation and biochemical processes. Therapeutic processes also seek to integrate cognition, emotion, sensory input, and behavior (Cozolino, 2017).

Psychotherapy has been proposed as an enriched environment that promotes neuronal growth and integration through sensory stimulation, new experiences, learning, safety, and nurturing relationships. These experiences promote neuroplasticity and neural change through a mix of mild-to-moderate stress, nurturance, and activation of relevant neural circuitry (Cozolino, 2017). The canine, through coevolution, domestication, and the distinct human–animal relationship is the personification of an enriched environment. The psychotherapy working dog can create safety, a welcoming, stimulating milieu, a model of healthy relationships and new, enriching experiences.

DOI: 10.4324/9781003217534-14

As the field of animal-assisted psychotherapy evolves, more complex concerns and dilemmas will arise. Animal welfare used to be based on health and safety, but current research and enlightened attitudes that acknowledge saliency, emotions, and individual interests in animals requires increased attention, advocacy, and action. The AAP field has also struggled to establish standardized criteria for dogs that work in therapeutic environments, yet debate continues on what constitutes an appropriate, safe, *and* effective dog. Nancy Parish-Plass (2022), an internationally respected animal-assisted clinician, author, and researcher is clear when she says that she wants a dog *with* her in therapy, not a 'therapy dog'. Her reasoning follows the logic that it is the authenticity, honesty, and natural behavior in canines that validates their ability to effect change in children, adolescents, and adults. Some experts fear that humans tend to 'train the dog out of the dog.' That can be interpreted as striving to make the dog exceedingly compliant, obedient, tolerant, accepting, and at our 'beck and call.' Dogs have worked for decades 'in the service' of humans, in law enforcement, rescue, and medical assistance. They have clearly identified criteria, expectations, traits, and skills that are recognized as necessary for proficient performance of well-defined roles. Our field *will* succeed in establishing criteria for specific roles of working psychotherapy dogs, but first, those roles need to be identified and clarified. The confusion over the use of the word 'therapy' reflects our lack of certainty. What is a 'therapy' dog and what does that mean they can do?

It is a daunting endeavor that is complicated by the wide range of ages of clientele and mental health conditions that we serve; and the diversity of incorporated species, models, and settings. There *should* be different expectations for a dog who visits fragile or ill seniors for the purpose of improving well-being versus a working psychotherapy dog that is required to interact in complicated situations that stem from traumatic experiences. The latter role requires authenticity and natural behavior, as healing trauma requires a relational context that can be experienced as natural, honest, and genuine.

The potency of the canine species for children with dysregulation lies in their now innate capacity for relationships, social cognition, and cooperative nature. While humans take credit for 'making the dog more human,' we need to recognize that it is also their differences from humans that source their effectiveness. The very fact that they are *not* human sidesteps the distrust and suspicion that trauma provokes; the dog feels much safer to a victim of interpersonal betrayal. The canine mind is also unencumbered by a complex belief system, history, details, and the opinions of others. They exist in the present, in a space and state that is safe, elemental, and uncomplicated. It is this 'therasphere' that can host a pure and uncontaminated relationship that will protect, reregulate, and heal.

Through coevolution, humans have changed the canine species and they have also changed us, yet this unique relationship cannot be reduced to categorizations of 'like me' or 'unlike me'. It is the relationship *between* humans and canines that is the secret ingredient, the dash or 'hyphen' (Horowitz, 2009). That is where the synergism lies.

Many fear that humans have been distancing themselves from the natural world, and that we could lose the evolutionarily encoded primordial guide that decrees our cooperation with Earth's resources to sustain the environment and its populations. If we fail to sustain our connections with other animals, we can forget our innate biological responsibilities and obligations and somehow lose our humanity. Throughout literature, it is frequently mentioned that humans require other humans to 'become human.' Others suggest that animals make humans 'more humane.' Perhaps humans and animals *need each other* to optimize our individual and collective potential on Earth, a process we might call '*humanimity*.' If we listen, we can hear them, but first, we must listen.

References

Cozolino, L. (2017). *The Neuroscience of Psychotherapy*. New York, NY: W.W. Norton & Co.

Horowitz, A. (2009). *Inside of a Dog: What Dogs See, Smell, and Know*. New York, NY: Schribner.

Kandel, E. (1998). A new intellectual framework for psychiatry. *The American Journal of Psychiatry*; 155(4): 457–469. https://doi.org/10.1176/ajp.155.4.457

Parish-Plass, N. (2022). Personal Communication

Index

For Product Safety Concerns and Information please contact our EU
representative GPSR@taylorandfrancis.com Taylor & Francis Verlag GmbH,
Kaufingerstraße 24, 80331 München, Germany

Printed and bound by CPI Group (UK) Ltd, Croydon, CR0 4YY
08/06/2025
01897009-0002